ASSESSMENT IN COGNITIVE THERAPY

Also Available

assessment in
COGNITIVE
THERAPY

edited by
Gary P. Brown
David A. Clark

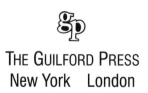

THE GUILFORD PRESS
New York   London

© 2015 The Guilford Press
A Division of Guilford Publications, Inc.
72 Spring Street, New York, NY 10012
www.guilford.com

Printed in the United States of America

This book is printed on acid-free paper.

Last digit is print number: 9 8 7 6 5 4 3 2 1

The authors have checked with sources believed to be reliable in their
efforts to provide information that is complete and generally in accord
with the standards of practice that are accepted at the time of publication.
However, in view of the possibility of human error or changes in behavioral,
mental health, or medical sciences, neither the authors, nor the editors and
publisher, nor any other party who has been involved in the preparation or
publication of this work warrants that the information contained herein is
in every respect accurate or complete, and they are not responsible for any
errors or omissions or the results obtained from the use of such information.
Readers are encouraged to confirm the information contained in this book
with other sources.

Library of Congress Cataloging-in-Publication Data

Assessment in cognitive therapy / edited by Gary P. Brown and David A. Clark.
    p. ; cm.
  Includes bibliographical references and index.
  ISBN 978-1-4625-1812-8 (hardcover : alk. paper)
  I. Brown, Gary P., editor.   II. Clark, David A., 1954– , editor.
  [DNLM: 1. Cognition Disorders—diagnosis.   2. Cognitive Therapy.
  3. Psychological Techniques.   4. Psychological Tests.   WM 425.5.C6]
  RC489.C63
  616.89′1425—dc23
                                                          2014024407

About the Editors

Gary P. Brown, PhD, is Senior Lecturer in the Psychology Department at Royal Holloway, University of London, United Kingdom, and Director of Research for the Clinical Psychology Doctoral Program. Dr. Brown has published extensively in the area of cognitive therapy for depression and anxiety. His particular focus has been on assessment and measurement, and he has been involved in the development of a number of the key measures used in the field. He has also been active in helping to develop the system of cognitive-behavioral training in the United Kingdom.

David A. Clark, PhD, is Professor of Psychology at the University of New Brunswick in Canada. Dr. Clark's research on the cognitive basis of anxiety and depression has appeared in numerous scientific journals. He is the author of several books, including *Scientific Foundations of Cognitive Theory and Therapy of Depression* (with Aaron T. Beck and Brad A. Alford), *Cognitive Therapy of Anxiety Disorders* (with Aaron T. Beck), *The Anxiety and Worry Workbook* (with Aaron T. Beck), and, most recently, *The Mood Repair Toolkit*. Dr. Clark is a Founding Fellow of the Academy of Cognitive Therapy and a recipient of its Aaron T. Beck Award for Significant and Enduring Contributions to Cognitive Therapy. He is also a Fellow of the Canadian Psychological Association. His website is *www.davidclarkpsychology.ca*.

Contributors

Alison Alden, BA, Department of Psychology, Northwestern University, Evanston, Illinois

John Baranoff, MClinPsych, School of Psychology, University of Adelaide, Adelaide, South Australia, Australia

Peter J. Bieling, PhD, Department of Psychiatry and Behavioural Neurosciences, McMaster University and St. Joseph's Healthcare Hamilton, Hamilton, Ontario, Canada

Simon E. Blackwell, DClinPsy, MRC Cognition and Brain Sciences Unit, Cambridge, United Kingdom

Gary P. Brown, PhD, Psychology Department, Royal Holloway University of London, Egham, Surrey, United Kingdom

Timothy A. Brown, PsyD, Department of Psychology and Center for Anxiety and Related Disorders, Boston University, Boston, Massachusetts

David A. Clark, PhD, Department of Psychology, University of New Brunswick, Fredericton, New Brunswick, Canada

Martina Di Simplicio, PhD, MRC Cognition and Brain Sciences Unit, Cambridge, United Kingdom

David J. A. Dozois, PhD, CPsych, Clinical Psychology Graduate Program, Department of Psychology, University of Western Ontario, London, Ontario, Canada

Katherine Elliott, BA, School of Psychology, University of Ottawa, Ottawa, Ontario, Canada

Lyndsay E. Evraire, MSc, Department of Psychology, University of Western Ontario, London, Ontario, Canada

Leila Guller, MS, Department of Psychology, University of Kentucky, Lexington, Kentucky

David A. F. Haaga, PhD, Department of Psychology, American University, Washington, DC

Susie Hales, DClinPsy, Department of Psychiatry, University of Oxford, Oxford, United Kingdom

Nick Hawkes, DClinPsy, Eating Disorders Unit, St Ann's Hospital, London, United Kingdom

Elizabeth P. Hayden, PhD, Department of Psychology and the Brain and Mind Institute, University of Western Ontario, London, Ontario, Canada

Emily A. Holmes, PhD, MRC Cognition and Brain Sciences Unit, Cambridge, United Kingdom, and Department for Clinical Neuroscience, Karolinska Institutet, Stockholm, Sweden

Jorg Huijding, PhD, Faculty of Social Sciences, Erasmus University Rotterdam, Rotterdam, The Netherlands

John Hunsley, PhD, CPsych, School of Psychology, University of Ottawa, Ottawa, Ontario, Canada

Lalitha Iyadurai, DClinPsy, Department of Psychiatry, University of Oxford, Oxford, United Kingdom

Anita T. M. Jansen, PhD, Department of Psychological Science, Faculty of Psychology and Neuroscience, Maastricht University, Maastricht, The Netherlands

Brenda Key, PhD, Department of Psychiatry and Behavioural Neurosciences, McMaster University, and Mood Disorders Program and Anxiety Treatment and Research Centre, St. Joseph's Healthcare Hamilton, Hamilton, Ontario, Canada

Colin M. MacLeod, PhD, Department of Psychology, University of Waterloo, Waterloo, Ontario, Canada

Kristin Naragon-Gainey, PhD, Department of Psychology, University at Buffalo, The State University of New York, Buffalo, New York

Peter J. Norton, PhD, Department of Psychology, University of Houston, Houston, Texas

Tian Po S. Oei, PhD, School of Psychology, University of Queensland, Brisbane, and CBT Unit, Toowong Private Hospital, Toowong, Queensland, Australia

Chelsea G. Ratcliff, MA, Department of Psychology, University of Houston, Houston, Texas

Anne Roefs, PhD, Department of Psychological Science, Faculty of Psychology and Neuroscience, Maastricht University, Maastricht, The Netherlands

Angela H. Smith, MA, Department of Psychology, University of Houston, Houston, Texas

Gregory T. Smith, PhD, Department of Psychology, University of Kentucky, Lexington, Kentucky

Fren T. Y. Smulders, PhD, Department of Cognitive Neuroscience, Faculty of Psychology and Neuroscience, Maastricht University, Maastricht, The Netherlands

Ari Solomon, PhD, Department of Psychology, Williams College, Williamstown, Massachusetts

Amanda A. Uliaszek, PhD, Department of Psychology, University of Toronto Scarborough, Toronto, Ontario, Canada

Kerry Young, DipClinPsychol, Department of Psychiatry, University of Oxford, Oxford, United Kingdom, and Forced Migration Trauma Service, Central and North West London NHS Foundation Trust, London, United Kingdom

Richard E. Zinbarg, PhD, Department of Psychology, Northwestern University, Evanston, Illinois

Preface

The great American essayist and poet Henry David Thoreau once wrote, "Do not worry if you have built your castles in the air. They are where they should be. Now put the foundations under them." In many respects, this apt statement describes the current state of cognitive-behavioral therapy (CBT). It could be said that we have built castles in the air. Our "castles" are hypothetical constructs about the nature of meaning generation or knowledge representation and involve concepts like schemas, processing biases, conditional assumptions, interpretations, judgments, and the like. A basic proposition of the CBT perspective is that our cognitive concepts are key mediators in the etiology, persistence, and treatment of disturbed emotions and behavior. The importance of cognitive mediation has been emphasized since the inception of CBT (Beck, 1967; Mahoney, 1974; Meichenbaum, 1977), although this fundamental tenet continues to be challenged even today (Longmore & Worrell, 2007). But any "castle," whether a metaphorical one or a physical entity, requires a foundation. And the foundation for our "cognitive castles" is assessment.

In its earliest days, assessment was at the forefront of developing the new clinical science of CBT. In his book *Cognitive-Behavior Modification*, Meichenbaum (1977) devotes the final chapter to the development of explicit assessment of affect, cognition, and volition, and the promotion of cognitive–functional case formulation. Mahoney (1974) elaborated a measurement theory for cognitive mediational models, and a significant aspect of Beck's research agenda over the decades has been the development of cognitive assessment instruments such as the Cognitions Checklist, the Dysfunctional Attitudes Scale, and the Beck Hopelessness Scale. Throughout the 1980s, several books appeared that specifically targeted cognitive assessment, such as Kendall and Hollon's *Assessment Strategies for Cognitive-Behavioral Interventions* (1981) and Merluzzi, Glass, and Genest's *Cognitive Assessment* (1981). Special journal issues and review articles were published on cognitive measurement and assessment as well (see Chapter 1 for a review). These progenitors of contemporary CBT repeatedly emphasized the importance and complexity of cognitive assessment as the foundation for cognitive clinical research and treatment. Kihlstrom and Nasby (1981), for example, argued for criterion-referenced assessment over standardized normative instruments and discussed how assessment procedures from experimental cognitive science could be creatively adapted to meet the measurement challenges of cognitive clinical psychology.

But these innovative ideas failed to take hold, and so advances in cognitive assessment theory and research appeared to stall. CBT clinical researchers seemed content to rely on standardized retrospective self-report questionnaires, especially in treatment-based studies. Moreover, interest in cognitive assessment more generally seems to have waned over the last 20 years, with the trail to innovation and development gone cold. Or has it? What is the state of cognitive assessment in the first two decades of the 21st century? Is it true that little progress is evident, that cognitive clinical researchers are stuck in an assessment "time-warp," with the very foundation of cognitive clinical science now threatened?

When we began our conversations about the current state of cognitive clinical assessment, our assumption was that little recent progress was evident. The status of CBT and the thorny issues raised by one of us 18 years ago are equally applicable today (Clark, 1997). We proposed writing this book in order to understand the source of the stagnation and to offer a fresh, in-depth, and critical analysis of current approaches to cognitive measurement and case formulation as viewed from the perspective of the clinical researcher, practitioner, and student of CBT. Although chapters diverge in their clinical versus research focus, we encouraged contributors to the book to take an integrative perspective by listing key points of interest to researchers, students, and clinicians. As you will see, they have done that. Furthermore, it turns out that there have been more advances, more innovation, and more creative clinical applications of cognitive clinical assessment than we thought possible. While inferred states remain a particular challenge for assessment, the contributors have documented real progress and promising leads in the measurement of thought content, process, and structure. Our cognitive assessment foundation may be shaky in places, but it is far from crumbling.

In the first chapter, Clark and Brown provide the historical context for the succeeding chapters by tracing the history of CBT assessment from its early years until the present, noting the parallel overall trends of a diminishing emphasis on concerns with measurement and assessment and an increasingly uncritical reliance on a single-method, respondent self-report. Part I draws together in-depth discussions of time-honored approaches, such as endorsement (Brown and Clark) and production (Haaga and Solomon) methods, along with newer approaches, such as imagery-based assessment (Hales et al.), and considers how these approaches can be applied both to a current symptomatic episode and to enduring vulnerabilities across episodes (Evraire et al.). A central thread running through these chapters is the perennial challenge of how to apply general (nomothetic) knowledge to the individual (idiographic) target of assessment, which is the focus of the chapter by Hunsley and Elliott on evidence-based assessment.

Given that assessment in mental health is inherently bound up with diagnosis, Part II grapples with the dichotomy between categorical diagnosis and dimensional measurement, delving within (Baranoff and Oei), across (Uliaszek et al. and A. H. Smith et al.), and beyond (Key and Bieling) diagnoses. Concerns with validity are central to the book, and the final part, Part III, addresses these concerns explicitly. Hawkes and Brown outline a validity framework for CBT assessment anchored in general cross-discipline validity standards. Guller and G. T. Smith show how these standards have evolved and discuss what implications current developments have for CBT assessment. Roefs et al. offer a close examination of implicit measurement as a springboard for considering whether experimental methods are inherently more valid, as is sometimes assumed, or whether they complement the more common explicit self-report methods of clinical assessment. Naragon-Gainey and T. A. Brown provide a survey of current state-of-the-art structural equation modeling and suggest ways that this technique and others may help unravel some of the more perplexing validity challenges facing the field. In the final chapter, Brown and Clark present an integrative summary that seeks to weigh both the shortcomings and achievements of CBT assessment to date and what implications these have for the practicing clinician, and conclude with a proposed set of benchmarks of future progress.

We are indebted to all of the contributing authors who provided valuable insights into and understanding of cognitive clinical assessment in their outstanding chapters. The strength of this book is entirely dependent on the knowledge and expertise expressed in their work. Both of us had the great privilege of working with Dr. Aaron T. Beck earlier in our careers. He taught us a great deal about the value of assessment and its role in cognitive clinical research and treatment. We are grateful for his wisdom, generosity, and continuing support in our work on assessment. We also want to acknowledge the significant contributions to cognitive assessment made by past clinical researchers and clinicians like Drs. Diane Arnkoff, John Cacioppo, Carol Glass, Steve Hollon, Philip Kendall, Michael Mahoney, Donald Meichenbaum, and Robert Schwartz, to name but a few. I (GPB) would like to express my gratitude to Chiara for her patience and support. And I (DAC) want to acknowledge with deep appreciation the ongoing support and encouragement of my spouse—and fellow academic and author—Nancy Nason-Clark. Last, but not least, we are grateful for the guidance, advice, and support of the staff at The Guilford Press, especially Jim Nageotte, Senior Editor, and Jane Keislar, Assistant Editor. Without their encouragement and understanding, our dissemination efforts truly would have faltered.

GARY P. BROWN
DAVID A. CLARK

REFERENCES

Beck, A. T. (1967). *Depression: Causes and treatment.* Philadelphia: University of Pennsylvania Press.

Clark, D. A. (1997). Introduction to the special section on measuring cognitive products in research and practice. *Journal of Consulting and Clinical Psychology, 65,* 907–910.

Kendall, P. C., & Hollon, S. D. (1981). Assessing self-referent speech: Methods in the measurement of self-statements. In P. C. Kendall & S. D. Hollon (Eds.), *Assessment strategies for cognitive-behavioral interventions* (pp. 85–118). New York: Academic Press.

Kihlstrom, J. F., & Nasby, W. (1981). Cognitive tasks in clinical assessment: An exercise in applied psychology? In P. C. Kendall & S. D. Hollon (Eds.), *Assessment strategies for cognitive-behavioral interventions* (pp. 287–317). New York: Academic Press.

Longmore, R. J., & Worrell, M. (2007). Do we need to challenge thoughts in cognitive behavior therapy? *Clinical Psychology Review, 27,* 173–187.

Mahoney, M. J. (1974). *Cognition and behavior modification.* Cambridge, MA: Ballinger.

Meichenbaum, D. (1977). *Cognitive-behavior modification: An integrative approach.* New York: Plenum Press.

Merluzzi, T. V., Glass, C. R., & Genest, M. (Eds.). (1981). *Cognitive assessment.* New York: Guilford Press.

Contents

CONCLUSION

INTRODUCTION

1

Cognitive Clinical Assessment

Contributions and Impediments to Progress

David A. Clark and Gary P. Brown

The cognitive revolution in clinical psychology and psychotherapy, launched in the 1970s and early 1980s by pioneers such as Aaron T. Beck, Albert Ellis, Donald Meichenbaum, Michael Mahoney, and Philip Kendall, has long since come of age. Cognitive-behavioral therapy (CBT) is now recognized as an empirically supported therapy and first-line treatment for a variety of psychological disorders, especially anxiety and depression, and has been included in the practice guidelines of the American Psychiatric Association (e.g., American Psychiatric Association, 2010) and the British National Institute for Health and Clinical Excellence, now the National Institute for Health and Care Excellence (e.g., National Institute for Health and Clinical Excellence, 2005). Moreover, it continues to be endorsed as an empirically supported treatment for many clinical disorders by the American Psychological Association (see Chambless & Ollendick, 2001) as well as other professional psychology organizations such as the Australian Psychological Society and the Canadian Psychological Association. Although practitioners consider CBT the most influential of the psychotherapies for adults (Cook, Biyanova, Elhai, Schnurr, & Coyne, 2010), it has achieved low levels of penetration as a fully implemented evidence-based treatment in real-world clinical practice delivered by fully certified CBT therapists (Stewart & Chambless, 2007). Thus, from one perspective the cognitive revolution has been hugely successful in spawning highly effective treatments for

3

the anxiety disorders, major depression, and eating disorders in particular, but the problem of limited access to effective treatment for mental health consumers is only beginning to be addressed (McHugh & Barlow, 2010). It is therefore incumbent upon those working in the area to continue to develop forms of CBT treatment that are compatible with the exigencies of health care delivery systems.

The last 30 years have also seen significant progress in cognitively based theoretical models and research on psychopathological conditions. A comparison of the early cognitive theories of anxiety and depression to more recent refinements and elaborations reveals considerable advance in ecological validity, integration, and predictive utility. We have seen substantial progress in elucidating the underlying cognitive structures and processes involved in the etiology and maintenance of clinical disorders. Findings from experimental clinical psychology have been incorporated into more recent cognitive-behavioral theories that better map the common and specific contributory processes to the etiology and maintenance of anxiety and depression (Clark & Beck, 2010; Gotlib & Joormann, 2010).

In contrast to these undeniable advances in theory, research, and treatment, the question needs to be asked: What has cognitive assessment contributed? Have our assessment approaches kept pace with the evolution of CBT, or has development in cognitive assessment stalled, so that we are left stuck in the methodology and perspectives of the pioneering days of CBT? Have we overcome barriers and challenges in cognitive assessment that could thwart innovation and development? Does cognitive assessment even matter to the day-to-day clinical service provided by those who consider themselves cognitive-behavioral therapists? And what are the critical issues for future research that could advance the case for cognitive assessment? These are some of the questions we begin to address in this chapter and that will continue to emerge throughout subsequent chapters in this volume. But before we begin, let's take a historical look at the critical role played by cognitive assessment in the early years of the paradigmatic shift in clinical psychology from a strictly response-based behavioral perspective to a stimulus-oriented information-processing paradigm.

BOUNDARIES AND ORIGINS
OF COGNITIVE CLINICAL ASSESSMENT

It could be argued that the term "cognitive assessment" is an all-encompassing concept that refers to all attempts to measure any aspect of information processing. From this perspective, any research on the cognitive basis of psychopathology would by necessity involve assessment methodology, and any treatment that targets cognitive change would require some method to measure this change. Given such breadth, it is important to define the boundaries of cognitive clinical assessment for the purposes of the present volume. Thus, in the current context, the term "cognitive clinical assessment" refers to *systematic empirically derived protocols, procedures, or instruments intended to measure the frequency, intensity, and salience of meaningful information comprising the thoughts, images, and beliefs that characterize psychopathological states.* This definition focuses on the measurement of "cognitive products," which according to the earlier taxonomic classification proposed by Ingram and Kendall (1986), are the thoughts, images, self-statements, or internal dialogue that represents output from the information-processing system, and cognitive propositions that are the content of underlying beliefs or schemas. Moreover, a diverse set of methodologies used to assess thought and belief content fall under our definition of cognitive clinical assessment, such as recording, production, sampling, and endorsement methods. However, for purposes of the present discussion we exclude various experimental paradigms derived from cognitive experimental psychology that assess the structure and operation of the information-processing system, such as dot-probe tasks, emotional Stroop color-naming tasks, the Implicit Association Test (IAT), the Self-Referent Encoding Task, and the like. Although these information-processing methodologies clearly fall under the rubric of "cognitive assessment" and account for much of the innovation and advance seen in cognitive clinical research in the last two decades (see Dunkley, Blankstein, & Segal, 2010, for review), their impact and implication for cognitive-behavioral treatment and practice is not as evident as cognitive assessment of content or products. Since our objective is to review cognitive assessment with more direct implications for both research and practice, restricted focus on the content of cognitive clinical assessment predominates in the present volume.

The advent of cognitive clinical assessment can be traced to an article published by Kendall and Korgeski (1979) in *Cognitive Therapy and Research*, followed in quick succession by two edited volumes that appeared in the same year (Kendall & Hollon, 1981a; Merluzzi, Glass, & Genest, 1981). In the last 30 years, review articles (e.g., Clark, 1988) and chapters (e.g., Dunkley et al., 2010) have appeared on cognitive assessment as well as special issues in the *Journal of Consulting and Clinical Psychology* (Haaga, 1997) and *Journal of Rational-Emotive Cognitive-Behavior Therapy* (McDermut & Haaga, 2009). There have also been major conceptual (e.g., McFall & Townsend, 1998) and methodological (e.g., Chamberlain & Haaga, 1999; Hunsley & Meyer, 2003) papers specific to cognitive clinical assessment or psychological assessment more generally.

What progress has been made in cognitive clinical assessment is reflected in the scores of published empirical articles over the years (1) describing the development of new assessment instruments for an expanding number of cognitive-emotive constructs, (2) establishing the psychometric properties of existing cognitive clinical measures, (3) determining treatment sensitivity and clinical utility of cognitive measures, and (4) introducing new statistical methodologies for determining construct validity. Despite these noteworthy gains, the momentum evident in the early years of cognitive clinical assessment appears to have evaporated. Compared to the substantial changes evident in cognitive clinical research and treatment, the advances in cognitive clinical assessment seem tepid. Why we have seen less progress in cognitive clinical assessment will be addressed in the chapters that follow in this volume.

In the early years of CBT, assessment issues were considered integral for further advances in theory, research, and treatment. Kendall and Korgeski (1979), for example, argued that progress in cognitive theory and treatment would be impeded without concomitant advances in the assessment of cognitive constructs. Kendall (1981) noted that advances in cognitive assessment are critical to research on (1) the role of cognition in emotion and behavior, (2) the cognitive basis of etiology and maintenance of psychological disorders, (3) the effects of treatment, and (4) the manipulation of cognitive processes in experimental research. And yet it has always been recognized that the assessment of cognition presents special challenges to researcher and practitioner alike. The most obvious is the private, internal, unobservable nature of cognitive content. Kendall (1981) argued that although the unobservable nature of cognition makes it "troublesome to assess," this does not make it any less important in understanding psychopathology and its treatment. Related issues raised by Kendall (1981) concern accuracy and accessibility. "Accuracy" refers to whether individuals report the actual cognitions they experienced, whereas "accessibility" refers to whether individuals have access to, that is, can report on the cognitions requested in the assessment. As seen in the following chapters, these core issues of cognitive clinical assessment (i.e., internality, accuracy, and accessibility) are confronted again and again whenever we attempt to measure cognitive content. Furthermore, the issues of reliability and validity are no less relevant for cognitive clinical assessment than they are for measurement of behavior, intellectual performance, or physical response. Admittedly, it is more challenging to demonstrate validity and reliability in measures of cognition due to the private nature of cognition, but its necessity is no less diminished by the challenges we face.

Kendall and Hollon (1981b) proposed a methodologically based system for organizing measures of cognitive content that has proven most useful over the intervening years. It is an organization that is followed by many of the authors in this book. Cognitive content can be assessed by "recording methods," which involve audiotaping and subsequent content analysis of an individual's spontaneous or task-related verbalizations. "Production methods" instruct individuals to retrospectively produce, either in oral or written form, their thoughts during a preceding time interval (e.g., engage in a role play and then write down all thoughts that occurred during the role play). "Thought-sampling procedures" instruct individuals to report their current thought whenever cued by a device, usually delivered on a random basis. Finally, "endorsement methods" provide individuals a predetermined list of cognitions (i.e., in question-naire format) and instruct them to indicate the frequency of occurrence or some other characteristic of the cognition, usually over a specified time period. By far the most common method to assess cognitive content has been via questionnaire, that is, endorsement methodology. As we will see, this method of assessment has also been subject to the most intense criticism by cognitive clinical researchers.

RECENT DEVELOPMENTS IN CBT

To determine whether cognitive clinical assessment has kept pace with the changing face of CBT research and treatment, it is important to rec-ognize some of the major developments that are occurring in the field. Several of these innovations and developments are discussed in greater depth by the chapter authors.

CBT Expansion to a Wide Array of Conditions

Cognitive-behavioral theory and treatment has now been applied to an ever expanding variety of psychological conditions and disorders such as personality disorders, anger and stress management, psychosis and schizophrenia, mania, addictions, obesity, relationship problems, parent management, and the like. Although much of the CBT research and treat-ment development continues to focus on the emotional disorders (anxiety and depression), each time the model is applied to a new problem it neces-sitates the development of a new suite of cognitive clinical measures. To date, there has been a tendency to utilize the same assessment method-ologies as we've seen in the measurement of cognitive content in anxiety and depression. That is, research in these new areas has primarily carried on the tradition of developing new retrospective self-report measures of cognitive content that seek to provide an adequate representation of the key cognitive features of the new psychological condition.

More Elaborated but Inaccessible Cognitive Constructs Proposed by Newer CBT Formulations

More recent iterations of CBT theory and treatment emphasize "deeper," more complex cognitive constructs that are probably more inaccessible to awareness, representing an even greater challenge for cognitive clinical assessment. For example, Cartwright-Hatton and Wells (1997) developed the Meta-Cognitions Questionnaire (MCQ; see also Wells & Cartwright-Hatton, 2004, for a shortened version) to assess key constructs of Wells's metacognitive theory, including beliefs about worry, cognitive confidence, and cognitive self-consciousness. The latter two constructs refer to individuals' self-efficacy beliefs in their memory and attentional functioning, and the extent that they focus on their own thinking (Cartwright-Hatton & Wells, 1997). Both constructs are meta-cognitive in nature; that is, they assume insight into how one thinks— the very cognitive processes that Nisbett and Wilson (1977) so long ago questioned as accessible to the introspective process.

Another example is the long form of the Young Schema Questionnaire, Third Edition, a 205-item self-report questionnaire that asks individuals the degree of self-descriptiveness of item statements assumed to represent early maladaptive schemas (Young & Brown, 2003). Some of the statements refer to behavioral responses, others self-referent beliefs, and still others specific emotion states. However, early maladaptive schemas (EMSs) are construed at the deepest cognitive level and are thought to emerge from childhood adverse or traumatic experiences (Martin & Young, 2010). They are the earliest and most central schemas that are automatic, temporally stable, affect-laden, and highly resistant to change, representing an interaction between temperament and early environmental experiences and reinforced by subsequent life experiences (Young, 1990). Martin and Young (2010) noted that EMSs are major determinants of thought, feeling, and behavior, are generally accepted as a priori truths, and are outside of awareness. Given these characteristics, how accurately can highly conscious, deliberate responses to questionnaire items tap into deeply embedded core structures like EMSs? Other cognitive clinical researchers have focused on assessing specific characteristics of thought that transcend content, such as the Perseverative Thinking Questionnaire (Ehring et al., 2011). We can assume that individuals have even less awareness of "how they think" (i.e., process) than "what they think" (i.e., content).

Greater Emphasis on Case Formulation

In recent years CBT clinicians have emphasized the importance of developing a cognitive case formulation as a guide to the treatment process

(J. S. Beck, 2011; Kuyken, Padesky, & Dudley, 2008; Persons, 2008). However, empirical support that case formulation has a significant impact on treatment outcome has not been demonstrated (see Key & Bieling, Chapter 10, this volume), while others have argued for a more standard, manualized approach to CBT that does not place as much emphasis on individualized case conceptualization. Moreover, current cognitive assessment methods may not map onto the various models of case formulation since their development has not been driven by case formulation concepts. Even though proponents of case formulation advocate use of psychometrically sound cognitive measures, the utility of these for individualized cognitive case formulation remains unsubstantiated.

Development of Low-Intensity CBT

Efforts to bridge the gap between research and the limited availability of evidence-based treatment in health services has led to the development of brief, therapist-limited CBT protocols for mild psychological disturbance (Bennett-Levy, Richards, & Farrand, 2010). Low-intensity CBT encompasses a fairly broad range of interventions, such as self-help books, Internet-based CBT, group psychoeducation programs, entry-level intervention in stepped care programs, and so on (Richards, 2010). Within low-intensity treatment, access to specialized mental health professionals may be limited to one or two contacts, so there is little scope for individualized case formulation. At most, assessment may be reduced to a structured clinical interview and a couple of brief standardized symptom ratings or questionnaires. Specific measures of cognitive content will be rarely employed due to time constraints. Moreover, it is not at all clear that existing cognitive clinical measures, which were developed for moderate to severe distress, would be valid in a downward extension to milder forms of emotional disturbance (see Hawkes & Brown, Chapter 11, this volume). It is likely that new measures of cognitive content will be needed to meet the distinctive demands of low-intensity CBT.

Transdiagnostic CBT

Recently, a number of prominent CBT clinical researchers have advocated transdiagnostic or unified treatment protocols as complementary to disorder-specific manualized treatment. Barlow and colleagues developed the unified treatment protocol for treatment of emotional disorders (Barlow, Allen, & Choate, 2004; Barlow et al., 2011); Norton introduced a transdiagnostic CBT for anxiety disorders (Norton, 2012; see Smith, Ratcliff, & Norton, Chapter 9, this volume); and Fairburn, Cooper, and Shafran (2003) developed transdiagnostic CBT for anorexia and bulimia nervosa. These approaches transcend the diagnostic boundaries of psychiatric classification systems such as the *Diagnostic and Statistical Manual of Mental Disorders* (DSM) and focus treatment on the common or shared features of psychological disorders (Mansell, Harvey, Watkins, & Shafran, 2009; McManus, Shafran, & Cooper, 2010). The rationale is that transdiagnostic protocols may be more effective in cases of multiple co-occurring disorders and eliminate the unrealistic expectation that therapists gain expertise in multiple disorder-specific treatment protocols, especially in rural or general mental health settings where practitioners deal with a wide range of conditions (see Smith et al., Chapter 9, this volume). In these treatment approaches, the case conceptualization is framed in terms of common and specific processes, with the former being the primary focus of treatment (Mansell et al., 2009).

Interestingly, our current measures of cognitive content may be easily applied to transdiagnostic treatments. Psychometric research on many of the most popular cognitive content measures has demonstrated good convergent validity but low discriminant validity. For example, measures of depressive and anxious cognitive content always correlate positively (see Baranoff & Oei, Chapter 8, this volume), which suggests they are tapping into the common or shared features of anxiety and depression. Even though unintended, if our current cognitive measures are highly saturated with common variance items, they may be more relevant for transdiagnostic interventions and easily adapted into transdiagnostic treatment protocols. Whether cognitive content measures have even greater treatment utility and predictive validity in transdiagnostic CBT compared to disorder-specific interventions remains to be seen.

PAST ISSUES AND CURRENT CHALLENGES

Many of the problems and challenges facing cognitive clinical assessment raised in the early years of CBT are as applicable today as they were in past decades. Many of these issues are taken up in greater detail in the following chapters. In this section, we highlight some of the more prominent concerns and whether progress has been made in the intervening years.

Insufficient Construct Validity

Without question, the most critical issue for any assessment measure is its "construct validity"—that is, the accuracy of judgments about a psychological phenomenon on the basis of test scores (American Psychological Association, 1999). For cognitive clinical assessment, construct validity depends to a greater degree on whether we can infer that responses on a measure reflect the individual's actual thought content (for a discussion of validity and veridicality, see Brown & Clark, Chapter 2, this volume).

Only a few cognitive clinical measures have been subjected to sufficient psychometric research to provide a firm evidence base for their construct validity. One of these measures is the Dysfunctional Attitude Scale (DAS). A 100-item version originally developed by Weissman and Beck (1978) to assess relatively stable prepotent schema content that Beck's cognitive model hypothesized as vulnerability to major depression has since been abbreviated to parallel 40-item versions (Cane, Olinger, Gotlib, & Kuiper, 1986) and an even briefer 9-item short form (Beevers, Strong, Meyer, Pilkonis, & Miller, 2007). Various factorial analyses conducted on the DAS-40 have found two highly reliable dimensions, need for approval from others (i.e., social dependency concerns) and performance evaluation/perfectionism (de Graaf, Roelofs, & Huibers, 2009), whereas the factorial structure for the 100-item DAS is less stable, depending on whether clinical or nonclinical samples are utilized (Beck, Brown, Steer, & Weissman, 1991; Calhoon, 1996). Generally the underlying dimensions of the DAS map onto the primary themes of Beck's cognitive model of depression.

In most studies, the DAS-40 has good internal consistency, and the perfectionism/performance factor in particular has a strong association with depressive symptoms (e.g., de Graaf et al., 2009; Dobson & Breiter, 1983). To determine the psychometric performance of individual DAS items, Beevers et al. (2007) conducted an item response theory analysis on the DAS-40 based on 250 patients with major depressive disorder. Twenty-two items failed to make sufficient discriminations, leaving 18 items that made adequate discriminations. The authors then divided these items into parallel 9-item DAS short forms. Further analysis of the 9-item and full 40-item DASs indicated that all versions significantly declined with treatment, correlated with other measures of depressive cognition, and higher pretreatment scores predicted less change in depression at posttreatment. In an earlier study, Zuroff, Blatt, Sanislow, Bondi, and Pilkonis (1999) employed structural equation modeling to show that the DAS-40 Need for Approval and Performance/Perfectionism dimensions exhibited both change and stability over the course of treatment for depression, and that high pretreatment DAS predicted poorer response to treatment. Moreover, depressive symptoms and dysfunctional attitudes tended to rise and fall together over the course of treatment. The authors concluded that dysfunctional attitudes are neither fixed nor enduring or mere consequences of the depressive state, but rather a mixed state–trait attribute that is entirely consistent with a vulnerability model. Hill, Oei, and Hill (1989) investigated the sensitivity and specificity of the DAS-40 and Automatic Thoughts Questionnaire (ATQ) in clinical and nonclinical samples representing a broad range of diagnostic groups. They concluded that the ATQ was more specific and sensitive to depression than the DAS-40, with the latter measure actually showing a far degree of nonspecificity. Other studies have also found that the DAS does not discriminate major depression from other diagnostic groups (e.g., Silverman, Silverman, & Eardley, 1984). Nevertheless, the DAS-40 has been used as a cognitive vulnerability measure in behavioral high-risk designs and shown to predict first onset of major depression (Alloy, Abramson, Keyser, Gerstein, & Sylvia, 2008). Moreover, increased DAS scores when primed by negative mood induction was shown to predict depressive relapse (Segal et al., 2006), although in a subsequent study posttreatment unprimed but not primed DAS scores predicted relapse over a 20-month follow-up period (Jarrett et al., 2012).

The DAS, then, provides an excellent example of a research literature building the case for construct validity through a variety of research methodologies involving psychometric analysis, clinical experimental research, and treatment outcome trials. In recent years, more sophisticated statistical tools such as structural equation modeling and item response theory analysis indicates that only a few DAS items possess sufficient discriminatory power and that dysfunctional attitudes possess both state and trait properties. Newer methods of analysis outlined by Naragon-Gainey and T. A. Brown (Chapter 12, this volume), such as the trait–state–occasion technique (e.g., LaGrange et al., 2011), hold promise for providing further clarification on this elusive but central issue of the relationship between constructs such as those measured by the DAS and symptoms over time.

The somewhat adequate sensitivity but poor specificity suggests that the DAS may be tapping into the more common features of emotional disorders, rather than structures specific to depression. As well, it is unclear whether the DAS requires priming (i.e., activation) in order to examine its effects. Nevertheless, we can infer that DAS responses do reflect schematic content that is characteristic of depression, given that these responses behave in ways predicted of cognitive vulnerability constructs; that is, they predict depressive onset, relapse and recurrence, and response to treatment. Thus, over the years progress has been made on the DAS, ensuring that clinical researchers will continue to use this instrument to assess cognitive vulnerability. It is hoped that the same sustained program of research can be conducted with other cognitive assessment measures in order to determine their construct validity.

Low Multimethod Convergence

An important aspect of construct validity is *convergent validity*, that is, confirmation of validity by different testing procedures (Campbell & Fiske, 1959). In the case of cognitive clinical assessment, a measure of, for example, negative self-referent thoughts of loss and failure should correlate with other measures of depressive cognition but also with measures of behavioral, emotional, somatic, and other characteristics of depression. Moreover, the various assessment methods of cognitive clinical assessment that differ along temporal and structural dimensions afford a special opportunity to investigate convergent validity (Dunkley et al., 2010).

Generally speaking, cognitive measures tend to exhibit moderate to high convergent validity with other measures of the same cognitive phenomena using the same methodology. For example, endorsement methods involving retrospective self-report responses to predetermined item statements tend to correlate well with other endorsement measures. The ATQ and DAS, for example, are strongly correlated with each other, and depression symptom measures (e.g., Hill et al., 1989). However, the correlations drop substantially when different methodologies of the same cognitive phenomena are compared in a multitrait–multimethod matrix (Campbell & Fiske, 1959). In their review, Chamberlain and Haaga (1999) concluded that the correlations between endorsement (i.e., self-report questionnaires) and production (i.e., articulated thoughts during simulated situations) methods tend to be quite low (see also Haaga & Solomon, Chapter 3, this volume; Clark, 1988). This low correlation, of course, raises concerns that endorsement, production, recording, and thought-sampling methods may be assessing different cognitive constructs (Dunkley et al., 2010). In their chapter, Haaga and Solomon suggest a number of ways that production methods can still be helpful in cognitive assessment, despite low convergent validity with self-report questionnaires.

Mumma (2004) provides an excellent example of utilizing items from standardized self-report measures of cognition and a structured clinical interview of core beliefs to construct an individualized daily questionnaire of cognitions that was then evaluated for convergent, discriminant, and incremental validity against variability in distress ratings and predictions of cognitive content specificity. The analysis was conducted on 90 days of data collected from an individual with major depressive disorder and demonstrates how nomothetic and idiographic methods of cognitive assessment can be integrated and used to validate cognitive case formulation in clinical practice (see Brown & Clark, Chapter 2, this volume, for a further discussion). It would be interesting to use Mumma's construct validation approach to compare the convergent and discriminant validity within individual cognitive case formulations for various types of assessment (i.e., thought sampling, production, endorsement methods). It would be informative to determine which of these assessment methods exhibits the most utility in validating the idiosyncratic core schemas featured in individual cognitive case formulations.

Overreliance on Questionnaire Methodology

It has been noted in earlier reviews there has been an overreliance on retrospective self-report questionnaires in cognitive clinical assessment (e.g., Clark, 1997). In the intervening years, little has changed in this regard. Endorsement methodology still continues to overwhelmingly dominate cognitive clinical assessment. Although the reasons for this are quite obvious (see Brown & Clark, Chapter 2, this volume), Glass and Arnkoff (1997) warn against the dangers of leaning so heavily on self-report cognition questionnaires given the lack of verdicality of retrospective cognitive self-report. Of course retrospective questionnaires are susceptible to the problems of selective memory biases and forgetting. After all, no one assumes that people keep track of their cognitions on a daily basis, except for the most fervent cognitive therapist. So, when an anxious individual endorses a self-statement like "I have thoughts of threat and danger," does that endorsement reflect frequent occurrence of that thought or the individual's sense that he or she frequently feels apprehensive and anxious?

These issues are elaborated further in subsequent chapters of this volume (Brown & Clark, Chapter 2; Hawkes & Brown, Chapter 11). In the meantime, it would be beneficial for clinical researchers and clinicians alike to place greater emphasis on collecting real-time cognitive content in the naturalistic setting (i.e., thought sampling), especially in light of the new opportunities afforded by apps and smartphone technology.

The Vulnerability Issue

Because cognitive theories postulate that particular cognitive structures, processes, and content play a causal role in emotional and behavioral disorders, the assessment of cognitive vulnerability is of paramount importance in empirical research on these models. In Beck's cognitive theory of depression (Beck, 1987; Clark, Beck, & Alford, 1999), for example, prepotent dysfunctional self-referent schemas derived from adverse childhood experiences, remain dormant until activated by a congruent negative life event. Once activated the schemas dominate the information processing system, creating a schema-congruent negativity bias in attention, memory, reasoning, and conscious thought. According to this diathesis–stress perspective, depressogenic schemas would remain undetected in vulnerable individuals until primed by an activating trigger.

In order for an instrument to qualify as a measure of vulnerability, certain parameters must be met by that measure. It must show temporal stability by reflecting a trait rather than state characteristic, although Ingram and Price (2010) suggest that having temporal stability does not mean the vulnerability factor is unchanging. They note that corrective experiences (i.e., treatment) could weaken the vulnerability factor, whereas certain life experiences might strengthen it. In addition to endurance, Ingram and Price (2010) include endogenous process (i.e., latent) and susceptibility to an activating stimulus as related characteristics.

One of the questions that have occupied cognitive clinical researchers for the past three decades is whether purported measures of schemas, such as the DAS, satisfy the criteria for vulnerability. Early studies comparing pretreatment to posttreatment of depression, or remitted and depressed patients, indicated that DAS scores returned to near normal levels once the depression remitted (e.g., Hamilton & Abramson, 1983; Hollon, Kendall, & Lumry, 1986), leading to the conclusion that the DAS, and possibly schemas themselves, do not satisfy the most basic requirement of vulnerability (i.e., stability) and so are probably a consequence rather than a cause of emotional disturbance (Barnett & Gotlib, 1988). However, cognitive theory predicts that vulnerability will not be evident unless underlying schemas are primed or activated. In fact, research over the last 20 years has generally supported this supposition. When measures of cognitive vulnerability (e.g., the DAS) are primed by an activating stimulus such as negative life event, negative mood state, and so on, they do tend to conform more closely to the parameters expected of vulnerability (see Evraire, Dozois, & Hayden, Chapter 5, this volume).

Although there are several important issues for cognitive assessment of vulnerability, two that are particularly important are highlighted by Evraire et al. (Chapter 5, this volume). One concerns the accuracy of self-report measures of vulnerability, with their proposal that inference-based experimental procedures like the Self-Referent Encoding Task or the IAT (see Roefs, Huijding, Smulders, Jansen, & MacLeod, Chapter 13, this volume, for a critical evaluation of the IAT) might prove more helpful in assessing vulnerability. The second issue concerns the necessity of priming. Although some have argued that priming is needed to adequately assess cognitive vulnerability (Ingram, Miranda, & Segal,

1998), it is not at all clear this is the case. Dozois (2007) demonstrated that schemas can be accessed without priming, and Jarrett et al. (2012) found that unprimed DAS predicted depressive relapse, whereas primed DAS was not a significant predictor. Thus two critical issues in cognitive vulnerability assessment are which method of assessment is most accurate and whether or not priming is necessary to determine the presence of vulnerability.

Incremental Validity and Treatment Utility

"Incremental validity" refers to the extent that "a measure adds to the prediction of a criterion above what can be predicted by other sources of data" (Hunsley & Meyer, 2003, p. 446). Within the context of cognitive clinical assessment, incremental validity would be the extent that a standardized measure of cognition would improve assessment of thoughts, beliefs, and other cognitive processes beyond what can be ascertained from a clinical interview or treatment process. The importance of incremental validity is readily apparent in the validation of new measures (Hunsley & Meyer, 2003). Cognitive clinical researchers are imaginative, energetic creators of an ever-expanding array of self-report cognition measures. Do we really need another measure of depressive cognitions? Instead of relying on our personal theoretical biases to answer this question, empirically based researchers should ask whether the new measure has incremental validity over existing depressive cognition measures. If the new measure significantly improves on the prediction of depression onset, relapse, response to treatment, cognitive reactivity, and so on, over existing cognitive measures, then it has sufficient incremental validity to justify its adoption in clinical research and practice. At the broader level, we could ask whether inclusion of an endorsement, production, or thought sampling method improves on clinical decision making, case formulation, or treatment outcome over clinical deductions drawn from unstructured interviews or inferences drawn from psychotherapy sessions (Hunsley, 2003). If incremental validity is demonstrated, then a stronger case could be made for incorporating more formalized cognitive clinical assessment in an evidence-based practice (see Hunsley & Elliott, Chapter 6, this volume). To date, however, cognitive clinical assessment research and development have tended to pay insufficient attention to incremental validity. Hunsley and Meyer (2003) made a number of recommendations that researchers could follow to rectify this deficiency, while acknowledging that for the practitioner there is no guidance on how incremental validity might be applied to individual cases.

"Treatment utility" refers to "the degree to which assessment is shown to contribute to beneficial treatment outcome" (Hayes, Nelson,

& Jarrett, 1987, p. 963). Typically, the treatment utility of assessment has been researched by determining whether assessment leads to treatment selection that results in a better client outcome or whether providing clinicians with assessment information leads to better outcomes (Nelson-Gray, 2003). In her review, Nelson-Gray (2003) concluded there is empirical evidence that functional analysis has treatment utility in linking behavioral assessment and treatment. Moreover, she speculated that use of diagnosis and semistructured interviews might have treatment utility if they are useful in accessing empirically supported treatments for particular disorders.

Studies employing specific measures of cognition or behavior have found that low scores, that is, individuals with a higher level of function, were associated with better treatment response (e.g., Jarrett et al., 2012; Rude & Rehm, 1991). This suggests that treatment utility of cognitive clinical assessment might operate contrary to expectations where low rather than high scores (i.e., having fewer negative cognitions) are predictive of more successful client outcome. (We might expect the opposite, that low measurement scores would be associated with less treatment change because of a more limited range of possible cognitive change.)

Unfortunately, little is known about the actual treatment utility of specific cognitive clinical measures in comparison to treatment outcome associated with a single clinician making clinical decisions based on monomethod assessment (i.e., clinical interview). Even though it is well-known that certain assessment methods such as self-monitoring can contribute to therapeutic change, it is likely that most clinicians expect that formal cognitive clinical assessment has low treatment utility, making it too inefficient and costly for real-world clinical practice. Thus, research demonstrating treatment utility could be helpful in persuading CBT practitioners to be more mindful of cognitive clinical assessment in the therapy setting.

Implications for Practice and DSM-5

A final issue concerns the low dissemination rate of empirically based cognitive clinical assessment among CBT practitioners. Historically, there has been a divide between treatment and assessment, with therapists utilizing limited systematic assessment when providing psychotherapy (Nelson-Gray, 2003). Butcher (2006) noted that the use of formal psychological testing, especially personality testing, in mental health settings declined with the advent of behavior therapy in the 1970s and then again in the 1990s with the rise of managed care and its concern with reducing mental health service costs. Although a small up-tick in formal assessment usage may be seen in certain sectors of clinical practice (such as court or some personnel settings), the reality is that the psychological tests developed in the 1940s—the Minnesota Multiphasic Personality Inventory and the Rorschach and Thematic Appreciation Tests—are still the most widely used today (Butcher, 2006). Despite evidence that psychological test validity is comparable to medical test validity and that single clinicians using single methods, like an interview, to obtain patient information will draw incomplete and biased conclusions about the patient (Meyer et al., 2001), assessment continues to be downplayed in clinical practice.

In a comparison of the 2010 survey of 549 clinical psychologists of the American Psychological Association's Division 12 membership with past membership surveys dating back to 1986, Norcross and Karpiak (2012) found a continuing decline in the proportion of clinical psychologists who routinely conduct diagnosis/assessment from 75% in 1986 to 58% in 2010. Moreover, the most popular theoretical orientations of respondents were cognitive (31%), eclectic/integration (22%), psychodynamic (18%), and behavioral (15%), with clinical interviews accounting for approximately half of all assessment time. Weiner (2012) in his commentary noted that the perceived decline of psychological assessment in clinical practice has led to reduced course offerings and assessment competency standards in many clinical psychology graduate programs.

It is increasingly recognized that therapist competency in evidence-based treatment does have a significant effect on patient outcome (Rakovshik & McManus, 2010), and CBT experts continue to emphasize assessment and case conceptualization in their training manuals (e.g., Antony & Barlow, 2010). However, given the rather dismal state of assessment in clinical practice, assessment competency may be deemphasized relative to therapy competency skills. As well, it is likely that the most common assessment methods employed in CBT practice are brief symptom measures like the Beck Depression Inventory, a clinically based self-monitoring form like the Daily Record of Dysfunctional Thoughts (Beck, Rush, Shaw, & Emery, 1979), and possibly a variant of a structured clinical interview. It is likely that few CBT practitioners routinely utilize the more empirically based cognitive clinical measures reviewed in this volume. Research is needed to (1) determine the current status of cognitive clinical assessment in CBT practice, (2) establish the policy and procedures needed to improve dissemination and training in cognitive clinical assessment, (3) develop standards of competency in cognitive clinical assessment and case formulation, and (4) demonstrate incremental validity and treatment utility of empirically grounded cognitive clinical assessment methods.

The publication of DSM-5 (American Psychiatric Association,

2013) has rekindled discussion of the role of diagnosis in assessment and treatment. Most CBT practitioners routinely utilize DSM diagnoses, if for no other reason than to meet administrative requirements or receive third-party compensation for clinical service. However, the link between psychiatric diagnosis and cognitive clinical assessment has remained tenuous at best. Diagnosis is often employed to determine the criterion-related validity of cognition measures, and cognitive measures are often developed with specific diagnostic groups in mind. However, actual measurement development in cognitive clinical assessment has been guided more by cognitive theory than diagnostic criteria. Thus, the implications of DSM-5 for cognitive clinical assessment may be minimal. Nevertheless, research is needed to determine if cognitive clinical assessment could be used to improve differential diagnosis, such as the inclusion of specific measures of thought content (see Baranoff & Oei, Chapter 8, this volume). Once again, the ultimate question for CBT clinical researchers and practitioners alike is whether empirically based cognitive clinical assessment can improve the accuracy of diagnosis and patient outcomes.

A GLANCE FORWARD

Many of the assessment issues touched on in this chapter are elaborated in the chapters that follow. We selected topics that are germane to the construct validity of cognitive assessment and its application to clinical practice. We asked the chapter authors to provide background information, a critical review of relevant empirical research, an overview of advances and impediments to progress, and implications for cognitive assessment research and practice.

In Chapter 2, on endorsement methods, we (Brown & Clark) tackle the thorny issue of retrospective questionnaire validation, setting out the parameters that should be met before a cognition questionnaire can be considered valid and incorporated into clinical practice. Subsequent chapters focus primarily on methodological or clinically based issues in cognitive assessment. Chapters 3, 7, and 11 through 14 deal with issues of measurement theory, with a particular emphasis on construct validity. Chapter 3, by Haaga and Solomon, discusses production-based cognitive assessment, noting how these methodologies could be modified to increase their clinical utility and improve convergent validity with other cognitive assessment methodologies. In Chapter 7, Uliaszek, Alden, and Zinbarg consider the perennial trade-off between dimensional and categorical assessment, the potential contribution of CBT to helping resolve the debate, and the implications for DSM-5. In Chapter 11, Hawkes and Brown consider whether and in what way a strict application of the general validity standards might help advance CBT assessment. In some instances, solutions to long-standing issues in research and practice depend on the development of suitable analytic techniques. In Chapter 12, Naragon-Gainey and T. A. Brown survey the latest development in structural equation modeling and item response theory and consider how these can be applied to issues of interest in CBT. Experimental paradigms are frequently held up as a more valid rigorous approach to the phenomena of interest in CBT research as an alternative to reliance on self-report scales. Roefs and colleagues focus on a particular experimental paradigm widely used in the field, the IAT, and consider their promise and their limitations in Chapter 13. Finally, in Chapter 14, Guller and G. T. Smith place CBT research within the historical context of developing conceptions of validity in the broader field.

Cognitive assessment issues pertinent to clinical practice are discussed in several chapters. In Chapter 4, Hales and colleagues provide a pragmatic guide to assessment of imagery, an area in which new ground is being broken and in which interventions such as imagery rescripting are being developed. Evraire, Dozois, and Hayden consider in Chapter 5 how cognitive assessment must be modified in order to deal with the unique features of vulnerability constructs such as their relative inaccessibility and inactive or latent state during asymptomatic time periods. In Chapter 6, Hunsley and Elliott provide a set of guidelines for establishing an evidence-based approach to cognitive assessment in clinical practice, with an illustrative reference to Dugas's CBT model for generalized anxiety disorder. Chapter 8 by Baranoff and Oei provides a comprehensive, critical review of empirical evidence for cognitive content-specificity, concluding that weak evidence for specificity, especially for anxiety, may be primarily due to measurement limitations, although weak conceptualization cannot be ruled out. A. H. Smith, Ratcliff, and Norton provide a broad conceptual and empirical overview of transdiagnostic CBT in Chapter 9, using a case illustration to highlight the transdiagnostic approach to cognitive assessment and case formulation. In Chapter 10, Key and Bieling discuss the pros and cons of cognitive case formulation including its limited empirical basis, while at the same time setting forth a series of recommendations that could improve its clinical utility and adaptation to "third wave" CBT.

The volume concludes with Chapter 15, which addresses two overarching questions that define the current state of cognitive clinical assessment: *What have we learned about cognitive assessment in the last 30 years? What are the impediments or challenges to further progress in CBT assessment, treatment, and its evaluation?* Answers to these questions, drawn from the preceding chapters, can set a course for cognitive clinical assessment in the coming years.

KEY POINTS

FOR PRACTITIONERS

- Reconsider the important role that cognitive assessment can play in strengthening an evidence-based cognitive-behavioral practice.
- Utilize cognitive assessment measures with high construct validity, especially methods that contribute to case formulation and that offer incremental treatment utility.
- Employ a greater mix of assessment methods that include production and sampling methodology as well as retrospective endorsement instruments. Thought sampling has greater potential for clinical use with the introduction of self-monitoring apps for smartphones.
- Priming methods can be adapted to the clinical setting in order to obtain a more accurate assessment of cognitive vulnerability.

FOR RESEARCHERS

- More research is needed at the item level using structural equation modeling and item response theory analysis to determine the veridicality of individuals' responses to item statements. It's at this more "microscopic," as opposed to "macroscopic" (i.e., total score), level that we will determine the validity of responses to cognitive assessment measures.
- The issue of low convergent validity between different methods of cognitive assessment is a critical problem in the field that has received scant research attention. Discovering the parameters of convergence could lead to the development of a more strategic approach to cognitive assessment.
- Most research on cognitive vulnerability has assumed that priming is critical to activate dormant cognitive structures. And yet there are a handful of studies that have demonstrated vulnerability effects without priming. At this point, little is known about the conditions under which priming is or is not necessary.
- New quick and efficient cognitive measures are needed for a whole array of innovative low-intensity CBT programs available over the Internet, as apps, or offered as minimal-therapist-contact self-help.
- Cognitive assessment researchers need to focus more on issues of incremental validity and treatment utility if their findings are to have any chance of significantly impacting clinical practice.

FOR STUDENTS AND EDUCATORS

- Given that training programs are spending less time on assessment more generally, it is likely that CBT training programs need to reconsider the quantity and quality of course content devoted to cognitive assessment.

- Training in cognitive case formulation should always include a module on cognitive clinical assessment and its role in case conceptualization.
- Competency standards in cognitive clinical assessment should be developed and these should be included in CBT certification programs.

REFERENCES

Alloy, L. B., Abramson, L. Y., Keyser, J., Gerstein, R. L., & Sylvia, L. G. (2008). Negative cognitive style. In K. S. Dobson & D. J. A. Dozois (Eds.), *Risk factors in depression* (pp. 221–236). Amsterdam: Elsevier.

American Psychiatric Association. (2010). Practice guideline for the treatment of patients with major depressive disorder, third edition. Retrieved January 29, 2013, from *PsychiatryOnline*.

American Psychiatric Association. (2013). *Diagnostic and statistical manual of mental disorders* (5th ed.). Arlington, VA: Author.

American Psychological Association. (1999). *Standards for educational and psychological testing*. Washington, DC: Author.

Antony, M. M., & Barlow, D. H. (Eds.). (2010). *Handbook of assessment and treatment planning for psychological disorders* (2nd ed.). New York: Guilford Press.

Barlow, D. H., Allen, L. B., & Choate, M. L. (2004). Toward a unified treatment of emotional disorders. *Behavior Therapy, 35*, 205–230.

Barlow, D. H., Ellard, K. K., Fairholme, C. P., Farchione, T. J., Boisseau, C. L., Allen, L. B., et al. (2011). *Unified protocol for transdiagnostic treatment of emotional disorders*. Oxford, UK: Oxford University Press.

Barnett, P. A., & Gotlib, I. H. (1988). Psychosocial functioning and depression: Distinguishing among antecedents, concomitants, and consequences. *Psychological Bulletin, 104*, 97–126.

Beck, A. T. (1987). Cognitive models of depression. *Journal of Cognitive Psychotherapy: An International Quarterly, 1*, 5–37.

Beck, A. T., Brown, G., Steer, R. A., & Weissman, A. N. (1991). Factor analysis of the Dysfunctional Attitude Scale in a clinical population. *Psychological Assessment: A Journal of Consulting and Clinical Psychology, 3*, 478–483.

Beck, A. T., Rush, A. J., Shaw, B. F., & Emery, G. (1979). *Cognitive therapy of depression*. New York: Guilford Press.

Beck, J. S. (2011). *Cognitive-behavior therapy: Basics and beyond* (2nd ed.). New York: Guilford Press.

Beevers, C. G., Strong, D. R., Meyer, B., Pilkonis, P. A., & Miller, I. H. (2007). Efficiently assessing negative cognition in depression: An item response theory analysis of the Dysfunctional Attitude Scale. *Psychological Assessment, 19*, 199–209.

Bennett-Levy, J., Richards, D. A., & Farrand, P. (2010). Low-intensity CBT interventions: A revolution in mental health care. In J. Bennett-Levy, D. A. Richards, P. Farrand, H. Christensen, K. M. Griffiths, D. J. Kavanagh, et al. (Eds.), *Oxford guide to low intensity CBT interventions* (pp. 3–18). Oxford, UK: Oxford University Press.

Butcher, J. N. (2006). Assessment in clinical psychology: A perspective on the past, present challenges, and future prospects. *Clinical Psychology: Science and Practice, 13,* 205–209.

Calhoon, S. K. (1996). Confirmatory factor analysis of the Dysfunctional Attitude Scale in a student sample. *Cognitive Therapy and Research, 20,* 81–91.

Campbell, D. T., & Fiske, D. W. (1959). Convergent and discriminant validity by the mulitrait–multimethod matrix. *Psychological Bulletin, 56,* 81–105.

Cane, D. B., Olinger, L. J., Gotlib, I. H., & Kuiper, N. A. (1986). Factor structure of the Dysfunctional Attitude Scale in a student population. *Journal of Clinical Psychology, 42,* 307–309.

Cartwright-Hatton, S., & Wells, A. (1997). Beliefs about worry and intrusions: The Meta-Cognitions Questionnaire and its correlates. *Journal of Anxiety Disorders, 11,* 279–296.

Chamberlain, J., & Haaga, D. A. F. (1999). Convergent validity of cognitive assessment methods. *Behavior Modification, 23*(2), 294–315.

Chambless, D. L., & Ollendick, T. H. (2001). Empirically supported psychological interventions: Controversies and evidence. *Annual Review of Psychology, 52,* 685–716.

Clark, D. A. (1988). The validity of measures of cognition: A review of the literature. *Cognitive Therapy and Research, 12,* 1–20.

Clark, D. A. (1997). Twenty years of cognitive assessment: Current status and future directions. *Journal of Consulting and Clinical Psychology, 65,* 996–1000.

Clark, D. A., & Beck, A. T. (2010). *Cognitive therapy of anxiety disorders: Science and practice.* New York: Guilford Press.

Clark, D. A., & Beck, A. T. (with Alford, B.). (1999). *Scientific foundations of cognitive theory and therapy of depression.* New York: Wiley.

Cook, J. M., Biyanova, T., Elhai, J., Schnurr, P. P., & Coyne, J. C. (2010). What do psychotherapists really do in practice?: An Internet study of over 2,000 practitioners. *Psychotherapy: Theory, Research, Practice and Training, 47,* 260–267.

de Graaf, L. E., Roelofs, J., & Huibers, M. J. H. (2009). Measuring dysfunctional attitudes in the general population: The Dysfunctional Attitude Scale (Form A) Revised. *Cognitive Therapy and Research, 33,* 345–355.

Dobson, K. S., & Breiter, H. J. (1983). Cognitive assessment of depression: Reliability and validity of three measures. *Journal of Abnormal Psychology, 92,* 107–109.

Dozois, D. J. A. (2007). Stability of negative self-structures: A longitudinal comparison of depressed, remitted, and nonpsychiatric controls. *Journal of Clinical Psychology, 63,* 319–338.

Dunkley, D. M., Blankstein, K. R., & Segal, Z. V. (2010). Cognitive assessment: Issues and methods. In K. S. Dobson (Ed.), *Handbook of cognitive-behavioral therapies* (3rd ed., pp. 133–171). New York: Guilford Press.

Ehring, T., Zetsche, U., Weidacker, K., Wahl, K., Schönfeld, S., & Ehler, A. (2011). The Perseverative Thinking Questionnaire (PTQ): Validation of a content-independent measure of repetitive negative thinking. *Journal of Behavior Therapy and Experimental Psychiatry, 42,* 225–232.

Fairburn, C. G., Cooper, Z., & Shafran, R. (2003). Cognitive-behavior therapy for eating disorders: A "transdiagnostic" theory and treatment. *Behaviour Research and Therapy, 41,* 509–528.

Glass, C. R., & Arnkoff, D. B. (1997). Questionnaire methods of cognitive self-statement assessment. *Journal of Consulting and Clinical Psychology, 65,* 911–927.

Gotlib, I. H., & Joormann, J. (2010). Cognition and depression: Current status and future directions. *Annual Review of Clinical Psychology, 6,* 285–312.

Haaga, D. A. F. (1997). Introduction to the special section on measuring cognitive products in research and practice. *Journal of Consulting and Clinical Psychology, 65,* 907–910.

Hamilton, E. W., & Abramson, L. Y. (1983). Cognitive patterns and major depressive disorder: A longitudinal study in a hospital setting. *Journal of Abnormal Psychology, 92,* 173–184.

Hayes, S. C., Nelson, R. O., & Jarrett, R. B. (1987). The treatment utility of assessment: A functional approach to evaluating assessment quality. *American Psychologist, 42,* 963–974.

Hill, C. V., Oei, T. P. S., & Hill, M. A. (1989). An empirical investigation of the specificity and sensitivity of the Automatic Thoughts Questionnaire and Dysfunctional Attitude Scale. *Journal of Psychopathology and Behavioral Assessment, 11,* 291–311.

Hollon, S. D., Kendall, P. C., & Lumry, A. (1986). Specificity of depressotypic cognitions in clinical depression. *Journal of Abnormal Psychology, 95,* 52–59.

Hunsley, J. (2003). Introduction to the special section on incremental validity and utility in clinical assessment. *Psychological Assessment, 15,* 443–445.

Hunsley, J., & Meyer, G. J. (2003). The incremental validity of psychological testing and assessment: Conceptual, methodological, and statistical issues. *Psychological Assessment, 15,* 446–455.

Ingram, R. E., & Kendall, P. C. (1986). Cognitive clinical psychology: Implications of an information-processing perspective. In R. E. Ingram (Ed.), *Information-processing approaches in clinical psychology* (pp. 3–21). Orlando, FL: Academic Press.

Ingram, R. E., Miranda, J., & Segal, Z. V. (1998). *Cognitive vulnerability to depression.* New York: Guilford Press.

Ingram, R. E., & Price, J. M. (2010). Understanding psychopathology: The role of vulnerability. In R. E. Ingram & J. M. Price (Eds.), *Vulnerability to psychopathology: Risk across the lifespan* (2nd ed., pp. 3–17). New York: Guilford Press.

Jarrett, R. B., Minhajuddin, A., Borman, P. D., Dunlap, L., Segal, Z. V., Kidner, C. L., et al. (2012). Cognitive reactivity, dysfunctional attitudes, and depressive relapse and recurrence in cognitive therapy responders. *Behaviour Research and Therapy, 50,* 280–286.

Kendall, P. C. (1981). Assessment and cognitive-behavioral interventions: Purposes, proposals, and problems. In P. C. Kendall & S. D. Hollon (Eds.), *Assessment strategies for cognitive-behavioral interventions* (pp. 1–12). New York: Academic Press.

Kendall, P. C., & Hollon, S. D. (Eds.). (1981a). *Assessment strategies for cognitive-behavioral interventions.* New York: Academic Press.

Kendall, P. C., & Hollon, S. D. (1981b). Assessing self-referent speech: Methods in the measurement of self-statements. In P. C. Kendall & S. D. Hollon (Eds.), *Assessment strategies for cognitive-behavioral interventions* (pp. 85–118). New York: Academic Press.

Kendall, P. C., & Korgeski, G. P. (1979). Assessment and cognitive-behavioral interventions. *Cognitive Therapy and Research, 3,* 1–21.

Kuyken, W., Padesky, C. A., & Dudley, R. (2008). The science and practice of case conceptualization. *Behavioural and Cognitive Psychotherapy, 36,* 757–768.

LaGrange, B., Cole, D. A., Jacquez, F., Ciesla, J., Dallaire, D., Pineda, A., et al. (2011). Disentangling the prospective relations between maladaptive cognitions and depressive symptoms. *Journal of Abnormal Psychology, 120*(3), 511–527.

Mansell, W., Harvey, A., Watkins, E., & Shafran, R. (2009). Conceptual foundations of the transdiagnostic approach to CBT. *Journal of Cognitive Psychotherapy: An International Quarterly, 23,* 6–19.

Martin, R., & Young, J. (2010). Schema therapy. In K. S. Dobson (Ed.), *Handbook of cognitive-behavioral therapies* (3rd ed., pp. 317–346). New York: Guilford Press.

McDermut, W., & Haaga, D. A. F. (2009). Assessment and diagnostic issues in rational emotive behavior therapy: Introduction to the special issue. *Journal of Rational-Emotive Cognitive-Behavior Therapy, 27,* 79–82.

McFall, R. M., & Townsend, J. T. (1998). Foundations of psychological assessment: Implications for cognitive assessment in clinical science. *Psychological Assessment, 10,* 316–330.

McHugh, K., & Barlow, D. H. (2010). The dissemination and implementation of evidence-based psychological treatments. *American Psychologist, 65,* 73–84.

McManus, F., Shafran, R., & Cooper, Z. (2010). What does a "transdiagnostic" approach have to offer the treatment of anxiety disorders? *British Journal of Clinical Psychology, 49*(Pt. 4), 491–505.

Merluzzi, T. V., Glass, C. R., & Genest, M. (Eds.). (1981). *Cognitive assessment.* New York: Guilford Press.

Meyer, G. J., Finn, S. E., Eyde, L. D., Kay, G. G., Moreland, K. L., Dies, R. R., et al. (2001). Psychological testing and psychological assessment: A review of evidence and issues. *American Psychologist, 56,* 128–165.

Mumma, G. H. (2004). Validation of idiosyncratic cognitive schema in cognitive case formulations: An intraindividual idiographic approach. *Psychological Assessment, 16,* 211–230.

National Institute for Health and Clinical Excellence. (2005). *Clinical guideline 26: Posttraumatic stress disorder: The management of PTSD in adults and children in primary and secondary care.* London: Gaskell and The British Psychological Society. Available at *http://guidance.nice.org/ CG26.*

Nelson-Gray, R. O. (2003). Treatment utility of psychological assessment. *Psychological Assessment, 15,* 521–531.

Nisbett, R. E., & Wilson, T. D. (1977). Telling more than we can know: Verbal reports on mental processes. *Psychological Review, 84,* 231–259.

Norcross, J. C., & Karpiak, C. P. (2012). Clinical psychologists in the 2010s:

50 years of the APA Division of Clinical Psychology. *Clinical Psychology: Science and Practice, 19*, 1–12.

Norton, P. J. (2012). A randomized clinical trial of transdiagnostic CBT for anxiety disorders by comparison to relaxation training. *Behavior Therapy, 43*, 506–517.

Persons, J. B. (2008). *The case formulation approach to cognitive-behavior therapy.* New York: Guilford Press.

Rakovshik, S. G., & McManus, F. (2010). Establishing evidence-based training in cognitive behavior therapy: A review of current empirical findings and theoretical guidance. *Clinical Psychology Review, 30*, 496–516.

Richards, D. A. (2010). Access and organization: Putting low-intensity interventions to work in clinical services. In J. Bennett-Levy, D. A. Richards, P. Farrand, H. Christensen, K. M. Griffiths, D. J. Kavanagh, et al. (Eds.), *Oxford guide to low-intensity CBT interventions* (pp. 19–33). Oxford, UK: Oxford University Press.

Rude, S. S., & Rehm, L. P. (1991). Response to treatments for depression: The role of initial status on targeted cognitive and behavioral skills. *Clinical Psychology Review, 11*, 493–514.

Segal, Z. V., Kennedy, S., Gemar, M., Hood, K., Pedersen, R., & Buis, T. (2006). Cognitive reactivity to sad mood provocation and the prediction of depressive relapse. *Archives of General Psychiatry, 63*, 749–755.

Silverman, J. S., Silverman, J. A., & Eardley, D. A. (1984). Do maladaptive attitudes cause depression? *Archives of General Psychiatry, 41*, 28–30.

Stewart, R. E., & Chambless, D. L. (2007). Does psychotherapy research inform treatment decisions in private practice? *Journal of Clinical Psychology, 63*, 267–281.

Weiner, I. B. (2012). Education and training in clinical psychology: Correcting some mistaken beliefs. *Clinical Psychology: Science and Practice, 19*, 13–16.

Weissman, A. N., & Beck, A. T. (1978). *Development and validation of the Dysfunctional Attitude Scale.* Paper presented at the annual meeting of the Association for Advancement of Behavior Therapy, Chicago.

Wells, A., & Cartwright-Hatton, S. (2004). A short form of the Meta-Cognitions Questionnaire: Properties of the MCQ-30. *Behaviour Research and Therapy, 42*, 385–396.

Young, J. E. (1990). *Cognitive therapy for personality disorders.* Sarasota, FL: Professional Resources Press.

Young, J. E., & Brown, G. (2003). The Young Schema Questionnaire—Long Version. Retrieved February 4, 2013, from *www.schematherapy.com/id53.htm*.

Zuroff, D. C., Blatt, S. J., Sanislow, C. A., Bondi, C. M., & Pilkonis, P. A. (1999). Vulnerability to depression: Reexamining state dependence and relative stability. *Journal of Abnormal Psychology, 108*, 76–89.

PART I

COGNITIVE ASSESSMENT STRATEGIES AND PRACTICES

2

"Better the Devil You Know"?

A Conceptual Critique of Endorsement Methods in Cognitive Therapy Assessment

Gary P. Brown and David A. Clark

ENDORSEMENT METHODS AND THE DEVELOPMENT OF COGNITIVE-BEHAVIORAL THERAPY

The rise of cognitive-behavioral therapy (CBT) as a dominant therapeutic approach was accompanied by an explosion of measurement instruments, and yet consideration is seldom given to what scores on these instruments can, with a reasonable degree of certainty, tell us with regard to clinical decision making and research inferences. The aim of this chapter is to focus on this question in the hopes of providing some guidance about what conclusions can be drawn from scores on "endorsement instruments," the name used in CBT assessment for the familiar self-report format in which respondents "endorse" a preset response option to a predetermined standardized item (Kendall & Hollon, 1981; see Clark & Brown, Chapter 1, this volume, for an explanation of other types of assessment in this classification). In practice, the term "self-report" typically refers to the endorsement approach.

It is not difficult to see why a proliferation of new instruments accompanied the rise of CBT to its present dominant position. The core clinical intuition that led Beck to develop CBT for depression grew out of the striking regularities he observed in the spontaneous "automatic thoughts" of depressed individuals, which appeared to mediate between the person's ongoing experiences and their emotional reactions. Arguably, CBT's core contribution has been to provide a framework for examining these thoughts systematically, and so it was natural for those working in this area to seek to exploit this knowledge by generalizing outward from the individual psychotherapy session. It was a short step from recording depressive automatic thoughts using the Daily Record of Dysfunctional Thoughts (DRDTs; Beck, Rush, Shaw, & Emery, 1979) within session to constructing thought inventories, such as the Automatic Thoughts Questionnaire (ATQ; Hollon & Kendall, 1980). Scores on scales such as the ATQ afforded a summary score of depressogenic cognition that permitted comparisons between individuals and the quantification of change within individuals over time, rooted in the same clinically potent phenomena captured by DRDTs. Rather than wait for these thoughts to be produced spontaneously in the therapy session, why not anticipate the occurrence of commonly encountered automatic thoughts and measure their perceived frequency and intensity, albeit from a retrospective viewpoint?

If automatic thoughts and other self-statements seemed to capture the immediate thought processes encountered by clinicians, a separate category of cognitive variable that also had a straightforward origin within day-to-day clinical experience appeared to be necessary to capture more enduring cognitive phenomena that, unlike automatic thoughts, persisted across therapy sessions and often across separate symptomatic episodes. As Beck et al. (1979) remarked, "It does not seem plausible to us that the aberrant cognitive mechanisms are created *de novo* every time an individual experiences a depression. It appears more credible that he has some relatively enduring anomaly in his psychological system" (p. 20). Within the CBT literature, this level of cognitive phenomena is seen as consisting of core beliefs (categorical attitudes toward the self, such as "I am unlovable") and associated underlying assumptions (if–then conditional propositions governing responses to arising circumstances—e.g., "If other people know what you are really like, they will think less of you"). The example of an underlying assumption is taken from the Dysfunctional Attitude Scale (DAS; Weissman & Beck, 1978), the main measure of enduring beliefs for depression. Over time, the schema became the central construct in Beck's cognitive model, with activation of schematic content (i.e., dysfunctional beliefs, assumptions) providing the guiding mechanism for operation of the information-processing system. Thus information congruent with schematic processing would be preferentially processed relative to schema-irrelevant information, whereas schema-incongruent material would be ignored or at least minimized (Beck, 1987; Clark, Beck, & Alford, 1999). Far fewer measures have been developed for schema content or structure than for automatic thoughts, which is likely due, among other reasons, to the fact that, unlike automatic thoughts, such beliefs are not as readily verbalized and can require skilled clinical investigation to elicit. Relatedly, a consensus has never formed around a standard terminology and clear delineation of more enduring constructs (see Kuyken, Padesky, & Dudley, 2009, pp. 12–16, for a recent summary of related issues).

Publication of Beck's (1976) *Cognitive Therapy and the Emotional Disorders* crystallized the theory first set out with reference to depression and laid the groundwork for the extension of both the psychotherapy and the accompanying research methods and instruments to the broad spectrum of clinical psychology phenomena. Two important features of the 1976 framework were the adoption of the general psychiatric nomenclature as a basis for investigating cognitive phenomenology and an unapologetic focus on subjective self-reports of thought content. The reliance on self-report was and, to some extent, still is controversial, given its definitive rejection by mainstream behaviorism. However, Beck maintained that cognitive content could provide an essential basis for distinguishing between diagnostic categories—a view formalized as the "cognitive content-specificity hypothesis" (Beck, Brown, Steer, Eidelson, & Riskind, 1987; Clark, Beck, & Brown, 1989; Baranoff & Oei, Chapter 8, this volume). The content-specificity hypothesis provided the seeds for thinking systematically about other disorders with the same approach that had been applied to depression, and, accordingly, similar self-statement questionnaires encompassing the distinctive expressed cognitive content of other disorders would soon follow (e.g., the Agoraphobic Cognitions Questionnaire [Chambless, Caputo, Bright, & Gallagher, 1984]). Likewise, scales measuring more enduring constructs also tracked the extension of CBT to different disorders, with the DAS joined, for example, by the Anxiety Sensitivity Index (Reiss, Peterson, Gursky, & McNally, 1986) for panic disorder and, somewhat later, the Obsessive Beliefs Questionnaire (OBQ; Obsessive Compulsive Cognitions Working Group, 2003) for obsessive–compulsive disorder (OCD).

The appearance of the *Diagnostic and Statistical Manual of Mental Disorders* third edition (DSM-III; American Psychiatric Association, 1980) formalized thinking about psychiatric phenomena across the mental health field in the same empirical, data-driven manner that had characterized the early development of CBT and provided even greater differentiation of the categories of interest, especially with regard to anxiety disorders. By this point, the shift in prevailing assessment and measurement practices had become pronounced. Lawyer and Smitherman (2004), using Lang's (1979) three-response-systems framework for anxiety (i.e., behavior, subjective report, and physiology), traced a discernible change in assessment approach, with the appearance of studies assessing more than one response system reaching a peak in the late 1970s and then declining steadily, overtaken by an increase in single-system assessment with an exclusive focus on self-report methodology. These monomethod self-report studies had always predominated, but by 2002 they represented 97.8% of research reports of anxiety disorders, compared to 85.5% during the 1970s, a trend tracking the rise of CBT for anxiety (e.g., Beck, Emery, & Greenberg, 2005). In summary, the burgeoning growth of assessment instruments, particularly those employing endorsement methods, reflected parallel developments in theory and therapy and compatible changes in the psychiatric nomenclature that served to amplify the already developing trends.

VERIDICALITY OF REPORTED THOUGHTS

As just outlined, the growth of CBT assessment benefited from an unusual convergence of facilitating circumstances within the broader mental health field and enthusiasm for a new treatment paradigm whose potential was just beginning to be realized. Where assessment was concerned, this enthusiasm was soon tempered, as doubts began to be expressed regarding what the scores on the newly developed instruments could provide in terms of supportable inferences of interest to practitioners and researchers. Experimental-behavioral clinical researchers who objected philosophically to any methodological reliance on subjectivity were particularly vocal in their objections. They regarded themselves, in common with CBT therapists and researchers, as beneficiaries of the "cognitive revolution," but adhered to a more traditionally strict behavioral perspective on the permissible targets of inquiry (e.g., Jacobson, 1997; Wilson, Hayes, & Gifford, 1997). These researchers shared the aims of enlarging the domain of investigation beyond associative learning but regarded the accompanying rise in use of methods which relied on subjective judgments as inimical to precise science.

The terms of debate were familiar, with self-report methods disparaged as examples of "introspectionism" and "mentalism," terms previously directed by behaviorists against psychoanalytic approaches. In the words of one leading researcher with reference to CBT endorsement methods, "developing an acceptable formal science of cognition requires adherence to rigorous methodological constraints that are at least as severe as those imposed by behaviourism. Conversely, the endorsement of the self-report data, yielded by introspection, as an acceptable source of information concerning mental processes, must place our discipline clearly outwith the boundaries of legitimate science" (MacLeod, 1993, p. 172). MacLeod went on to support his argument for the inherent fallibility of introspective self-report by referring to the influential criti-cal review by Nisbett and Wilson (1977), which documented demon-strably erroneous and confabulated accounts of self-report. In addition, MacLeod pointed to different types of learning that can take place with-out awareness and adduced this as a further basis for holding self-report evidence suspect.

MacLeod's critique combined the time-honored behavioral indict-ment of subjective report with contemporary supporting evidence from cognitive science. However, researchers with scientific interests that depended on the validity of subjective verbal reports had already begun to make use of the same new understandings of cognition and informa-tion processing to strengthen the conceptual basis for regarding subjec-tive reports as potentially valid data. Ericsson and Simon's (1980) main conclusion in their landmark rejoinder to Nisbett and Wilson (1977), following an extensive review of the relevant literature, had been that the invalidity of verbal reports arose mainly from tasks that required respondents to infer rather than directly report their responses: "The inaccurate reports found by other research are shown to result from requesting information that was never directly heeded, thus forcing subjects to infer rather than remember their mental processes" (p. 215). They argued that verbal reports can be potentially valid sources of data when these are direct reports of what is or has been attended to, whereas reports based on inferences are unlikely to be valid in the sense of being a veridical account of the relevant thought processes. Accordingly, direct verbal reports of the ongoing content of thought as it is being attended to would have the strongest claim to validity, whereas inferences about the reasons for having particular thoughts would be less reliable. As stated by McNally (2001), "people can often provide answers to what-questions, but often cannot provide answers to how-questions" (p. 520).

In this way, Ericsson and Simon (1980) established distinct parame-ters of validity that were supported with well-accepted research evidence for regarding verbal reports as an admissible target of scientific study. Contrary to strict behaviorism, these validity parameters can be used to establish a level of confidence in whether specific self-reported informa-tion can be relied upon as veridical. The greater the departure from these criteria, the more susceptible the task in question is of asking respon-dents to "tell more than they can know"—that is, to provide responses based on inference rather than on direct report. These criteria can be straightforwardly applied to the cognitive variables introduced above that are typically targeted by endorsement methods, and are particularly pertinent to automatic thoughts, as measured by instruments such as the ATQ, which are regarded as manifestations of actual thought processes.

Automatic thoughts, which in psychopathology normally involve some form of evaluation of the self, others, or the future, are discrete occurrences inherently bound to specific episodes. Accordingly, calling upon a respondent to accurately rate how frequently they have the precise thought "There must be something wrong with me" (ATQ item 22), consistent with Ericsson and Simon framework, would depend on the successful recall of specific episodes during which the thought was attended to. This is clearly a prohibitive standard for self-report scales, but it provides a useful benchmark against which to gauge the veridicality of such self-report tasks. Accordingly, it has long been recognized by CBT researchers that such reports are likely to be substantially based on inference. As noted by Haaga (1997), "an item on an inventory may be endorsed, not because the respondent actually had that thought but because she or he agrees with the thought, had some thought generally like it, or is in a mood captured by the thought" (p. 907; see Haaga & Solomon, Chapter 3, this volume, for a similar discussion). Indeed, it has also been noted that it cannot even be assumed that the relevant experience has been verbalized as a discrete thought. According to Glass and Arnkoff (1982), it is unlikely that people have precisely the thoughts that they endorse on a questionnaire, because actual thought processes are probably highly idiosyncratic, automatic, not in the form of complete sentences, and heavily based in imagery and not just language. In light of this fact, the argument typically made for the use of production methods (see Haaga & Solomon, Chapter 3, this volume) in preference to endorsement instruments echoes Ericsson and Simon's line of reasoning in that they "do not restrict participants to a predetermined set of experimenter-derived questionnaire items nor do they rely on participants' ability to recall their own thought processes." Rather, they "assess cognitions in 'real time' and, therefore, provide a more accurate representation of what individuals are actually thinking in particular situations" (Clark, 1997, p. 998).

Aside from the degree of inference required to make a relevant judgment, veridicality is diminished further by the limited item choices available to the respondent completing a self-report scale. Arguably, the hallmark of endorsement measures is that the respondent is constrained to choose a response from a predetermined range of possible responses relating to a rating scale (e.g., frequency for cognitions and degree of agreement for beliefs) chosen by the authors of the instrument. These represent a further substantial distancing of the output of the measurement procedure from the respondent's natural thinking. As Glass and Arnkoff (1997) note, "It is also highly unlikely, even if the individual is aware of having had the particular thoughts, that she or he has counted or tallied them and knows exactly how frequently they occurred" (p. 917). They go on to consider what respondents might be drawing upon in responding if not an estimated frequency of occurrence of the thought, proposing that they may be (1) gauging the impact, salience, or importance of the thought and inferring that a particularly pertinent thought must have occurred frequently; (2) translating from idiosyncratic or fragmented actual thoughts to the grammatically complete sentences on the inventories; (3) translating affective experience into a language-based self-statement format; or (4) conveying that the item on the questionnaire matches their self-concept, indicating "That's like me" by endorsing the item. The first three of these possibilities relate to the aptness of the thought in question; the respondent in each case is translating a response that cannot be conveyed directly in terms of frequency into the available (frequency) metric. It is for this reason that certain automatic thought scales also provide for a separate rating of believability in addition to frequency. Aside from this, the last possibility, that the respondent is indicating "That's like me," warrants separate consideration, because the respondent answering on this basis is relating to a qualitatively different question of aptness, not about the occurrence of particular thoughts, no matter how inexact or incomplete a match with their actual thoughts, but rather about their ongoing disposition as a person to respond in a particular way, potentially without ever having actually responded in that way. The person who responds on this basis is saying "I'm the kind of person who would have thoughts like that" rather than "I have frequently had thoughts like that." In effect, she is spontaneously reporting on their enduring beliefs rather than on her momentary thoughts, and so is crossing over into what is considered a separate category of constructs within cognitive-behavioral theory and assessment. The relationship between momentary thoughts and enduring beliefs is a central idea in CBT that has a bearing on ongoing susceptibility for further difficulties; a closer examination of this relationship within the context of assessment is the focus of the following section.

OCCURRENT AND DISPOSITIONAL BELIEFS

A putative measure of automatic thoughts that only elicits enduring beliefs would, by definition, not be valid as a measure of automatic thoughts. However, by the same token, an automatic thoughts scale that was *not* closely associated with an ongoing disposition to depression, as potentially reflected in enduring beliefs, would also not be suitable for its intended purpose. Consider, for example, a person not particularly predisposed to depression completing the ATQ. Such a person just might happen to be in the habit of chastising themselves for minor mistakes with a thought similar to the ATQ item "There must be something wrong with me" and so would accordingly provide a high rating of the frequency of the thought. However, this person would likely have an absence of an accompanying broader depressive picture that included the presence of more enduring beliefs and so would likely have a low DAS score. The high frequency score rating on the ATQ item would appear to be idiosyncratic, and it would be unlikely that this person would respond to many other items in this way, producing a low ATQ total score. However, a high ATQ *total* score would be suspect in the absence of evidence of a more general depressive cognitive picture, and so a measure of automatic thoughts reflecting enduringness to some degree would not be a fatal threat to validity.

In contrast, a putative measure of enduring beliefs that is temporally unstable or in other respects appears to reflect more transitory sources of variance, such as automatic thoughts, would be lacking its defining feature and so could not be considered to have construct validity (see Evraire, Dozois, & Hayden, Chapter 5, this volume, for a discussion of measurement stability with regard to vulnerability). For this reason, it is expected that authors of such scales would wish to be clear about the intention of measuring more enduring, dispositional constructs as opposed to closely associated transitory variables such as automatic thoughts and mood. For example, with regard to anxiety sensitivity, McNally (1994) noted, "Anxiety sensitivity denotes beliefs about the harmfulness of bodily sensations . . . anxiety sensitivity is a dispositional, not an occurrent concept. . . . In contrast, . . . catastrophic misinterpretations are occurrent (i.e., episodic) concepts" (p. 117). He later added, "As an inferred dispositional construct, anxiety sensitivity must not be confused with anticipatory anxiety, an occurrent construct denoting an increase in distress occasioned by the prospect of imminent threat" (McNally, 2002, p. 938). Here McNally is drawing on terms used within philosophy to distinguish momentary (occurrent) and enduring (dispositional) beliefs: "A dispositional claim is a claim, not about anything that is actually occurring at the time, but rather that some particular thing is prone to occur, under certain circumstances. . . . The occurrent belief comes and goes, depending on whether circumstances elicit it; the dispositional belief endures" (Schwitzgebel, 2006; see Fridhandler, 1986, for a general discussion of the relevance of this distinction to psychology). One reason the ASI might be susceptible to the assertion that it measures transitory rather than enduring phenomena is evident in such items as "When my chest feels tight, I get scared that I won't be able to breathe properly." The item is intended to index an ongoing propositional belief about an if–then contingency between a body sensation and a catastrophic outcome but employs the temporal term "when" instead of the logical "if," potentially cuing respondents to draw on their memories of relevant episodes to base their responses. Moreover, the general instructions potentially reinforce a focus on episodic memory by asking the respondent to "answer all items on the basis of your own experience" (see Hawkes & Brown, Chapter 11, this volume, for a broader analysis of validity issues with regard to the ASI and similar scales).

Aside from the requirement that a belief measure should reflect enduring rather than transitory beliefs, considerations of veridicality do not appear to be as critical to the validity of belief measures. For these measures, the scale used is almost always degree of belief; as such, the main vehicle for responding relates directly to the aptness of the belief. Veridicality—that is, correspondence or lack of correspondence to actual beliefs—can be reflected in the rating and is germane to what is being measured. Moreover, given that it is assumed that the belief is ongoing and enduring, whether and when the belief came into consciousness as an occurrent thought is not critical. Indeed, the assumption is that the respondent can be asked about a belief that they may not have previously explicitly thought about as this can be readily synthesized from existing general knowledge, an implicit premise in the practice of surveys and polling. There is still some ambiguity about what a rating actually means—if a respondent chooses "slightly agree" as a rating, does that reflect their small degree of belief in the stated item or perhaps the fact that they "agree very much" with a loosely related belief? With an if–then format item (e.g., item 8 of the OBQ-44: "If I don't act when I foresee danger, then I am to blame for any consequences") is a given rating that falls short of "agree completely" due to a mismatch with respect to the condition (the "if") or the consequence (the "then") or the contingency between the two (as intended) or some combination of these? However, none of these possibilities fundamentally threatens the inference that the rating reasonably reflects the respondent's degree of belief in the proposition being set forth in the item.

With reference to Ericsson and Simon's standards, it seems reasonable to conclude that endorsement methods for dispositional constructs such as enduring beliefs have a stronger inferential basis than occurrent constructs such as automatic thoughts, as they depend less on episodic recall. This might be at odds with subjective experience, because automatic thoughts are experienced consciously, whereas beliefs are more stable but potentially implicit until explicitly brought to consciousness. Indeed, in this regard, it is important to note that the actual endorsement of an item on a dispositional scale such as the DAS—the literal thought "I agree with this belief very much"—is an expression of an occurrent belief. This point should not be overlooked, as it once again brings into play all of the factors that threaten verbal reports when these are over-reliant on inference. Whereas, in theory, a respondent should not need to engage in inference to form a response, there is nothing to prevent them from doing so. This relates to the important matter of what episodic factors might have a bearing on the responses provided on a putative dispositional scale such as the DAS, which is presumed to be stable (see Evraire et al., Chapter 5, this volume, for a discussion of stability and vulnerability). It also points up the need for means to validate self-reported beliefs through other response paradigms.

A well-established non-self-report paradigm for studying strength of beliefs and attitudes makes use of response latency (e.g., Bassili, 1996). Consistent with this view, Sheppard and Teasdale (2000) note that "attitudes have traditionally been conceptualized as precomputed evaluations of objects in memory, which become automatically activated and retrieved in the presence of an appropriate cue" (p. 768) and have been shown to be better predictors of subsequent behavior in particular contexts. They adapted DAS items to a speeded response paradigm, and found that depressed patients were significantly quicker to respond to DAS beliefs than were matched controls. This type of paradigm, in which strength of belief is not based on a conscious, controlled response, often under speeded conditions, can be regarded as accessing beliefs implicitly. Because they are not subject to the inferential influences of explicit report, it is tempting to regard these as being "truer" indices of beliefs. However, as Roefs et al. (Chapter 13, this volume) demonstrate, such a conclusion is not justified by a broad review of the literature.

Finally, with regard to beliefs, there is a more pragmatic impetus for accepting the essential veridicality of self-reported beliefs, and that is, as asserted by McNally (2001) that "many aspects of psychopathology do not have overt behavioral manifestations other than self-reports of phenomenal states" (p. 519). McNally gives the example of obsessions, which are defined entirely in terms of introspectively ascertainable features. Like the DAS respondent endorsing a perfectly matching belief, the individual with obsessions who fears contamination does not need to infer a response to the belief "If I touch something unclean, I will be contaminated."

VALIDITY FOR DIFFERENT ASSESSMENT TARGETS: SIGNS, SAMPLES, AND CONSTRUCTS

CBT self-report instruments were developed to systematize and quantify the phenomena clinicians were encountering in their day-to-day clinical experiences in the hopes of producing generalizable and objective knowledge that could further inform clinical research and practice.

However, it would appear that the available means for accomplishing this aim was arguably highly qualified and attenuated, at least to the extent that validity is seen to be based to some extent on veridicality. In view of the discussion to this point, automatic thoughts measures particularly need to be regarded as susceptible to responding based on inference rather than on direct report, and both cognition and belief measures are constrained by preset measurement scales. These limitations need to be weighed against the obvious strengths and advantages of endorsement methods relative to the context and pragmatic aims of assessment.

An important determination in considering how strictly measures need to be held to the requirement of veridicality is whether responses are viewed as *samples* of behavior or *signs* of latent constructs. Where test items are viewed as samples, the items are meant to be essentially similar to the behavior they are intended to predict. Where they are viewed as signs, they are regarded as representing and indicating the presence of traits and other behaviors which they do not resemble (Loevinger, 1957, p. 644). Loevinger argued that all scale items are both signs and samples given the fact that the aim is always to make inferences about behavior outside of the test situation but that there is an expectation that items bear a resemblance on some basis to the phenomenon of interest. In the foregoing discussion, particularly with regard to automatic thoughts, lack of veridicality in the sense of not faithfully capturing clinical material has clearly been a concern within the literature. It is also evident from early writings in the area that those working on developing assessment methods regarded sampling behavior as their aim (e.g., "Whereas traditional personality tests have typically taken the sign approach to interpretation, behavioral procedures approach test interpretation with the sample orientation" [Goldfried & Kent, 1974, p. 413]). Moreover, as detailed above, the impetus for rejecting the strictures of behaviorist epistemology was to enable the direct study of intervening cognitive mechanisms instead of relying on inferring such mechanisms from patterns of objectively verifiable responses. This only makes sense if measures are aimed at literally measuring the mechanisms in question rather than being indirect indicators of other constructs. Finally, as stated previously, some of the key phenomena CBT researchers were interested in (beliefs, mental symptoms such as fears and obsessions) can only be studied through self-report and necessarily represent the actual phenomena of interest rather than signs of indirectly measured constructs.

The idea that CBT measure scores are signs has also been expressed in the literature from time to time (e.g., "Self report assessment procedures are commonly interpreted as signs of behaviour or other responses; that is, although they do not directly enable observation or real-life processes, they approximate these processes" [Dobson & Segal, 1992, p. 279]; "Although inventories cannot hope to include all possible thoughts, they sample a range of such thoughts and thus assess the presence or absence of overall positive and negative thinking" [Glass & Arnkoff, 1997, p. 917]). This is a more prudent position in certain respects and establishes a basis for validity that does not depend on veridicality. However, greater emphasis is then necessarily placed on other preconditions for establishing validity, such as strong theoretical predictions, and use of tests in this sense would need to entail caution about drawing inferences about actual thought processes if evidence of veridicality is not supported. On balance, CBT assessment typically seeks to find out about the cognitive phenomena actually encountered in clinical settings and veridicality is therefore an inescapable consideration in most instances.

It is clear that the aim of systematically gathering clinical material through endorsement methods is subject to significant limitations on what can be inferred. Even when the content of assessment instruments is carefully chosen to faithfully reflect what is encountered spontaneously in clinical interactions, the use of preset item content and fixed rating scales imposes an unavoidable distance between the instrument and the target of assessment. In research applications and where more abstract constructs are the targets of investigation, the challenges of demonstrating construct validity in general become an additional focus (see Guller & Smith, Chapter 14, this volume, for a detailed discussion of construct validity). Where theory and methodology are not developed to a sufficient level to enable strong empirical tests, the status of a particular measure as a marker of a latent construct is likely to be inconclusive.

An instructive case in point is the study of cognitive vulnerability to depression. As previously discussed, responses to belief statements on a self-report measure like the DAS were considered behavioral referents of latent schematic processing, although, crucially, a specific mechanism linking DAS beliefs to schematic processing has never been satisfactorily established (see Segal, 1988, and Guller & Smith, Chapter 14, this volume, for a discussion). In the absence of such a mechanism, the validity of the DAS as a sign or marker of schematic processing needed to be established by inference. Early criticisms of the DAS noted that mere correlations with depressive symptoms were inadequate evidence that DAS scores represented a predisposition to depression (e.g., Coyne & Gotlib, 1983). Subsequent promising findings were drawn from longitudinal designs, but these, too, appeared to be insufficient for excluding the possibility that scores on measures such as the DAS were concomitants rather than precursors of depression (see Barnett & Gotlib, 1998, for a discussion). More recent research, summarized by Clark and Brown (Chapter 1, this volume), has made use of methodological advances such as item response theory (Beevers, Strong, Meyer, Pilkonis, & Miller, 2007), structural equation modeling (Zuroff, Blatt, Sanislow, Bondi, & Pilkonis, 1999), behavioral high-risk designs (Alloy, Abramson, Keyser, Gerstein, & Sylvia, 2008), and priming designs (Segal et al., 2006) to support the DAS as a marker of schematic processing. Although encouraging, the more recent findings need to be considered in the broader context as representing additional strands in the inferential narrative about the DAS and its putative role as a cognitive marker of vulnerability to depression that do not directly call into dispute or otherwise override the previous negative findings, which therefore also remain strands in the narrative.

In a similar vein to the discussion of veridicality relative to clinical phenomena, confidence in a measure of a latent construct is enhanced when scores on the measure reflect variation in the target construct (see discussions of the concept of "construct representation" [e.g., Embretson, 1983] in Hawkes & Brown, Chapter 11, this volume, and Guller & Smith, Chapter 14, this volume). In this regard, it was not self-evident how variation in scores on the DAS could be regarded as tracking change in schematic processing of ongoing experience, and this became more of a focus with the accumulation of contradictory findings. Segal (1988) carefully examined descriptions of the schema concept in the CBT literature and concluded that scales of negative self-statements, such as the DAS, were not credible means for testing the theory and operationalizing the central constructs. This has added impetus to the development of alternative measures based on experimental paradigms which, from time to time, have shown results that address one of the main gaps in vulnerability research (mainly being detectable outside of symptomatic periods without priming), but these have arguably not been robust enough to achieve any greater levels of sustained success as self-statement measures and are even further removed from the clinical phenomena they are intended to shed light on (see Evraire et al., Chapter 5, this volume).

NOMOTHETIC AND IDIOGRAPHIC ASSESSMENT

A final important consideration with respect to endorsement methods concerns the fact that, typically, scale scores are aggregates of related items. Where the aim of assessment is nomothetic (namely, to order and rank a sample of individuals along a dimension), it is appropriate to do so using a fixed set of items for all respondents. Such a measure needs to be sufficiently precise for broadly distinguishing individuals from each other in a meaningful way, similar to assigning a diagnosis. Where the aim is idiographic (namely, to be able to characterize the unique features of an individual), the set of constituent items that contribute to the total score will vary in their degree of relevance to a given respondent. This is a consideration separate from but related to veridicality in that particular items might faithfully capture a respondent's thought content but be drowned out or at least obscured by other items contributing to the same score which are not pertinent. Indeed, any number of items on a scale may be wholly inapplicable to a respondent. Hawkes and Brown (Chapter 11, this volume) discuss the impact inapplicability can have on measurement. However, where the goal is accurately characterizing a given individual on a dimension of interest even a modest degree of irrelevance can mean that a large component of the score obtained for that individual can justifiably be regarded as error variance (Haynes, Mumma, & Pinson, 2009).

An obvious way to manage these apparently contradictory assessment aims is to employ a sequential approach by which aggregate scores are used for broad diagnostic purposes followed by a detailed case conceptualization in the course of which scale items are disaggregated and considered individually on the basis of their salience to the individual. For example, automatic thought scales (the ATQ, the Agoraphobic Cognitions Questionnaire, etc.) and belief scales (the DAS, the ASI, and the OBQ) specific to particular disorders might be administered at the diagnostic stage and then items with relative elevations identified and incorporated into the individual case conceptualization. Such a procedure has been followed informally by CBT practitioners and is often described in discussions of case formulation (e.g., Kuyken et al., 2009).

The move from the nomothetic to the idiographic level has typically been assumed to imply moving from a systematic, objective approach to a more anecdotal and subjective one. However, new experimental and quantitative methods for use at the individual level have appeared recently in the literature that can potentially bridge this divide. Mumma and colleagues (Mumma, 2004; Mumma & Mooney, 2006, 2007) have described a method for designing individualized CBT assessment batteries and accompanying psychometric techniques. These approaches can potentially provide a systematic link between assessment and case conceptualization. Compatible approaches have also been described in psychometrics (e.g., Bornstein, 2011) and personality assessment (e.g., Cervone, 2004). The availability of objective methods at the level of the individual also opens the possibility for improving the validity of nomothetic approaches wherein a basis can be established for aggregating cases with meaningful similarities at the idiographic level—for example, by grouping together individuals who attach similar meanings and engage in similar processing within a given situation (see Mischel, 2004). D. M. Clark's (1986) panic model provides an example of a relatively rare instance in which such a pattern is identifiable at the aggregate level owing to the striking uniformity of both the situational factors present and processing engaged in by individuals during the panic cycle. The one-to-many movement from idiographic to nomothetic level of analysis may be capable of identifying rarer patterns that are nevertheless equally useful to know about clinically. The link between the self-report of beliefs, such as are included in scales like the DAS, and the sort of schematic processing described by the CBT model, which Segal (1988) found lacking, are among the other important functional relationships that can only be established at the level of the individual and not in aggregate.

THE PRESENT AND FUTURE OF ENDORSEMENT METHODS

As Lawyer and Smitherman (2004) showed, trends in the types of methodologies that appear in empirical journals can plausibly track corresponding trends in theory development. An updated survey of the sorts of methods currently in use would likely be similarly informative. It would not be surprising to find that levels of use of endorsement methods have remained near their maximum levels, given their ease of use and their straightforward grounding in clinical phenomena. On the other hand, a key motivation for devising measures of automatic thoughts was that these measures were seen to hold the promise of complementing and extending the standard phenomenology taken into account in the understanding of emotional disorders in conjunction with affective and behavioral markers established in the official nomenclature. It seems self-evident that the importance of cognitive content in clinical assessment has now been established and basic studies of this type are arguably no longer warranted, which could lead to a marginal decrease in their use. The situation is somewhat different for measures of enduring constructs. Whereas the efficacy of CBT interventions for a great many disorders has been established and the importance of cognitive content such as automatic thoughts is not controversial, some perceive an "efficacy ceiling" (Foa & Kozak, 1997) that can only be penetrated by a broader and deeper understanding of etiological factors (e.g., McNally, 2007). As previously discussed, the basis for regarding belief scales as reflecting etiological factors has not been established definitively, both in terms of empirical findings and in terms of construct-representation-based validity. However, experimental methods, aside from addressing the subjective report flaws of self-report, have not been shown conclusively to be appreciably more valid. Moreover, they appear to be imperfect, at best, as proxies for subjectively ascertainable thought content (e.g., Roefs et al., Chapter 13, this volume; De Houwer, 2011; Van den Hout, 1999). Referring back to MacLeod's (1993) critique, a central aspect of this not referred to in the previous discussion was MacLeod's issue with the use of introspection-derived measures as dependent variables. This almost never appears to be the case, at least currently, and the measures of putative etiological factors are instead used as independent variables to explain other phenomena of interest, usually symptoms and symptom states, either concurrently or over time. Moreover, newer analytic methods are making it possible to tease apart the temporal sequencing of variance due to cognition and affect (see Naragon-Gainey & T. A. Brown, Chapter 12, this volume, and Evraire et al., Chapter 5, this volume), a problem that previously hindered research in this area (for a review, please refer to Barnett & Gotlib, 1998).

Ultimately, a complete account of the role of endorsement methods will need to account for their surprising relative lack of use in actual day to day clinical practice. Even in the time of an earlier round of reviews of CBT assessment practices, Glass and Arnkoff (1997) noted that "in spite of the fact that a large number of self-statement assessment instruments have now been developed, most have been used mainly in research and not in clinical practice, leaving the external validity of these measures an unresolved issue" (p. 917). Indirect evidence for the fact that this must be true is that very few cognitive scales have published norms, which would be standard for instruments routinely used in practice. The scales that do have formally published norms are typically symptom outcome scales, which often serve as the dependent variables in research employing cognitive predictor variables. In addition, as noted previously, CBT endorsement measures scales are frequently used idiographically to inform case formulation. Here, individual items are typically employed, a use for which norms are not critical.

Although everyday use of CBT endorsement scales in practice appears to be the exception, practice is still informed by models developed in research using these scales. We should therefore not understand assessment research as a predominantly academic activity removed from practice. The lesson to be taken away is that practice follows policy. If the predominant paradigm is diagnosis, assessment will follow it, and the assessment measures used will, for pragmatic reasons, be ones that settle questions of diagnosis. Dimensional assessment in CBT might stimulate use of dimensionally based cognition measures and make it more likely that practitioners will see fit to augment their diagnosis-based categorical assessment with dimensional assessment that is theory-based, with cognitive prognostic variables offering more precision in tailoring treatment, predicting course of therapy, and identifying etiological factors. Given the centrality of endorsement methods to research and practice, an empirical study of patterns of usage both clinically and in research would be illuminating.

KEY POINTS

FOR PRACTITIONERS

- In light of their strengths and shortcomings, endorsement methods are most effectively used as part of a nomothetic–idiographic assessment sequence whereby elevated scores can identify problem areas, which are then followed up clinically on an item-by-item basis.
- Measures of cognition should not be taken as literal reports, but rather as indicative of a general clinical picture consistent with the thought content of a particular emotional problem.
- Clients might be less aware of their enduring beliefs, but regarding responses on endorsement belief measures as reflections of actual beliefs has a stronger theoretical basis than that of automatic thought measures.

FOR RESEARCHERS

- Use of endorsement methods should be grounded in the types of inferences that research seeks to support.
- Scales that are based on the reports of frequency or intensity of thoughts should not be relied upon as veridical measures of these dimensions, but may still hold useful information.
- Means need to be developed to implement construct-representation-based validity, which will first require an understanding of what construct representation implies for CBT research.
- Idiographic case series studies have potential for providing a basis for documenting the sorts of functional relationships that are not possible to establish with aggregate measures.

FOR STUDENTS AND EDUCATORS

- Use of endorsement methods depends on carefully weighing their strengths and weaknesses. Decisions about their use should not be oversimplified.
- There is a great need for efforts devoted to improving endorsement methods—an area that has been neglected for several decades.
- Because of their incomparable utility, strengthening the basis for using endorsement methods could have a considerable impact on the field.

REFERENCES

Alloy, L. B., Abramson, L. Y., Keyser, J., Gerstein, R. K., & Sylvia, L. G. (2008). In K. S. Dobson & D. J. A. Dozois (Eds.), Negative cognitive style. *Risk factors in depression* (pp. 221–236). New York: Academic Press.

American Psychiatric Association. (1980). *Diagnostic and statistical manual of mental disorders* (3rd ed.). Washington, DC: Author.

Barnett, P. A., & Gotlib, I. H. (1998). Psychosocial functioning and depression: Distinguishing among antecedents, concomitants, and consequences. *Psychological Bulletin, 104*(1), 97–126.

Bassili, J. N. (1996). Meta-judgmental versus operative indexes of psychological attributes: The case of measures of attitude strength. *Journal of Personality and Social Psychology, 71*(4), 637–653.

Beck, A. T. (1976). *Cognitive therapy and the emotional disorders*. New York: International Universities Press.

Beck, A. T. (1987). Cognitive models of depression. *Journal of Cognitive Psychotherapy, 1*, 5–37.

Beck, A. T., Brown, G., Steer, R. A., Eidelson, J. I., & Riskind, J. H. (1987). Differentiating anxiety and depression: A test of the cognitive content-specificity hypothesis. *Journal of Abnormal Psychology, 96*(3), 179–183.

Beck, A. T., Emery, G., & Greenberg, R. L. (2005). *Anxiety disorders and phobias: A cognitive perspective* (15th anniversary ed.). Cambridge, MA: Basic Books.

Beck, A. T., Rush, A. J., Shaw, B. F., & Emery, G. (1979). *Cognitive therapy of depression*. New York: Guilford Press.

Beevers, C. G., Strong, D. R., Meyer, B., Pilkonis, P. A., & Miller, I. W. (2007). Efficiently assessing negative cognition in depression: An item response theory analysis of the Dysfunctional Attitude Scale. *Psychological Assessment, 19*(2), 199.

Bornstein, R. F. (2011). Toward a process-focused model of test score validity: Improving psychological assessment in science and practice. *Psychological Assessment, 23*(2), 532–544.

Cervone, D. (2004). Personality assessment: Tapping the social-cognitive architecture of personality. *Behavior Therapy, 35*(1), 113–129.

Chambless, D. L., Caputo, G. C., Bright, P., & Gallagher, R. (1984). Assessment of fear in agoraphobics: The Body Sensations Questionnaire and the Agoraphobic Cognitions Questionnaire. *Journal of Consulting and Clinical Psychology, 52*(6), 1090–1097.

Clark, D. A. (1997). Twenty years of cognitive assessment: Current status and future directions. *Journal of Consulting and Clinical Psychology, 65*(6), 996–1000.

Clark, D. A., Beck, A. T., & Alford, B. A. (1999). *Scientific foundations of cognitive theory and therapy of depression*. New York: Wiley.

Clark, D. A., Beck, A. T., & Brown, G. (1989). Cognitive mediation in general psychiatric outpatients: A test of the content-specificity hypothesis. *Journal of Personality and Social Psychology, 56*(6), 958–964.

Clark, D. M. (1986). A cognitive approach to panic. *Behaviour Research and Therapy, 24*(4), 461–470.

Coyne, J. C., & Gotlib, I. H. (1983). The role of cognition in depression: A critical appraisal. *Psychological Bulletin, 94*(3), 472–505.

De Houwer, J. (2011). Why the cognitive approach in psychology would profit from a functional approach and vice versa. *Perspectives on Psychological Science, 6*(2), 202–209.

Dobson, K. S., & Segal, Z. V. (1992). Reflections on consensus building and cognitive models of depression. *Psychological Inquiry, 3*(3), 278–282.

Embretson, S. E. (1983). Construct validity: Construct representation versus nomothetic span. *Psychological Bulletin, 93*(1), 179–197.

Ericsson, K. A., & Simon, H. A. (1980). Verbal reports as data. *Psychological Review, 87*(3), 215–251.

Foa, E. B., & Kozak, M. J. (1997). Beyond the efficacy ceiling?: Cognitive behavior therapy in search of theory. *Behavior Therapy, 28*(4), 601–611.

Fridhandler, B. M. (1986). Conceptual note on state, trait, and the state–trait distinction. *Journal of Personality and Social Psychology, 50*(1), 169–174.

Glass, C. R., & Arnkoff, D. B. (1982). Think cognitively: Selected issues in cognitive assessment and therapy. *Advances in Cognitive-Behavioral Research and Therapy, 1*, 35–71.

Glass, C. R., & Arnkoff, D. B. (1997). Questionnaire methods of cognitive self-statement assessment. *Journal of Consulting and Clinical Psychology, 65*(6), 911–927.

Goldfried, M. R., & Kent, R. N. (1972). Traditional versus behavioral personality assessment: A comparison of methodological and theoretical assumptions. *Psychological Bulletin, 77*(6), 409–420.

Haaga, D. A. F. (1997). Introduction to the special section on measuring cognitive products in research and practice. *Journal of Consulting and Clinical Psychology, 65*(6), 907–910.

Haynes, S. N., Mumma, G. H., & Pinson, C. (2009). Idiographic assessment: Conceptual and psychometric foundations of individualized behavioral assessment. *Clinical Psychology Review, 29*(2), 179–191.

Hollon, S. D., & Kendall, P. C. (1980). Cognitive self-statements in depression: Development of an automatic thoughts questionnaire. *Cognitive Therapy and Research, 4*(4), 383–395.

Jacobson, N. S. (1997). Can contextualism help? *Behavior Therapy, 28*(3), 435–443.

Kendall, P. C., & Hollon, S. D. (Eds.). (1981). *Assessment strategies for cognitive-behavioral interventions.* New York: Academic Press.

Kuyken, W., Padesky, P. C. A., & Dudley, D. R. (2009). *Collaborative case conceptualization: Working effectively with clients in cognitive-behavioral therapy.* New York: Guilford Press.

Lang, P. J. (1979). A bio-informational theory of emotional imagery. *Psychophysiology, 16*(6), 495–512.

Lawyer, S. R., & Smitherman, T. A. (2004). Trends in anxiety assessment. *Journal of Psychopathology and Behavioral Assessment, 26*(2), 101–106.

Loevinger, J. (1957). Objective tests as instruments of psychological theory. *Psychological Reports, 3*(3), 635–694.

MacLeod, C. (1993). Cognition in clinical psychology: Measures, methods or models? *Behaviour Change, 10,* 169–195.

McNally, R. J. (1994). *Panic disorder: A critical analysis.* New York: Guilford Press.

McNally, R. J. (2001). On the scientific status of cognitive appraisal models of anxiety disorder. *Behaviour Research and Therapy, 39*(5), 513–521.

McNally, R. J. (2002). Anxiety sensitivity and panic disorder. *Biological Psychiatry, 52*(10), 938–946.

McNally, R. J. (2007). Mechanisms of exposure therapy: How neuroscience can improve psychological treatments for anxiety disorders. *Clinical Psychology Review, 27*(6), 750–759.

Mischel, W. (2004). Toward an integrative model for CBT: Encompassing behavior, cognition, affect, and process. *Behavior Therapy, 35*(1), 185–203.

Mumma, G. H. (2004). Validation of idiosyncratic cognitive schema in cognitive case formulations: An intraindividual idiographic approach. *Psychological Assessment, 16*(3), 211–230.

Mumma, G. H., & Mooney, S. R. (2006). Incremental validity of cognitions in a clinical case formulation: An intraindividual test in a case example. *Journal of Psychopathology and Behavioral Assessment, 29*(1), 17–28.

Mumma, G. H., & Mooney, S. R. (2007). Comparing the validity of alternative cognitive case formulations: A latent variable, multivariate time series approach. *Cognitive Therapy and Research, 31*(4), 451–481.

Nisbett, R. E., & Wilson, T. D. (1977). Telling more than we can know: Verbal reports on mental processes. *Psychological Review, 84*(3), 231–259.

Obsessive Compulsive Cognitions Working Group. (2003). Psychometric validation of the Obsessive Beliefs Questionnaire and the Interpretation of Intrusions Inventory: Part I. *Behaviour Research and Therapy, 41*(8), 863–878.

Reiss, S., Peterson, R. A., Gursky, D. M., & McNally, R. J. (1986). Anxiety sensitivity, anxiety frequency and the prediction of fearfulness. *Behaviour Research and Therapy, 24*(1), 1–8.

Schwitzgebel, E. (2006). Belief. Retrieved from *www.science.uva.nl/~seop/entries/belief/#2.1.*

Segal, Z. V. (1988). Appraisal of the self-schema construct in cognitive models of depression. *Psychological Bulletin, 103*(2), 147–162.

Segal, Z. V., Kennedy, S., Gemar, M., Hood, K., Pedersen, R., & Buis, T. (2006). Cognitive reactivity to sad mood provocation and the prediction of depressive relapse. *Archives of General Psychiatry, 63*(7), 749.

Sheppard, L. C., & Teasdale, J. D. (2000). Dysfunctional thinking in major depressive disorder: A deficit in metacognitive monitoring? *Journal of Abnormal Psychology, 109*(4), 768–776.

Van den Hout, M. (1999). Armies of idiots and idiosyncrasies: On reductions in experimental psychopathology. *Behaviour Research and Therapy, 37*(Suppl. 1), S135–S145.

Weissman, A. N., & Beck, A. T. (1978). Development and validation of the

Dysfunctional Attitude Scale: A preliminary investigation. Retrieved from *www.eric.ed.gov/ERICWebPortal/contentdelivery/servlet/ERICServlet? accno=ED167619.*

Wilson, K. G., Hayes, S. C., & Gifford, E. V. (1997). Cognition in behavior therapy: Agreements and differences. *Journal of Behavior Therapy and Experimental Psychiatry, 28*(1), 53–63.

Zuroff, D. C., Blatt, S. J., Sanislow, C. A., III, Bondi, C. M., & Pilkonis, P. A. (1999). Vulnerability to depression: Reexamining state dependence and relative stability. *Journal of Abnormal Psychology, 108*(1), 76–89.

3

Production-Based Assessment in Cognitive-Behavioral Therapy

David A. F. Haaga and Ari Solomon

What are you thinking at this moment? Could you capture all of your thoughts for us in writing or aloud? *Would* you, if we asked you to do so for a research study? What if some of your thoughts were embarrassing, upsetting, frightening, or illicit—could we still count on you to share all of them with us? Might your spoken or written version of your thoughts lack sufficient coherence or context for us to interpret them?

Such questions provide a sense of the challenges associated with the "production methods" of cognitive assessment. In all such methods, written or spoken thought samples are analyzed to identify cognitive constructs of theoretical or clinical importance. Well-known examples of production methods include thought sampling via probes at random moments during daily life (Hurlburt, 1979), thought listing (Cacioppo & Petty, 1981), the articulated thoughts in simulated situations (ATSS) paradigm (Davison, Robins, & Johnson, 1983), and the application of lexical coding rules to transcripts (e.g., Pennebaker & Francis, 1999). All of these techniques form a clear contrast to the "endorsement method" of cognitive assessment, in which participants are simply asked to review and rate predetermined options (e.g., "How strongly do you believe each of the following statements about your self-worth?").

The ATSS approach, which we have used in our own research, illustrates many of the issues surrounding production methods. In the

ATSS paradigm, an imaginary scenario is presented to participants in very short audio or video segments; participants are instructed to imagine, as vividly as possible, that they are personally experiencing the depicted situation. As the scenario unfolds it is interrupted frequently, so that participants may think aloud for approximately 30 seconds in reaction to the latest developments, and those spoken thought samples are recorded for subsequent content analysis. Detailed instructions and practice scenarios are used to identify and remediate common misunderstandings, such as commenting on a scene as though it did not personally involve oneself (e.g., "I guess this would have been a tough situation for somebody to handle"). Participants with such misunderstandings are reminded to instead fully immerse themselves in the scenes, to imagine they are personally experiencing the events, and to then report what actually goes through their minds in response to the scenes. For a detailed review of ATSS procedure, theory, and research findings, see Zanov and Davison (2010).

POTENTIAL ADVANTAGES OF PRODUCTION METHODS

The development and ongoing use of production methods in cognitive assessment were motivated by several apparent advantages of these methods relative to endorsement methods. First, production methods may lend themselves better to studies of the situational specificity of cognition. In the case of ATSS, situations are typically manipulated by the investigator. For example, in a study by Solomon, Haaga, Brody, Kirk, and Friedman (1998), participants imagined themselves in a series of upsetting scenarios of differential relevance to two personality styles described in Beck's (1983) cognitive theory of depression—for example, being rejected by a romantic partner in one scenario (a particular stressor for the sociotropic personality), and being audited by the IRS (a particular stressor for the autonomous personality) in another. In Rayburn and Davison (2002), participants spoke their thoughts aloud while imagining overhearing a conversation between two students conspiring to commit either (1) an anti-gay hate crime or (2) a non-hate crime. This kind of "stimulus matching" allows for clearer causal inferences about the impact of situational variables on thinking than do studies of what people typically think or believe. Moreover, use of simulations makes it feasible to study situations that are of high interest or impact but may be extremely private (e.g., sexual), sensitive (e.g., dating violence), or statistically rare and difficult to anticipate the timing of (e.g., a first lapse after cessation of substance use).

Random thought sampling and similar methods such as the

experience-sampling method (ESM; Csikszentmihalyi & Larson, 1987) relinquish experimental control of situational stimuli for the presumptively higher ecological validity of real situations. Many such studies also require participants to report their situational context whenever they are prompted for a response (e.g., with other people, at a meal, in an argument), so that questions pertaining to situational specificity can be addressed.

A second potential advantage for production methods is decreased reliance on participants' recall of earlier thoughts. On endorsement measures, the timeframe usually is either completely general or at least covers a long period (e.g., on the Dysfunctional Attitude Scale [Weissman & Beck, 1978] the instructions emphasize "Remember that your answer should describe the way you think *MOST OF THE TIME*"), whereas the Hopelessness Scale [Beck, Weissman, Lester, & Trexler, 1974] calls for consideration of "your attitude for the past week"). Production methods, on the other hand, generally call for a respondent to say or write what he or she is thinking at that very moment. In light of significant discrepancies in reporting cognitive coping tactics between momentary reports and reports based on recall of periods as brief as 2 days (Stone et al., 1998), *in situ* self-report methods appear to have an important advantage.

Third, cognitive responses elicited via production methods may have greater credibility simply by virtue of their having been produced rather than endorsed. As a thought experiment, picture asking your young child, "What is 12 divided by 4?" and getting "3" as a response. Presumably this response would give you more confidence in the child's arithmetic knowledge than if you had led with "Could you agree that 12 divided by 4 is 3?" and received in reply an "I guess so." Similarly, if thought listing is conducted after a role-played conversation, and a socially anxious participant writes down, "I'm such an idiot. I sounded like I had no idea what I was talking about," it seems relatively likely that these ideas actually occurred to the person at that time. If, on the other hand, a young mother chooses "2" ("Sometimes") to indicate how frequently she thinks "I'm a social failure" in the context "When I have to attend a social occasion" (an item on the Cognition Checklist [CCL]; Beck, Brown, Steer, Eidelson, & Riskind, 1987), it is not known when or how often she had that thought. Her response of "Sometimes" might mean any of the following: (1) she recollects having had that exact thought sometimes but not other times; (2) she recollects having had a thought that was somewhat like that thought on almost every social occasion; (3) she recollects having had the exact thought every time to only a partial degree ("sort of a failure, but not a *complete* failure"); (4) she cannot recall her exact thoughts in social situations; (5) she is uncertain about the meaning of some aspect of the statement ("Do our office's team-building work retreats, which I dread, count as 'social occasions'? Do our parent effectiveness training classes count?"); or, most simply, (6) she has not attended any social events in recent months.

Fourth, production methods may hold greater potential than do endorsement methods for yielding novel and unexpected findings. For example, if one simply asks participants in a smoking cessation program to complete an endorsement measure such as the Smoking Self-Efficacy Questionnaire (Colletti, Supnick, & Payne, 1985), it is possible to determine whether their self-efficacy to resist the temptation to smoke in various high-risk-for-most-smokers situations is high, medium, or low, whether it correlates with the number of years they have been smoking, whether it predicts treatment outcome, and so on. But such a measure would not reveal whether, left to her own devices, a particular participant does not tend to think about self-efficacy in such situations at all. Such a measure also could not have discovered the existence of self-efficacy in the first place. In contrast, production methods are good at revealing these kinds of things.

Indeed, the cognitive constructs and contextual parameters revealed by such studies can genuinely surprise the researcher. In one ATSS study, for instance (Haaga, 1990), some recent ex-smokers showed evidence of gender-schematic parapraxes in that they mistook the biological sex of speakers in audiotaped scenarios, seemingly on the basis of stereotypes about the roles they were playing The study had not been designed to assess gender-related perceptions, but use of an open-ended production method of cognitive assessment made it possible to detect them.

Descriptive experience sampling, a variant of thought sampling, has been used with this potential in the foreground. In descriptive experience sampling studies, participants are signaled at random intervals to make notes on their immediate subjective experience—exactly what they are thinking, feeling, and sensing in the moment. Subsequent interviews with the investigator are used to gain as much clarity as possible on the specific details of these inner experiences. The potential of this method to yield novel or surprising results was noted by Hurlburt and Akhter (2006): "We throw the net widely at the concept of inner experience on the possibility that individual subjects may have features of inner experience that we have never before encountered" (p. 275).

LIMITATIONS OF PRODUCTION METHODS

Balanced against this array of potential advantages for production methods are noteworthy disadvantages. First, whereas requiring participants to *produce* cognitive responses enhances credibility, *failure* to produce a particular response is ambiguous. For example, if a man was randomly prompted for a thought sample at a point when his mind was jumping around from a work project to a weekend plan to a book he is reading to the London 2012 Olympics and recorded only the Olympics and book-related thoughts, it would not mean that thoughts about work were absent. Cognitive assessment researchers have acknowledged that it is very unlikely that respondents produce a complete sample of their thoughts (e.g., Zanov & Davison, 2010), so are the data that production methods yield representative enough?

A creative experiment on this subject by Kashima and Davison (1989) found a high positive correlation ($r = .73$) for an ATSS indicator of irrational beliefs across two presentations of the same scenarios in a condition in which the participants had been instructed to report *different* thoughts the second time. Content analysis revealed that, as instructed, these participants had indeed reported more topographically dissimilar thoughts than had participants in a separate condition who were assessed twice but not asked to report different thoughts the second time. This result suggests that, at least for irrationality, the incompleteness of ATSS responses may not be a critical problem; the (usually unmeasured) other thought content the participant did not report the first time through the scenario was similar from the standpoint of level of irrational belief. Further studies along these lines with different inferential coding schemes would be useful with respect to gauging the seriousness of this disadvantage of production methods.

Second, production methods of cognitive assessment tend to be more time-consuming and labor-intensive than are endorsement methods. This is the case to a small degree for participants; it is more cumbersome to write out what one was thinking for a thought-listing exercise than to circle numbers indicative of varying levels of agreement with preselected thoughts. It is the case to a very large degree for assessors. In particular, content analysis of production measure data is much more difficult than scoring endorsement questionnaires. Depending on the details of the production method, there may be a need to transcribe spoken text into written material for content analysis. Even if the material presents itself in the first place in written form (e.g., with thought listing), there is still the need to develop an explicit coding scheme for inferring cognitive variables of interest from the responses. Perhaps as a result, we are not aware of any regular use of such methods in day-to-day clinical practice of cognitive behavior therapists.

In research contexts, time may be less constrained than it is in clinical practice, but still an important consideration. One must, for instance, train independent raters in a measure's use, help the raters to complete the content analysis, evaluate interrater reliability, and recycle through this process if initial results are not satisfactory.

Third, for lab-based production methods such as ATSS, though not for *in vivo* methods such as experience sampling, the concern of generalizability arises. That is, if someone thinks in a particular way in a simulated situation, can we be confident that they think the same way when analogous situations arise in the natural environment? There is little empirical evidence directly on this point, but it may be possible to derive hypotheses from the literature on lab-based behavioral and psychophysiological assessment. Some studies in these areas have shown advantages for individualizing assessment scenarios. For instance, concurrent validity (correlation with depressive symptoms) was stronger for behaviorally assessed social skills when role-play content was tailored to the individual depressed patient to maximize personal relevance than when the content was standardized (Chiauzzi, Heimberg, Becker, & Gansler, 1985). Similarly, heart rate reactivity to audiotaped descriptions of the particular motor vehicle accident (MVA) a participant had survived distinguished those with posttraumatic stress disorder (PTSD) from MVA survivors without PTSD, whereas reactivity did not differ across groups in response to a standard MVA stimulus (Blanchard et al., 1996).

Tailoring simulated situations to the individual respondent would detract from the meaningfulness of between-person comparisons; if I think more hostile thoughts after being fired from a job than you do after getting a slightly smaller merit pay increase than you had hoped, it does not necessarily imply that I am across the board a more hostile person than you are, but could instead reflect a situational effect. However, in some circumstances (e.g., clinical practice), comparison of scores with those of other respondents might be a lower priority, and individualization could be worthwhile for maximizing realism and situational generalizability. That is, patients might be asked to think aloud while imagining themselves in situations the general properties of which are stipulated by the assessor (e.g., "interpersonal stressor," "assertion challenge") but the specific details of which are generated by the respondent.

PSYCHOMETRIC EVALUATION OF PRODUCTION METHODS OF COGNITIVE ASSESSMENT

A general review of the psychometrics of all production methods is beyond the scope of this chapter, but to illustrate the sorts of questions cognitive assessment researchers have addressed, we focus on two especially salient concerns regarding production methods: interrater reliability of scoring them and convergent validity with endorsement methods.

Interrater Reliability

Interrater reliability is perhaps the main distinguishing feature of the psychometric evaluation of production versus endorsement measures. Scoring endorsement measures is easy and generally not subject to judgment. If the respondent hit "Y" for "yes" on a computer, or circled the number 5 to correspond to "sometimes" on a written form, the scoring of that response follows automatically. For production measures, on the other hand, translating a spoken or written statement into a numerical score involves judgment, and it therefore makes sense to ask how consistent versus idiosyncratic that judgment is.

For the most part researchers have been able to achieve high interrater reliability. For example, in an ATSS study that compared maritally violent to nonviolent men, after 30 hours of training raters were able to score transcripts reliably for such indicators as a desire to commit physical aggression (intraclass correlation = .88) or belligerence toward a provocative person in the simulated situation (intraclass correlation = .76) (Eckhardt, 2007).

There have been exceptions to this rule of high interrater reliability in the production methods, and more may be buried in file drawers as unpublishable false starts toward a coding scheme. One above-ground report of difficulty came from an ATSS study by Chamberlain and Haaga (2001), who noted that articulated thoughts in response to three simulated situations (romantic breakup, stressful job-application scenario, positive job-search outcome) were for the most part coded as "inconclusive" in relation to indicators of self-accepting thoughts. Perhaps the coding scheme or coder training process was faulty, or perhaps self-acceptance in the wake of a stressful experience is a tacit process rather than something clearly reflected in people's verbalized cognitive responses. Standardized coding schemes are not readily available or are completely nonexistent as in the case of the ATSS. Thus researchers are required to generate idiosyncratic production coding schemes for each new study.

Convergent Validity with Endorsement Methods

In light of the substantial procedural differences between endorsement and production methods in assessing cognitive variables, and conceptual and practical advantages for one versus the other type of assessment, it is natural to ask whether, in the end, they yield similar data. Accordingly, numerous studies have examined the convergent validity of endorsement and production methods. Several reviews have drawn the conclusion that convergent validity has been quite low (Chamberlain & Haaga, 1999;

Clark, 1988). For example, in a social anxiety study, state-of-mind ratio scores (Schwartz, 1986) derived from endorsement measures correlated just $r = .19$ with the same ratio scores derived from production methods (Heimberg, Bruch, Hope, & Dombeck, 1990). Relatedly, thought listing state-of-mind scores proved less sensitive to treatment effects for social anxiety than were state-of-mind scores derived from questionnaires (Heinrichs & Hofmann, 2005). This desynchrony between a performance measure and what Donald Campbell (1950) called "voluntary self-description" (p. 15) is hardly limited to the case of production and endorsement methods of cognitive variables. For example, questionnaire measures of experiential avoidance correlated nonsignificantly ($r = .08–.16$) with behavioral indicators of persistence or distress tolerance hypothesized to reflect similar processes (Schloss & Haaga, 2011).

On the face of it, lack of convergent validity is a clear negative outcome. If there is one stable underlying construct reflecting the respondent's self-efficacy for approaching feared stimuli, or depressotypic attributional style, or achievement-related irrational beliefs, then multiple measures ought to converge in assessing that construct. However, these low correlations can be seen instead as opening up additional potential uses for production methods. If such measures always correlated highly with endorsement measures that are far simpler and quicker to administer and score, then production methods might be restricted to serving as initial validation measures for newly developed endorsement methods. But with more independence from traditional measures, other possibilities arise.

POTENTIAL USES OF PRODUCTION METHODS IN VIEW OF LOW CONVERGENT VALIDITY

One way production methods can be used in combination with endorsement measures is at a preliminary stage of *developing content to be included on endorsement measures*. That is, open-ended production instructions can be used to solicit cognitive responses, which can then be translated to an endorsement format and subjected to further psychometric testing. In principle, such a test development process will enhance the content validity of the resulting endorsement measures because the content originated in respondents' reports of their actual thoughts. As an example, Huntley and Juliano (2012, Study 1) generated an initial set of items for a caffeine expectancy questionnaire by asking two separate samples (one of people in treatment for caffeine dependence; one of community adults) to list all the positive and negative effects caffeine has on them, effects of caffeine on health, and effects of abstaining from caffeine. This amounts to using a written thought listing as a preliminary step in development of an endorsement measure of a specific cognitive variable, expectancies for caffeine. If instead the test authors had generated initial-item content solely off the tops of their heads or by consulting other caffeine researchers, there would have been no assurance that the items captured expectancies actually held by laypeople.

A second potential use of production methods in conjunction with endorsement methods is for *identifying the respondents for whom endorsement methods should be especially valid*. For example, one concern raised in relation to endorsement methods of attributional style is that in assessing *what* people consider to be the main cause of various hypothetical events, and how they classify these causes along various theoretically relevant dimensions, these measures take for granted *that* people routinely ponder the causes of what happens to them at all (e.g., Davison & Neale, 1994; Downey, Silver, & Wortman, 1990). If someone is disinclined to analyze causes, her or his responses on an attributional style measure might be less meaningful.

A production measure that does not compel causal thinking could be used to gain an independent assessment of whether someone tends to make attributions. A study testing this line of reasoning applied the Content Analysis of Verbatim Explanations (CAVE; Peterson, Luborsky, & Seligman, 1983) coding scheme to transcripts of cognitive therapy sessions from a clinical trial of treatments for depression (Haaga et al., 1995, Study 1). Participants whose transcripts yielded more frequent causal attributions tended to show the strongest correlations between (1) the stability and globality of their attributions for negative events, as measured before treatment using an endorsement method (Attributional Style Questionnaire; Peterson et al., 1982); and (2) change in depressive symptoms over the course of therapy. See also Haaga (1989) for an example involving self-efficacy among cigarette smokers, with the production method being ATSS. If this effect applies widely, it could point to a fruitful method of combining cognitive assessment methods: use production methods to determine *who* thinks about a particular issue (e.g., danger level, causality, self-efficacy), and then more efficient endorsement methods to determine *what* in particular those respondents think.

A third possible use of production methods in a context of low convergent validity is to help determine the nature of subtle differences in the actual constructs being indexed by different measures. Ordinarily, low convergent validity must mean that at least one of the measures is low in construct validity, but an alternative possibility is that each is validly measuring something slightly different. This interpretation is of course much more useful if the nature of the difference can be determined. Research on measurement of subjective well-being provides a possible model. Using their Day Reconstruction Method, in which people report on their experiences in detail from the prior day, Kahneman and colleagues found that women's reported affect while taking care of their children was (1) more favorable than when they were commuting or doing housework but (2) less favorable than for numerous other activity categories, including socializing, relaxing, eating, exercising, watching TV, and preparing food (Kahneman, Krueger, Schkade, Schwarz, & Stone, 2004).

This result rests uneasily beside not only most parents' self-images, but also beside data indicating that parents describe interacting with their children as the most enjoyable from a long list of activities of daily life (e.g., Juster, 1985). Kahneman et al. (2004) argue that the generic statements about enjoying being with one's kids are based on beliefs and prototypical experiences accruing over a period of time, while the Day Reconstruction Method taps specific, recent, episodic memories. Neither method is simply invalid, and each is likely to correlate with important dependent measures (e.g., beliefs may relate to the decision to have another child, while recent episodic memories may relate to sleep quality that night), but they are not the same. Such distinctions may be relevant for understanding differing results with cognitive assessment methods, but the key step would be using theory and research to figure out the exact nature of the distinctions rather than using the possibility of subtle construct distinctions as more of an all-purpose excuse for low convergent validity.

MODIFYING PRODUCTION METHODS TO INCREASE EFFICIENCY

As noted earlier, some inefficiencies associated with production measures may limit their use in clinical or even research settings. For some such measures, the inefficiencies include a need for time-intensive expert rating of thought samples; a need for time-intensive data collection, including practice trials, coaching participants, and so on; a need for individual sessions so that privacy of thoughts can be assured; a need for special safeguards for highly sensitive archival data containing personally identifiable features; and more. However, it might be possible to retain some of the advantages of production assessments while reducing such complexities of administration and scoring.

One strategy is to combine essential features of production methods with advantageous features of a conventional questionnaire. For example, participants might be asked to witness a scenario and then simply circle all of the categories of thoughts or beliefs about the self that they are aware of having "right now" in response to the video (e.g., "Are you having thoughts about . . . Expecting to be rejected? Expecting to be welcomed? Feeling like you don't 'fit in here'? Feeling like you do 'fit in here'?").

Some researchers have indeed developed measures that attempt to retain some of the advantages of both the production and endorsement methods. For example, Hedlund and Rude (1995) used a scrambled sentence task to infer that depression-prone individuals experience a uniquely high rate of depressotypic automatic thoughts, due to an underlying depressotypic cognitive bias. Each sentence in the task had two possible unscrambled solutions, with only one of the solutions reflecting a depressotypic belief. This task retains some important features of a production method, including that participants must generate an interpretation at the moment of assessment ("This sentence makes immediate sense to me"), rather than attempt to report their historical thoughts or beliefs. On the other hand, the scrambled sentence task retains many of the efficiency advantages of a traditional self-report questionnaire: It can be completed quickly, silently, and in a group setting, and scoring it is as simple as any traditional questionnaire.

For another example, Solomon, Arnow, Gotlib, and Wind (2003) hypothesized that conventional rational-emotive behavior therapy (REBT; Ellis, 1994) self-report measures of self-demandingness, such as the Belief Scale (Malouff & Schutte, 1986), had repeatedly failed to correlate with depression-proneness because they forced participants to reject or endorse very abstracted, even stereotypical, self-belief statements like "To be a worthwhile person, I must be thoroughly competent in everything I do," and "To be happy, I must maintain the approval of all the persons I consider significant" (Belief Scale; Malouff & Schutte, 1986). Solomon et al. noted that

> Such broad and absolute items certainly resemble the statements Ellis himself has used traditionally to define irrational beliefs in sentence form. . . . However, they seem unlikely to reflect how demandingness is expressed in remitted depressed or similar high-functioning populations. Indeed, REBT practitioners recognize that high-functioning clients often frame their key psychological demands in narrow, idiosyncratic terms, such as, "I won't be able to live with myself if I lose this particular job opportunity," rather than "It is intolerable for me to fail at anything important". . . . If so, an individualized measure might reveal demandingness in depression-prone populations where traditional questionnaires have failed. (2003, p. 442)

As an alternative, Solomon et al. instructed participants to indicate whether there was anything about their experience or behavior that prevented them from "feeling completely worthwhile and acceptable to myself," within each of 15 normative self-domains (e.g., anything about "my mental abilities," "my physical abilities," "my physical appearance," "my actions from the past," and so on). To ensure that non-normative self-domains were also captured, a 16th category was included: "something else about me that hasn't been listed yet." Thus participants' scores were based on their *own* idiosyncratic self-demands in each domain. Depression-prone and never-depressed participants differed dramatically on the idiographic self-demands measure: The interquartile ranges of the groups did not even overlap, whereas their interquartile ranges on the Belief Scale were nearly identical.

Another way to enhance the efficiency of production methods is to borrow or adapt an automated coding methodology that has already been extensively validated in other research programs. One example of this is the use of Pennebaker's text analysis program Linguistic Inquiry and Word Count (LIWC; Pennebaker & Francis, 1999) to test hypotheses that bear on cognitive theory. The LIWC software automatically analyzes transcripts, sorting the thousands of words in its lexicon into hundreds of theoretically and empirically meaningful categories, including some cognitive categories (e.g., self-discrepancies, causal statements, etc.). Additional categories can be developed by a researcher or clinician. Rude, Gortner, and Pennebaker (2004) used the LIWC to explore whether remitted-depressed students differed from never-depressed students in self-focus, as defined by frequency of using first-person singular words ("I," "me," "my," "myself") in essays concerning their deepest feelings and thoughts about being in college. Intriguingly, these groups did not differ in their use of the first person early in their essays, but remitted-depressed students began using the first person more as their essays progressed. This finding may fit with other theories and research on reinstating core schemas via mood or cognitive priming in remitted depression (Miranda, Gross, Persons, & Hahn, 1998; Rude, Valdez, Odom, & Ebrahimi, 2003).

Importantly, it remains an empirical question whether scores for a particular construct on a "hybrid" measure assess the same thing as scores for that construct using cleaner production methods. A stepwise approach to developing hybrid instruments would begin by establishing the validity of a benchmark production method such as the ATSS, integrate any serendipitous findings using that method, and then develop a hybrid measure that converges well with the benchmark. Eventually, all such measures would ideally be positioned within a nomologic network that includes traditional production measures, endorsement measures, and hybrid measures of the same putative construct.

PRODUCTION METHODS IN CLINICAL PRACTICE

As noted earlier, cognitive therapists have not generally incorporated the ATSS, LIWC, thought listing, or random thought sampling into their clinical practice. Likely obstacles to adoption of these techniques include the added complexity and cost of training a client in a specialized methodology, confidentiality concerns regarding spoken thought recordings, and lack of training.

Still, cognitive therapists are no strangers to the logic of production methods. Examples of in-session production-oriented cognitive therapy methods include the so-called downward arrow technique for identifying core dysfunctional beliefs (e.g., Burns, 1999), and the "empty-chair" technique and very similar "friend-dispute" technique for identifying positive coping beliefs (e.g., DiGiuseppe, Doyle, Dryden, & Backx, 2014; Walen, DiGiuseppe, & Dryden, 1992, p. 94). In each case a client is asked to notice and report the idiosyncratic core meanings of a crucial life scenario, event, or context. Most generally, of course, all cognitive therapists learn to notice sudden shifts in affect or tone so as to inquire as to thoughts that went through their client's mind "just now." Such inquiries often serve as a production method that generates data about automatic thoughts, biases, and core beliefs that inform the therapist's ongoing cognitive case formulation (Persons, 1989).

Accordingly, some researchers have taken advantage of therapy session transcripts as a source of cognitive assessment data. For instance, DeRubeis, Tang, and colleagues investigated shifts in patients' thoughts and beliefs immediately before large, sustained symptomatic improvements during cognitive therapy for depression. Independent raters coded therapy session transcripts for patient statements that disavowed or contradicted an earlier depressotypic thought, belief, or distortion—for example, "How could I [have] let him decide if I am attractive or not?" (Tang & DeRubeis, 1999, p. 899). Using a cognitive change score based on such statements, these researchers repeatedly found that pronounced in-session endorsement of cognitive change tended to occur immediately before pronounced symptomatic improvements (Tang, DeRubeis, Beberman, & Pham, 2005).

Process research outside the cognitive therapy framework has likewise used coding of session transcripts to understand changes in patients' self-views during treatment. Goncalves and colleagues (e.g., Matos, Santos, Goncalves, & Martins, 2009) have identified as a key process marker the occurrence in sessions of so-called "innovative moments," in which patients show evidence of assigning new personal meanings to aspects of their self-narrative that have long been associated with dysfunctional personal meanings. Goncalves and colleagues have reliably coded such moments in the self-narratives of patients in several forms of psychotherapy and demonstrated that the frequency of innovative moments is associated with clinical improvement.

Supplementing in-session assessments, cognitive therapists have used variants of production methods as homework assignments. For example, cognitive therapists typically ask their clients to monitor thoughts during periods of distress in daily life and synopsize those thoughts and stressful circumstances on the Daily Record of Dysfunctional Thoughts (DRDTs; e.g., DeRubeis, Webb, Tang, & Becker, 2010); therapists analyze those thought samples informally for various kinds of theoretically relevant content. Several research teams have coded DRDTs more systematically for use in descriptive or treatment process–outcome studies. For example, Riskind, Castellon, and Beck (1989) found, consistent with the reformulated learned helplessness theory of depression, that thoughts listed on DRDTs by patients with major depressive disorder proved more consistent with a depressotypic attributional style than did the thoughts listed on the DRDTs of anxiety-disordered patients. Persons and Burns (1985) reported that cognitive therapy clients' changing degree of belief in their negative DRDT statements was closely correlated with changes in their mood symptoms; and determined (Persons & Burns, 1986), via a series of cognitive therapy cases, that the first dysfunctional thought listed by clients on their DRDT forms consistently proved to be the most difficult to change, regardless of the order in which the thoughts were challenged with a therapist. Finally, Neimeyer and Feixas (1990) asked patients who had completed cognitive therapy to complete a blank DRDTs while thinking about a highly relevant stressful situation. Responses were scored for several key cognitive skills: "Objectively describing upsetting situations, articulating the nature and intensity of their affective reaction, identifying the associated automatic thoughts, developing more adaptive alternatives, [and] recording the emotional outcome of their attempt at rational restructuring" (p. 285). Mere assignment to a homework-intensive therapy condition was not associated with 6-month clinical status, but cognitive skill scores at posttest were.

CONCLUSION AND FUTURE DIRECTIONS

The methods and findings we have summarized show that CBT practitioners and researchers have been creative in developing a range of production methods for assessing cognition. These methods can help us make new discoveries, or test established theories, about the very basic issue of what is going on in others' minds, which is of the utmost importance to CBT research and practice. Probably the main impediment to their more widespread use is the sheer laboriousness of collecting spoken or written thought samples and then conducting content analysis of them by well-trained and supervised human judges. One development that might substantially increase activity in this area is increased automation of content analysis. A "bottom-up" (deriving coding categories from the text itself rather than from a priori conceptualizations) scheme for automating content analysis of psychotherapy transcripts was described recently by Salvatore, Gennaro, Auletta, Tonti, and Nitti (2012), and it will be fascinating to see whether such systems are validly applied to verbal samples collected via the production methods of cognitive assessment reviewed in this chapter.

KEY POINTS

FOR PRACTITIONERS

- Production methods can be used to decrease reliance on faulty long-term recall in assessment of patients' thoughts and beliefs.
- Idiographic tailoring of the situational context of cognitive assessment detracts from standardization, but may maximize the validity of cognitive assessment of the individual patient.
- Session transcripts and between-session self-monitoring assignments can serve as the raw data for cognitive assessments.

FOR RESEARCHERS

- Production methods can be used either experimentally (e.g., with articulated thoughts in simulated situations) or in correlational studies in the natural environment (e.g., with random thought sampling) to investigate situational effects on cognitive variables.
- Production methods are likely to be very useful in exploratory research.
- More studies are needed of the validity implications of the *incompleteness* of thought samples.
- More research is also needed to determine the generalizability of findings from lab-based production assessment methods.
- Production methods can be used to solicit content for developing new endorsement methods of cognitive assessment or to identify the types of respondents for whom endorsement methods may be especially likely to be valid.
- Production methods can be adapted in ways that make scoring more structured or even perhaps automated.

FOR STUDENTS AND EDUCATORS

- Production methods of cognitive assessment may have greater credibility than do measures requiring only endorsement of preselected thoughts because the content originates entirely with the subject or patient responding to the assessment.
- Interrater reliability of coding of production methods tends to be high, but convergent validity with endorsement methods has been weaker.
- Less labor-intensive methods of scoring production methods are likely to be needed before these procedures will become widely used in routine clinical practice.

ACKNOWLEDGMENTS

We thank Rob DeRubeis, Miguel Goncalves, Wendy Lichtenthal, Robert Neimeyer, and Jackie Persons for comments and suggestions regarding assessment methods discussed in this chapter.

REFERENCES

Beck, A. T. (1983). Cognitive therapy of depression: New perspectives. In P. J. Clayton & J. E. Barrett (Eds.), *Treatment of depression: Old controversies and new approaches* (pp. 265–291). New York: Raven Press.

Beck, A. T., Brown, G., Steer, R. A., Eidelson, J. I., & Riskind, J. H. (1987). Differentiating anxiety and depression: A test of the cognitive content-specificity hypothesis. *Journal of Abnormal Psychology, 96,* 179–183.

Beck, A. T., Weissman, A., Lester, D., & Trexler, L. (1974). The measurement of pessimism: The Hopelessness Scale. *Journal of Consulting and Clinical Psychology, 42,* 861–865.

Blanchard, E. B., Hickling, E. J., Buckley, T. C., Taylor, A. E., Vollmer, A., & Loos, W. R. (1996). Psychophysiology of posttraumatic stress disorder related to motor vehicle accidents: Replication and extension. *Journal of Consulting and Clinical Psychology, 64,* 742–751.

Burns, D. D. (1999). *Feeling good: The new mood therapy.* New York: Harper.

Cacioppo, J. T., & Petty, R. E. (1981). Social psychological procedures for cognitive response assessment: The thought-listing technique. In T. V. Merluzzi, C. R. Glass, & M. Genest (Eds.), *Cognitive assessment* (pp. 309–342). New York: Guilford Press.

Campbell, D. T. (1950). The indirect assessment of social attitudes. *Psychological Bulletin, 47,* 15–38.

Chamberlain, J., & Haaga, D. A. F. (1999). Convergent validity of cognitive assessment methods. *Behavior Modification, 23,* 294–315.

Chamberlain, J. M., & Haaga, D. A. F. (2001). Unconditional self-acceptance and psychological health. *Journal of Rational-Emotive and Cognitive-Behavior Therapy, 19,* 163–176.

Chiauzzi, E. J., Heimberg, R. G., Becker, R. E., & Gansler, D. (1985). Personalized versus standard role plays in the assessment of depressed patients' social skill. *Journal of Psychopathology and Behavioral Assessment, 7,* 121–133.

Clark, D. A. (1988). The validity of measures of cognition: A review of the literature. *Cognitive Therapy and Research, 12,* 1–20.

Colletti, G., Supnick, J. A., & Payne, T. J. (1985). The Smoking Self-Efficacy Questionnaire: Preliminary scale development and validation. *Behavioral Assessment, 7,* 249–260.

Csikszentmihalyi, M., & Larson, R. (1987). Validity and reliability of the experience-sampling method. *Journal of Nervous and Mental Disease, 175,* 526–536.

Davison, G. C., & Neale, J. M. (1994). *Abnormal psychology* (6th ed.). New York: Wiley.

Davison, G. C., Robins, C., & Johnson, M. K. (1983). Articulated thoughts during simulated situations: A paradigm for studying cognition in emotion and behavior. *Cognitive Therapy and Research, 7,* 17–40.

DeRubeis, R. J., Webb, C. A., Tang, T. Z., & Beck, A. T. (2010). Cognitive therapy. In K. S. Dobson (Ed.), *Handbook of cognitive-behavioral therapies* (3rd ed., pp. 277–316). New York: Guilford Press.

DiGiuseppe, R. A., Doyle, K. A., Dryden, W., & Backx, W. (2014). *A practitioner's guide to rational emotive behavior therapy* (3rd ed.). New York: Oxford University Press.

Downey, G., Silver, R. C., & Wortman, C. B. (1990). Reconsidering the attribution-adjustment relation following a major negative event: Coping with the loss of a child. *Journal of Personality and Social Psychology, 59,* 925–940.

Eckhardt, C. I. (2007). Effects of alcohol intoxication on anger experience and expression among partner assaultive men. *Journal of Consulting and Clinical Psychology, 75,* 61–71.

Ellis, A. (1994). *Reason and emotion in psychotherapy.* New York: Birch Lane.

Haaga, D. A. F. (1989). Articulated thoughts and endorsement procedures for cognitive assessment in the prediction of smoking relapse. *Psychological Assessment: A Journal of Consulting and Clinical Psychology, 1,* 112–117.

Haaga, D. A. F. (1990). Gender schematic parapraxes in the articulated thoughts of ex-smokers. *Social Behavior and Personality: An International Journal, 18,* 261–266.

Haaga, D. A. F., Ahrens, A. H., Schulman, P., Seligman, M. E. P., DeRubeis, R. J., & Minarik, M. L. (1995). Metatraits and cognitive assessment: Application to attributional style and depressive symptoms. *Cognitive Therapy and Research, 19,* 121–142.

Hedlund, S., & Rude, S. S. (1995). Evidence of latent depressive schemas in formerly depressed individuals. *Journal of Abnormal Psychology, 104,* 517–525.

Heimberg, R. G., Bruch, M. A., Hope, D. A., & Dombeck, M. (1990). Evaluating the states of mind model: Comparison to an alternate model and effects of method of cognitive assessment. *Cognitive Therapy and Research, 14,* 543–557.

Heinrichs, N., & Hofmann, S. G. (2005). Cognitive assessment of social anxiety: A comparison of self-report and thought listing methods. *Cognitive Behaviour Therapy, 34,* 3–15.

Huntley, E. D., & Juliano, L. M. (2012). Caffeine Expectancy Questionnaire (CaffEQ): Construction, psychometric properties, and associations with caffeine use, caffeine dependence, and other related variables. *Psychological Assessment, 24*(3), 592–607.

Hurlburt, R. T. (1979). Random sampling of cognitions and behavior. *Journal of Research in Personality, 13,* 103–111.

Hurlburt, R. T., & Akhter, S. A. (2006). The Descriptive Experience Sampling method. *Phenomenology and the Cognitive Sciences, 5,* 271–301.

Juster, F. T. (1985). Preferences for work and leisure. In F. T. Juster & F. P. Stafford (Eds.), *Time, goods, and well-being* (pp. 397–414). Ann Arbor, MI: Institute for Social Research.

Kahneman, D., Krueger, A. B., Schkade, D. A., Schwarz, N., & Stone, A. A. (2004). A survey method for characterizing daily life experience: The Day Reconstruction Method. *Science, 306,* 1776–1780.

Kashima, K., & Davison, G. C. (1989). Functional consistency in the face of topographical change in articulated thoughts. *Journal of Rational-Emotive and Cognitive-Behavior Therapy, 7,* 131–139.

Malouff, J. M., & Schutte, N. S. (1986). Development and validation of a measure of irrational beliefs. *Journal of Consulting and Clinical Psychology, 54,* 860–862.

Matos, M., Santos, A., Goncalves, M., & Martins, C. (2009). Innovative moments and change in narrative therapy. *Psychotherapy Research, 19,* 68–80.

Miranda, J., Gross, J. J., Persons, J. B., & Hahn, J. (1998). Mood matters: Negative mood induction activates dysfunctional attitudes in women vulnerable to depression. *Cognitive Therapy and Research, 22,* 363–376.

Neimeyer, R. A., & Feixas, G. (1990). The role of homework and skill acquisition in the outcome of group cognitive therapy for depression. *Behavior Therapy, 21,* 281–292.

Pennebaker, J. W., & Francis, M. E. (1999). *Linguistic Inquiry and Word Count: LIWC* [software]. Mahwah, NJ: Erlbaum.

Persons, J. B. (1989). *Cognitive therapy in practice: A case formulation approach.* New York: Norton.

Persons, J. B., & Burns, D. D. (1985). Mechanisms of action of cognitive therapy: The relative contributions of technical and interpersonal interventions. *Cognitive Therapy and Research, 9,* 539–551.

Persons, J. B., & Burns, D. D. (1986). The process of cognitive therapy: The first dysfunctional thought changes less than the last one. *Behaviour Research and Therapy, 24,* 619–624.

Peterson, C., Luborsky, L., & Seligman, M. E. P. (1983). Attributions and depressive mood shifts: A case study using the symptom-context method. *Journal of Abnormal Psychology, 92,* 96–103.

Peterson, C., Semmel, A., von Baeyer, C., Abramson, L. Y., Metalsky, G. I., & Seligman, M. E. P. (1982). The Attributional Style Questionnaire. *Cognitive Therapy and Research, 6,* 287–301.

Rayburn, N. R., & Davison, G. C. (2002). Articulated thoughts about antigay hate crimes. *Cognitive Therapy and Research, 26*, 431–447.

Riskind, J. H., Castellon, C. S., & Beck, A. T. (1989). Spontaneous causal explanations in unipolar depression and generalized anxiety: Content analyses of dysfunctional-thought diaries. *Cognitive Therapy and Research, 13*, 97–108.

Rude, S. S., Gortner, E.-M., & Pennebaker, J. W. (2004). Language use of depressed and depression-vulnerable college students. *Cognition and Emotion, 18*, 1121–1133.

Rude, S. S., Valdez, C., Odom, S., & Ebrahimi, A. (2003). Negative cognitive bias predicts depression. *Cognitive Therapy and Research, 27*, 415–429.

Salvatore, S., Gennaro, A., Auletta, A. F., Tonti, M., & Nitti, M. (2012). Automated method of content analysis: A device for psychotherapy process research. *Psychotherapy Research, 22*, 256–273.

Schloss, H. M., & Haaga, D. A. F. (2011). Interrelating behavioral measures of distress tolerance with self-reported experiential avoidance. *Journal of Rational-Emotive and Cognitive-Behavior Therapy, 29*, 53–63.

Schwartz, R. M. (1986). The internal dialogue: On the asymmetry between positive and negative coping thoughts. *Cognitive Therapy and Research, 10*, 591–605.

Solomon, A., Arnow, B. A., Gotlib, I. H., & Wind, B. (2003). Individualized measurement of irrational beliefs in remitted depressives. *Journal of Clinical Psychology, 59*, 439–455.

Solomon, A., Haaga, D. A. F., Brody, C., Kirk, L., & Friedman, D. G. (1998). Priming irrational beliefs in recovered-depressed people. *Journal of Abnormal Psychology, 107*, 440–449.

Stone, A. A., Schwartz, J. E., Neale, J. M., Shiffman, S., Marco, C. A., Hickcox, M., et al. (1998). A comparison of coping assessed by ecological momentary assessment and retrospective recall. *Journal of Personality and Social Psychology, 74*, 1670–1680.

Tang, T. Z., & DeRubeis, R. J. (1999). Sudden gains and critical sessions in cognitive behavioral therapy for depression. *Journal of Consulting and Clinical Psychology, 67*, 894–904.

Tang, T. Z., DeRubeis, R. J., Beberman, R., & Pham, T. (2005). Cognitive changes, critical sessions, and sudden gains in cognitive-behavioral therapy for depression. *Journal of Consulting and Clinical Psychology, 73*, 168–172.

Walen, S. R., DiGiuseppe, R., & Dryden, W. A. (1992). *A practitioner's guide to rational-emotive therapy* (2nd ed.). New York: Oxford University Press.

Weissman, A., & Beck, A. T. (1978, November). *Development and validation of the Dysfunctional Attitude Scale.* Paper presented at the annual convention of the Association for Advancement of Behavior Therapy, Chicago.

Zanov, M. V., & Davison, G. C. (2010). A conceptual and empirical review of 25 years of cognitive assessment using the articulated thoughts in simulated situations (ATSS) think-aloud paradigm. *Cognitive Therapy and Research, 34*, 282–291.

4

Imagery-Based Cognitive-Behavioral Assessment

Susie Hales, Simon E. Blackwell, Martina Di Simplicio, Lalitha Iyadurai, Kerry Young, and Emily A. Holmes

A BRIEF, SELECTED REVIEW OF IMAGERY RESEARCH

What is mental imagery? Mental imagery occurs when perceptual information is accessed from memory, giving rise to the experience of "seeing with the mind's eye," "hearing with the mind's ear," and so on. By contrast, perception occurs when information is directly registered from the senses. Mental images need not result simply from the recall of previously perceived objects or events; they can also be created by combining and modifying stored perceptual information in novel ways (see review by Kosslyn, Ganis, & Thompson, 2001). Thus, mental imagery can occur in any sensory modality, although in psychopathology we often focus on visual images. In psychopathology, problematic images typically have the qualities of being highly emotional and of intruding into consciousness unbidden. This involuntary property has led to the idea that images can "flash" to mind. "Flashbacks" are the hallmark of posttraumatic stress disorder (PTSD; see box on page 83 for description). However, images of negative past events are not the only ones that can spring to mind with high levels of emotion. Our group coined the term "flashforwards" to refer to intrusive imagery of the future (Holmes, Crane, Fennell, & Williams, 2007), which has now been used by other researchers (e.g., Engelhard, van den Hout, Janssen, & van der Beek, 2010).

The importance of mental imagery in day-to-day functioning and its potential usefulness for effecting change has been recognized beyond the world of clinical practice—for example, in cognitive neuroscience (e.g., Addis, Pan, Vu, Laiser, & Schacter, 2009; D'Argembeau, Renaud, & Van der Linden, 2011; Schacter, Addis, & Buckner, 2008) and social psychology (Crisp, Birtel, & Meleady, 2011). The use of mental imagery in cognitive-behavioral therapy (CBT) was recognized early by Beck (1971), and researchers such as P. J. Lang (1979) developed pioneering theories of the role that imagery may play in human behavior. However, it is only in the last decade that clinical research concerning imagery has truly gathered momentum. Indeed, it is now regarded as a "hot topic" and a new frontier for development in CBT.

Our clinical research group called EPaCT (Experimental Psychopathology and Cognitive Therapies) has been intrigued by the role of mental imagery in psychopathology (Holmes, James, Blackwell, & Hales, 2011). Mental imagery has been described richly and widely in the literature (for reviews, see Edwards, 2007; Holmes & Mathews, 2010; and Arntz, 2012). It is beyond the scope of this chapter to discuss the whole field of mental imagery research and practice to date, and therefore the focus of this chapter is restricted to the imagery work that has been conducted within EPaCT. There are various key issues that the EPaCT lab have been concerned with. One is the impact of imagery on emotion. Our work has shown that imagery has a more powerful impact on our emotions than thinking in words about the same topic (Holmes, Mathews, Mackintosh, & Dalgleish, 2008). If this is the case, then it seems particularly important to ask about the presence of any imagery at assessment.

Another key issue that fascinates us is the occurrence of emotional imagery in disorders where it hitherto may have been neglected. Assessing the content of intrusive, emotional imagery can reveal useful clinical insights. For example, we have identified and described imagery in suicidal thinking (e.g., Hales, Deeprose, Goodwin, & Holmes, 2011), in agoraphobia (Day, Holmes, & Hackmann, 2004), in bipolar disorder (Holmes, Geddes, Colom, & Goodwin, 2008) and in chronic pain (Berna et al., 2011). Identifying and characterizing the presence of imagery across a range of psychological disorders have been the focus of various special issues in recent years—see Holmes and Hackmann (2004) and Holmes, Arntz, and Smucker (2007). More recently, research has been investigating imagery-related treatments too (see special issues by Hagenaars & Holmes, 2012; Krans, 2011; and Moulds & Holmes, 2011).

A third key area is thus how to harness the properties of imagery for our clinical work. We have been developing treatment innovations using imagery and imagery techniques. These may involve CBT techniques such as imagery rescripting (Giesen-Bloo et al., 2006; Hackmann, Bennett-Levy, & Holmes, 2011). However, new techniques may also consist of more novel forms, such as positive imagery promotion (T. J. Lang, Blackwell, Harmer, Davison, & Holmes, 2012) and imagery interference (Holmes, James, Coode-Bate, & Deeprose, 2009). While mental imagery research is exciting and has plenty of room for further development, imagery treatment techniques are beyond the scope of the current chapter. The main purpose of this chapter is to focus on the assessment of imagery within a CBT framework.

Why is it important to assess for imagery? There are many reasons. Imagery helps us build a fuller understanding of the content of people's concerns. Imagery is important to know about, as it has a strong impact on behaviors and beliefs (see Holmes & Mathews, 2010). Perhaps the pivotal reason, however, relates to the research discussed above: Imagery has been found to have a greater impact on emotion than verbal thoughts. We have proposed that imagery acts as an "emotional amplifier" across emotional disorders (Holmes, Geddes, et al., 2008). If imagery heightens our emotions, then clearly we need to consider how it may impact on emotional disorders.

COGNITION, VERBAL THOUGHTS, AND MENTAL IMAGERY

Cognition is defined as "the mental process by which external or internal input is transformed, reduced, elaborated, stored, recovered, and used. As such, it involves a variety of functions such as perception, attention, memory coding, retention, and recall, decision-making, reasoning, problem-solving, imaging, planning and executing actions" (Neisser, 1967, p. 4). We argue that imagery is different from verbal thinking and so needs a different assessment approach. When we recall events from the past or imagine something happening in the future, we recruit mental imagery. Mental imagery has been described as comparable to having a sensory experience in the absence of a physical sensory stimulus (Kosslyn et al., 2001). Although mental imagery frequently consists of visual images, it can also refer to images in any of the five senses. When we think in verbal thoughts, we tend to use words and verbal language of the sort we would use when we speak. Verbal thoughts are thus very different in nature from images.

In the course of CBT, we routinely ask our patients, "What is going through your mind?" The awareness of this type of cognition can take the two forms described above: verbal thoughts or mental images. When we think in verbal thoughts, we use verbal language of the sort we would use when we speak. For example, a verbal thought of someone with social anxiety about giving a presentation might be "There will be so many people! I will be awful." This would be experienced as a mental phenomenon in the form of words, that is, a verbal representation. In contrast, when we think in mental images, these are sensory impressions. So, for the same person with social anxiety, an associated mental image about giving a presentation might be seeing oneself walk on stage, shaking and as red as a tomato. We will argue that compared to verbal thoughts, images have a greater impact on emotion and may contain extra information. Images should, therefore, form a critical part of assessment (Di Simplicio, McInerney, Goodwin, Attenburrow, & Holmes, 2012). Henceforth in this chapter we consider imagery as a subset of cognitive processes and as different from verbal thought.

HOW HAS IMAGERY BEEN ASSESSED IN CBT RESEARCH AND PRACTICE?

Imagery is a natural part of all human experience. Therefore, when it comes to assessing imagery, commonalities can be found across laboratory research, translational research, and clinical practice.

Laboratory Research

The experience of mental imagery can be measured experimentally in several ways. These can include computer tasks as well as pen-and-paper questionnaires. Various standardized measures are summarized in a recent review by Pearson and colleagues, which includes information about the validity and reliability of these measures (Pearson, Deeprose, Wallace-Hadrill, Burnett Heyes, & Holmes, 2013).

While the assessment of imagery has evolved independently in laboratory research and clinical practice, there is certainly an argument for bringing laboratory measures to the clinic. For example, the process of creating a mental image (image generation) is argued to be distinct from the process of mentally manipulating the image (image transformation). Computer-based assessment tasks such as the Image Generation Task (Dror & Kosslyn, 1994) and the Mental Rotation Task (Shepard & Cooper, 1982) can be used to assess these two processes, respectively. This may be clinically important when it comes to making decisions about the types of intervention techniques to use with a patient, so they are tailored to the patient's specific imagery abilities. In laboratory studies, physiological responses to imagery have been measured as a proxy for the emotionality of imagery (Cummings,

Olphin, & Law, 2007). This type of measurement could also have useful clinical applications.

A variety of pen-and-paper questionnaires can be used in both the laboratory and the clinic to measure trait and state levels of different kinds of imagery experience (see review by Pearson et al., 2013). In our experience, we have found the following measures particularly useful. The Spontaneous Use of Imagery Scale (SUIS; Reisberg, Pearson, & Kosslyn, 2003) is a 12-item measure assessing the extent to which an individual uses imagery in everyday life, and as such can be considered a measure of trait imagery use. It includes items such as "When I first hear a friend's voice, a visual image of him or her almost always springs to mind," each of which are rated on a 5-point Likert scale for the extent to which it occurs (1 = never, 5 = always). Other useful questionnaires, assessing state future imagery processes, are the Impact of Future Events Scale (IFES; Deeprose & Holmes, 2010)[1] and the Prospective Imagery Task (PIT; Holmes, Lang, Moulds, & Steele, 2008; Stöber, 2000). As previously stated, intrusive future imagery can be just as clinically significant as intrusive past imagery. The IFES is based on the Impact of Event Scale—Revised (IES-R; Weiss & Marmer, 1997) but reworded to reflect future rather than past events. Respondents are first required to identify three future events that they have been imagining over the past 7 days and then to state whether these imagined events were positive or negative. The remaining questionnaire items assess the impact of this future imagery on the respondents. The PIT is a measure of ability to generate mental imagery about future events. Participants are asked to form a mental image of 10 negative future scenarios and 10 positive future scenarios. These include events such as "You will have a serious disagreement with your friend," or "You will do well on your course." Each image is rated for vividness on a continuous 5-point Likert scale (1 = no image at all and 5 = very vivid). For the positive items of the PIT, the internal consistency is excellent (alpha = .92), and for the negative items, internal consistency is good (alpha = .87).

Translational Clinical Research

Experimental studies that investigate the effects of novel imagery-based therapeutic approaches (e.g., Jacob et al., 2011) in a controlled laboratory setting provide a natural link between assessment in the laboratory and assessment in clinical practice. One example of where laboratory-based assessment may have increasing clinical relevance is in the delivery of novel computerized interventions for depression that use mental

---

[1] Available on request.

imagery (Blackwell & Holmes, 2010; T. J. Lang et al., 2012). As depression is associated with a deficit in positive future imagery (Holmes et al., 2008; Morina, Deeprose, Pusowski, Schmid, & Holmes, 2011) and a negative interpretation bias (Butler & Mathews, 1983; Rude, Wenzlaff, Gibbs, Vane, & Whitney, 2002), these interventions aim to boost positive imagery and train positive interpretation. They involve repeated practice in generating positive mental imagery in the context of ambiguous cues, presented either as photos (e.g., Pictet, Coughtrey, Mathews, & Holmes, 2011) or as audio descriptions listened to via headphones (e.g., Holmes, Lang, & Shah, 2009). There is preliminary evidence that an individual's scores on imagery questionnaire measures may predict whether the intervention will be of benefit (T. J. Lang et al., 2012). This suggests that questionnaire measurement of imagery may be an important part of the assessment for these novel interventions, as it may identify people for whom the intervention may be less useful, or who may need additional preparation in generating imagery before embarking on the course of treatment.

In addition to this questionnaire assessment of mental imagery ability, an initial face-to-face introduction to the imagery training program offers the opportunity to assess patients' ability to engage in imagery in the way required for the intervention to be effective. By guiding patients through examples of the kinds of scenarios they will be required to imagine in the intervention, the researcher can pick up potential problems such as a tendency to switch into a verbal, analytical thinking style (Holmes, Lang, et al., 2009), or a tendency to imagine the scenarios from a detached "observer" perspective (Holmes, Coughtrey, & Connor, 2008). Noticing and correcting these cognitive styles may be crucial in increasing the chance of the intervention being effective. Patients with depression may be particularly sensitive to feeling that they are "doing it wrong," but if this exploration is carried out with genuine interest and encouragement from the researcher, the assessment becomes an opportunity to instill in patients a sense of curiosity about their experience of imagery. This turns the assessment into an interesting experience that will enhance their motivation to engage with the computerized intervention on their own over the forthcoming weeks.

Clinical Practice

However, we would not recommend the use of questionnaires alone to assess imagery, as these do not capture the full clinical presentation and are often designed to tap a single dimension of imagery experience. Nevertheless, questionnaires are useful in providing supplementary information or for outcome research, but should not be used as a standalone clinical assessment tool. Assessment and microformulation of patients' idiosyncratic imagery can be more informative in a clinic setting.

Assessment of Imagery with Disorder-Specific Questionnaires

There are a number of disorder-specific questionnaires that contain items about mental imagery, most notably for assessment of posttraumatic stress symptoms. The IES-R (Weiss & Marmer, 1997) is a questionnaire that measures the subjective response to a perceived traumatic event. It contains an Intrusions subscale, which includes items such as "Pictures about it [the trauma] popped into my mind," and "I had dreams about it [the trauma]." As such, it is a useful tool for clinicians and researchers wishing to assess for trauma-related imagery, though it should be noted that it is not a diagnostic instrument for PTSD. Another disorder-specific instrument that includes items about imagery is the Yale–Brown Obsessive Compulsive Scale (Goodman et al., 1989), which assesses symptoms of obsessive–compulsive disorder (OCD). Respondents are simply asked to indicate whether they have experienced each symptom on the scale currently or in the past. The scale contains four imagery symptom items: "violent or aggressive images," "intrusive (nonviolent) images," "forbidden or perverse sexual thoughts, images, or impulses," and "intrusive nonsense sounds, words, or music."

There are obvious limitations to the sole use of disorder-specific questionnaire measures to assess for imagery. The types of questionnaires administered can often be influenced by subjective clinician or researcher judgments about a respondent's likely diagnosis, rather than based on a full clinical diagnostic assessment, such as the Structured Clinical Interview for DSM-IV-TR (First, Spitzer, Gibbons, & Williams, 2002). A further issue is that respondents can only indicate the presence or absence of imagery included in the questionnaires; therefore, key imagery experiences may be missed. Indeed, many commonly used clinical questionnaires do not include items regarding imagery at all. Administration of imagery-specific questionnaires (as detailed below) may therefore be more useful in providing supplementary information for the clinical assessment of imagery than disorder-specific questionnaires.

Assessment of Imagery with Imagery-Specific Questionnaires

Another approach to imagery assessment is to administer questionnaires that assess general imagery processes, rather than specific imagery-related clinical symptoms. These are suitable for administering to both clinical and nonclinical participants and have been discussed in an earlier section on laboratory assessment of imagery. Such measures include the SUIS (Reisberg et al., 2003), the IFES (Deeprose & Holmes, 2010), and the PIT (Holmes, Lang, et al., 2008; Stöber, 2000).

Administration of both disorder-specific and imagery-specific questionnaires can certainly prove useful in assessing some aspects of mental imagery. However, questionnaire measures are unlikely to capture the "full picture" when it comes to assessing imagery.

A Phenomenological Approach to Assessment of Imagery

Phenomenological approaches are concerned with the study of experience from the perspective of the individual, and data are typically gathered through qualitative methods such as interviews. This type of research is suited to increasing understanding of subjective experience and gaining insights into people's motivations and actions. It is particularly useful in areas where there is a lack of an established knowledge base. In the past decade or so, a growing body of clinical research (see "A Brief, Selected Review of Imagery Research" on pp. 69–71) has used phenomenological methods to capture rich information about the content and qualities of mental imagery experienced by different clinical populations. An example of a useful interview assessment is the Mental Imagery Interview, as used, for example, by Day et al. (2004), which is drawn from previous work by Ann Hackmann. This interview allows the exploration of both quantitative measures of imagery experience (such as the frequency of mental images), but also asks participants to describe in detail the images they experience. A key part of the interview is identification of an image that is important to a participant. The participant is then asked to describe the image in detail before answering further questions about the image, including "How did [the image] make you feel?," "What did it mean to you?," "What did it make you want to do?" Identification of common themes of imagery experienced by different populations has led to the development of novel treatments targeting distressing image-based cognitions (e.g., Wheatley et al., 2007). Research of this kind may also pave the way for improved imagery assessment questionnaires.

Although developing an understanding of the types of imagery frequently present in different disorders is undoubtedly useful, mental imagery is also highly idiosyncratic in nature. In therapeutic work with a patient, an individualized approach to assessment is therefore likely to produce the most valid and clinically useful results. Next, we detail how to assess imagery and use the information gained to create an imagery "microformulation" with a patient.

Individual Assessment and "Microformulation" of Imagery

Some psychological models do emphasize the assessment and subsequent formulation of problematic mental imagery. Ehlers and D. M. Clark's (2000) model of PTSD and D. M. Clark and Wells's (1995) model of social phobia are two well-validated examples. However, the presence and impact of mental imagery can be neglected unless the researcher or clinician is working from a model within which maladaptive imagery processes are core features. In our experience, we have found it useful to assess imagery-based cognitions (in addition to verbal thoughts), regardless of the provisional or established diagnosis of a patient.

We suggest that the clinical assessment of imagery should contain the following steps:

1. Patients are first provided with a definition of what is meant by the term "mental imagery."
2. Clinicians then ask patient whether he or she experiences any mental images that have a strong impact on him or her—for example, ones associated with feeling afraid, or ashamed, or perhaps overly excited (in a bipolar population).
3. Once a significant image is identified, a clinician guides a patient to examine the image in detail. An imagery micro-formulation template (see Figure 4.1) is used to guide the assessment and "map out" the content and impact of the image.

Refer to the box on page 79 for a step-by-step guide of how to complete the imagery microformulation. Further information and a comprehensive guide to imagery assessment and practice can be found in the *Oxford Guide to Imagery in Cognitive Therapy* (Hackmann et al., 2011).

REASONS FOR NEGLECT OF IMAGERY ASSESSMENT

Perhaps the most fundamental reason that patients do not report imagery is that clinicians simply do not ask about its presence. We know that the majority of patients will not spontaneously report imagery; therefore, clinicians must take responsibility for including questions about imagery in their standard assessments. There are several reasons why patients do not report their experiences of imagery. We examine the key ones in more detail.

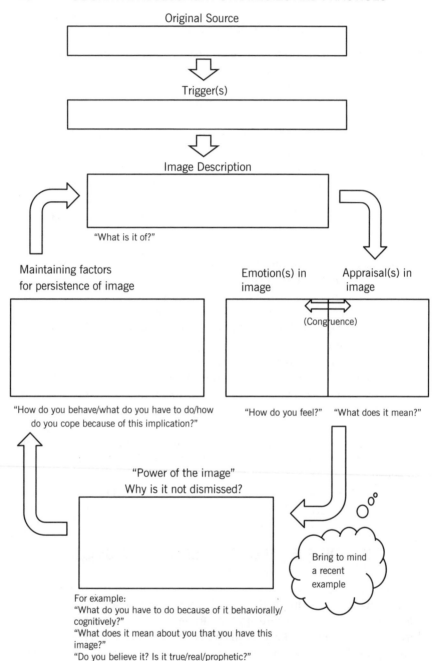

FIGURE 4.1. Microformulation template.

A Step-by-Step Guide
for How to Complete an Imagery Microformulation

General ethos. Completion of the microformulation should be a collaborative, curi-ous process, with responsibility for completion shared equally between a therapist and a patient. It is good practice to have the microformulation template where it can be seen by both the therapist and the patient and to encourage the patient to write on the template him- or herself.

Choosing an image to microformulate. A patient may report more than one significant image. The following may be helpful in selecting the image to start a microformulation on: choosing an image that seems directly connected to the treatment target identified by the patient, or an image that is relevant in the cur-rent clinical presentation and that has been present in the most recent week(s) preceding the session.

Image description. To aid the patient in describing the image selected, ask her to remember the last time she had the image, then ask her to bring it back to mind and describe it in as much detail as possible (keeping the eyes closed can be help-ful but is not necessary). Make sure you get to know from which perspective the image is seen: Is a patient in the picture, or is it seen from an observer position? Elicit details about dimensions, colors, if and how the image(s) changes, if there is any action going on, and so on. Remember to explore characteristics from sensory modalities other than visual, such as sounds, smells, and tactile sensations.

Emotion(s) in image. Ask the patient how she feels as she holds the image in mind and/or how she felt on the last occasion she experienced it. If this is difficult to grasp, you can try prompting the patient by summarizing the image description she gave you and asking how specific details and features in the image make her feel as you describe the image back to her. An image may often elicit more than one emo-tion; write down as many emotions as are present. Sometimes emotions will not be described using the standard labels but in more idiosyncratic ways. It is fine to keep the patient's exact words in this case, provided that you ask her to explain fully to you what she means so that you share the felt sense behind each word.

Appraisal(s)/meaning(s) in image. The next step is to understand what specific meaning is attributed to the image. You can find this out by asking the patient why she feels the various emotions she has just described—for example, "Why does this image make you anxious?" You can also ask what thoughts are present as she holds the image in mind. Note that images that elicit multiple emotions will tend to have a variety of appraisals attached, perhaps even contradictory ones.

"The power of the image." Once you have identified the main emotions and appraisals linked to the emotions, you want to explore further what implications and consequences these have. This can lead to discovering further and more general/deeper appraisals and also behaviors. Behaviors can also lead to or directly represent maintaining factors (see next step). Useful questions to obtain this information are "What does it mean to you that you have this image?", "What does it say about you?", "What does it make you think or do?" Answers to these questions will elucidate why the image(s) has such a "powerful" impact on a patient and why the patient is unable or unwilling to dismiss it. Often a patient comments that the image "feels so real" that she thinks that it must be "true" or prophetic in some way.

Maintaining factors. The last step is to identify what the patient does when she experiences the image—that is, actions and behaviors that contribute to the persistence of the image and related emotions, thus creating a vicious cycle. It is useful to ask directly, "What do you have to do when the image pops into your mind? For example, do you try to push it away? Or perhaps replay it in your mind's eye?" It is also useful to investigate not just the immediate reaction, but what further behaviors follow in different contexts and situations. Avoidance strategies ("Do you do anything so that the image does not happen to you again?") and/or engagement strategies ("Do you do anything to make the image come back or change it?") are often used to cope with imagery.

• *The patient doesn't understand what is meant by "mental imagery."* If the assessing clinician asks about mental imagery, then it is essential to provide a description. We have provided a technical definition of mental imagery at the beginning of this chapter (Kosslyn et al., 2001), but the following definition can be easier for patients to grasp:

"When we think in *mental images*, we imagine pictures in our mind's eye. A mental image of this assessment might be picturing in your mind's eye what the room looks like with us sitting in it. Although mental images often take the form of pictures, they can actually include any of the five senses. For example, you could 'hear' the sounds of us talking in your imagination. We can also have images that come in the form of smells, tastes, or bodily sensations. Images can be clear or unclear, fully formed or fleeting. When we talk about *mental images*, we are referring to *all* these types of imagining."

• *Not all images are visual.* Mental images comprise any type of sensory impressions; therefore it is essential that clinicians make this clear. For example, olfactory (smell) intrusions can be a feature of PTSD. Sometimes patients will report that they "don't have images." This may be true in a minority of cases, but it may be that further enquiry about all forms of mental imagery are warranted in this instance.

• *Patients may appraise their mental imagery as a sign that they are "really going mad."* Among the general public, the experience of "seeing things" has tended to become synonymous with severe mental health problems, such as psychosis. Patients may therefore have a real fear that if they discuss their mental imagery with health professionals, they will be appraised as severely ill and treated accordingly.

• *Patients may also find their mental imagery shaming.* Some intrusive images are particularly nasty, such as those involving violence, bestiality, or incest. The most repugnant and persistent imagery tends to be associated with OCD (Rachman & de Silva, 1978). Unsurprisingly, patients may find it extremely difficult to "admit" that they are experiencing socially inappropriate, ego-dystonic imagery.

In summary, imagery-based cognitions are unlikely to be elicited unless clinicians specifically ask their patients about them.

THE PLACE OF IMAGERY IN COGNITIVE CASE FORMULATION

The fundamentals of the cognitive case formulation approach have been described in detail elsewhere (Bieling & Key, Chapter 10, this volume; Kuyken, Padesky, & Dudley, 2009), and so these aspects are not repeated here. To illustrate how imagery assessment can be integrated into the cognitive case formulation approach, we present an example from our service, the Mood Action Psychology Programme (MAPP).

The MAPP Service

MAPP is a clinical psychology service for people with bipolar disorder, located within a psychiatric outpatient setting. We offer a detailed, four-session assessment to map out current presenting difficulties, using a cognitive-behavioral approach with an imagery focus. The aim of assessment is to identify a target for intervention that is distressing in its own right but also has impact on mood stability.[2]

Referral Information

Serena was offered an initial assessment with MAPP following referral from a psychiatrist at a community mental health team. She was a 45-year-old graphic designer living in inner London. She had a diagnosis of bipolar II disorder; that is, she experienced episodes of both depression and hypomania. She had a 20-year history of such mental health difficulties, having experienced approximately 10 episodes of depression and 15 episodes of hypomania during this period. Serena had a 9-year-old daughter for whom she provided most of the care. Serena's psychiatrist noted that she had prominent anxiety in addition to ongoing mood instability, for which she was seeking help. She declined medication but was open to trying a psychological approach.

---

[2] We typically have two therapists present at each assessment session.

MAPP Assessment

The following aspects are covered as part of a standard MAPP assessment.

Reported Priorities

Serena stated that she had two priorities for treatment. The first was to tackle the anxiety she experienced that she felt was associated with intrusive mental images of (1) real negative past events ("flashbacks") and (2) imagined negative future events ("flashforwards") (see box on the facing page). She reported that, as a result of these images, she constantly felt "stuck in fight/flight mode" and she wanted to find "respite" from this sense of ongoing agitation. Serena's second priority was to improve her mood stability, particularly when it interfered with her work or weekend activities with her daughter.

Reported Difficulties

At the initial assessment session, which directly asked about imagery, Serena stated that she "visualized everything." While this could be extremely useful for her—for example, in her work as a graphic designer—it could also cause her difficulties. She reported that the following types of imagery had a particularly negative impact on her:

1. Serena experienced frequent vivid intrusive imagery of a recent real event in which her daughter had nearly choked. She reported these image "flashbacks" to be highly anxiety-provoking, consistent with an early posttraumatic stress reaction.
2. In addition to experiencing images of past events, Serena also reported that she regularly experienced "horrible images of bad things happening to my daughter or me" in the future. The content of this "flashforward" imagery included finding her daughter dead in a local park or her daughter contracting a fatal illness. When these "flashforwards" occurred, they made her feel very anxious and agitated, and consequently unable to concentrate on her work or household chores.

In addition to the negative imagery symptoms described above, Serena had ongoing issues with general management of her bipolar disorder; for example, she reported that her mood was frequently unstable and her sleeping and eating patterns were often disturbed.

Definition of Flashbacks and Flashforwards

What is a "flashback"? A "flashback" is the term used to describe a mental image of a past real event—for example, of a traumatic situation—that springs to mind unbidden (involuntarily). "Flashbacks" are the hallmark of PTSD, but such negative intrusive images can occur across many disorders and be of a range of events.

What is a "flashforward"? A "flashforward" is a mental image of a simulated future event, that is, one that has not yet occurred. For example, someone with depression may experience a "flashforward" of being rejected by peers, or being unable to complete a work assignment; someone with bipolar disorder may have a "flashforward" of creating an amazing piece of art.

Scores on Mood and Imagery Measures Administered at Assessment

The key clinical issues for Serena related to the intrusive "flashbacks" and "flashforwards" that she experienced. Along with the detailed assessment and microformulation to be described next, supplementary information was gained through administration of a variety of mood and imagery measures at the first MAPP assessment session. Serena scored in the "severe" range of depression on the Quick Inventory of Depressive Symptomatology (QIDS; Rush et al., 2003) and in the "moderate" range of anxiety on the Beck Anxiety Inventory (BAI; Beck & Steer, 1993). No manic symptoms were present. Serena's scores on the SUIS (Reisberg et al., 2003), IES-R (Weiss & Marmer, 1997), and IFES (Deeprose & Holmes, 2010) indicated high trait use of imagery and a high impact of "flashback" and "flashforward" imagery.

Selection of Potential Intervention Targets

Two potential intervention targets were selected to microformulate: (1) intrusive imagery of past harm to her daughter (in the form of "flashbacks" to her daughter nearly choking) and (2) intrusive imagery of future harm to her daughter (in the form of "flashforwards" to bad events happening to her). These targets were selected as they were both distressing in their own right, but were also hypothesized to link with her mood stability. Serena noted that both the "flashbacks" and the "flashforwards" she experienced could have a strong impact on her mood and made it difficult for her to remain calm. Importantly, the problematic imagery symptoms were also ones which the MAPP team judged to be tractable via a cognitive intervention.

Microformulation of Each Potential Intervention Target

Once a potential imagery intervention target or targets have been identified, the next stage in the MAPP assessment procedure is to collaboratively map out the imagery process with the patient using a microformulation template as a guide. Note that the template provided in Figure 4.1 is a basic template that can be adapted for use with different types of disorders (e.g., anxiety, depression, bipolar disorder, OCD). The MAPP service has produced a more comprehensive template for use with people with bipolar disorder, highlighting imagery processes proposed to be particularly pertinent for this group.[3] This bipolar-specific template was used to microformulate both of the imagery targets that Serena identified.

The Next Stage: Formulation-Based Treatment

Once a thorough assessment and microformulation of imagery have been completed, clinicians can then choose from their general clinical skills "toolkit" to intervene with the problematic imagery process. A variety of intervention techniques may be appropriate, depending on the formulation of the problem. For example, imagery rescripting techniques may be used to actively modify and update the problematic imagery, attention retraining could be used to switch the focus of attention away from internal imagery and onto external targets, or metacognitive techniques could be applied to teach a patient that "an image is just an image." Note that it is not always necessary to work actively with imagery (e.g., in the form of imagery rescripting) to achieve therapeutic benefit. For a review of both "direct" and "indirect" ways of working with imagery, see Holmes, Arntz, and Smucker (2007).

MAPP Treatment and Outcome

After assessment, Serena was offered a brief treatment intervention. Following from the microformulations mapped out in the assessment process, imagery rescripting (IR) was chosen as an appropriate intervention to treat the "flashback" and "flashforward" images, as the meaning

---

[3] Available to download from our team website at *www.mrc-cbu.cam.ac.uk*.

contained within these images seemed to be maintaining the negative imagery processes.

MAPP delivered a six-session intervention consisting of two sessions of IR of the "flashback" image, two sessions of IR of the "flashforward" image, and two sessions of consolidation. The consolidation sessions included the creation of a video "blueprint"—a record of the strategies Serena used in therapy, which she could refer back to in the future. (We hypothesize that a visual form is more accessible to patients with bipolar disorder than verbal-based records, like the traditional paper-based "blueprints" used in CBT.)

At the end of the treatment period, Serena's image intrusions had decreased substantially in frequency. More important, when "flashback" and "flashforward" imagery did intrude, she did not rate it as distressing. In addition, a number of behavioral changes occurred across the treatment period: Serena ceased consuming cannabis, alcohol, and caffeine, and reported a more regular sleeping pattern. At 1-month follow-up, Serena's levels of anxiety, mania, and depression were all within the "nonclinical" range, and her mood had become more stable (as defined by the frequency with which her mood cycled up and down) compared with the pretreatment period. Thus, as predicted in the model, treating and modifying Serena's intrusive emotional imagery had a corresponding impact on her mood stability. At 18-month follow-up, Serena's improvements in mood and behavioral changes had been maintained, and she reported no difficulties related to the images that had been treated in the MAPP intervention.

DOES RESEARCH ON IMAGERY HAVE ANY IMPLICATIONS IN RELATION TO DSM-5?

Future directions in systematizing and diagnosing mental disorders—including the 2013 publication of the *Diagnostic and Statistical Manual of Mental Disorders*, fifth edition (DSM-5)—point to the fact that numerous symptoms and cognitive processes are reported across the traditional boundaries of diagnostic categories. Some of these symptoms and processes may not be tied to a patient's primary diagnosis, but still have a relevant clinical impact. Typical examples could be anxiety, insomnia, or anhedonia. It is important to recognize these to ensure adequate clinical care. Unsurprisingly, therefore, DSM-5 (in the new Section III) integrates dimensional assessments of cross-cutting symptom measures as an additional way to help clinicians (1) capture general functioning and the severity of mental illnesses and (2) track in a comprehensive way a patient's progress in treatment (American Psychiatric Association,

2013; Kupfer & Regier, 2011). Parallel to and informing this process of diagnostic review, the National Institute of Mental Health has also recently launched a research initiative based on a dimensional approach to the study of the genetic, neural, and behavioral features of mental disorders. This approach includes domains such as cognition, along with social processes, arousal/regulatory systems, and negative and positive valence (Insel et al., 2010). Imagery-based cognitions fit within this approach.

The majority of individuals experience imagery-based cognitions, but they will vary in the extent to which they use imagery rather than verbal thoughts, and in the intrinsic characteristics of this imagery (such as vividness, emotional arousal, etc.) and possibly in the subjective impact that imagery has on their feelings and behavior (Cui, Jeter, Yang, Montague, & Eagleman, 2007; Deeprose & Holmes, 2010; Holmes & Mathews, 2010). As already described in "A Brief, Selected Review ...," intrusive and clinically significant images are found across different mental disorders. Hence, imagery can be considered both a dimensional and a transdiagnostic phenomenon (see Smith, Ratcliff, & Norton, Chapter 9, this volume) similar to most of the other psychological processes that merge into psychiatric symptoms. This means that the presence of intrusive or disturbing images is not indicative of a specific diagnosis; however, imagery assessment can both clarify diagnosis and represent a valuable parameter of disease severity. For example, assessing the specific emotion and appraisal associated with an image can help elucidate affective states and behavioral responses, which might otherwise remain unclear.

Investigating imagery can directly contribute to differential diagnosis. In a case of first-onset psychosis, Marcus, a 38-year-old male, presented with paranoid ideation and persecutory voices. He denied visual hallucinations but described vivid images of his younger brother who had recently died of cancer, staring at him from the hospital bed. On further investigation, while Marcus was aware that this image was not real, he reported that to him it meant he should have looked after his brother better and been of greater comfort in his last days. The imagery assessment process led to the disclosure of deep guilt feelings and a sense of bereavement, allowing us to make a diagnosis of psychotic depression rather than delusional disorder.

In line with the more dimensional approach proposed in Section III of DSM-5 (American Psychiatric Association, 2013; Narrow & Kuhl, 2011) and by the most recent developments in the understanding of the neurobiological bases of mental disorders (Morris & Cuthbert, 2012), the level of intensity and frequency of imagery-based cognitions can also guide severity assessment and treatment decisions. For example, arousing and unstoppable imagery of future scenarios often occurs in patients with bipolar disorder and is associated with both anxiety and excitement. When such phenomena remain between full-blown manic–depressive episodes, they can signal partial remission of the overall mood instability and a potential for more frequent relapses. This has implications in terms of both medication management and additional psychological intervention (Perlis et al., 2010; Simon et al., 2007).

In conclusion, future directions in the diagnosis and assessment of mental disorder support the need to integrate a thorough investigation of imagery across all psychiatric disorders. This inquiry can serve as a tool to refine diagnosis, to identify comorbid syndromes, and to highlight additional isolated but clinically relevant symptoms. Moreover, a dimensional approach to imagery-based cognition can help capture residual risk and improve relapse prevention.

SUMMARY

Mental imagery can have a powerful impact on emotion, and dysfunctional mental imagery may play an important role in maintaining distress or problematic behavior in many psychological disorders. However, mental imagery is often neglected in assessment procedures. A variety of means can be used to assess mental imagery, including questionnaires, computer tasks, and interviews. A thorough assessment of mental imagery can aid development of a formulation to guide the application of powerful imagery-focused techniques in treatment. However, patients often do not spontaneously report mental images, and so it is crucial that clinicians inquire specifically about them in order to ascertain their presence and potential as a target for treatment.

KEY POINTS

FOR PRACTITIONERS

- Mental images typically take the form of static or moving pictures. However, it is important to remember that frequently they also involve "hearing" sounds in imagination, as well as "smelling," "tasting," or "feeling" bodily sensations.
- The ability and propensity to have mental images varies from person to person, but can be developed through practice.
- Mental images have been found to have a more powerful impact on mood than verbal thoughts.
- Patients tend not to spontaneously report mental images—so it is important that clinicians ask about them at assessment.

- Imagery-based cognitive-behavioral assessment should have five steps:
  - First, provide the patient with a definition of mental imagery that encompasses its multisensory nature.
  - Second, get a broad idea of the different types of images that the patient experiences and how often they occur. Use imagery questionnaires to provide supplementary information or as outcomes in research, but do not rely on them alone as assessment tools.
  - Third, with the patient, identify a particularly troublesome, pivotal, or tractable image.
  - Fourth, ask questions about this image so that together you are able to "microformulate" it—that is, to draw out a formulation describing the image and its meaning, why the patient does not simply dismiss/ignore it, and how the patient responds cognitively or behaviorally to it.
  - Fifth, repeat for other troublesome, pivotal, or tractable images. The microformulation(s) can then be integrated into the wider case formulation.

FOR RESEARCHERS

- It is important to remember that images can involve any of the five senses, alone or in combination; research participants may need to be prompted to think about this possibility, as most people associate images with the visual sense only.
- People's experiences of mental imagery can be measured experimentally in several ways: via computer tasks (e.g., Image Generation Task, Mental Rotation Task); questionnaires (e.g., Spontaneous Use of Imagery Scale [SUIS; measuring everyday imagery use], Prospective Imagery Task [PIT; measuring ability to generate images about future events], Impact of Future Events Scale [IFES; measuring intrusive future-related imagery]; or interviews (e.g., Mental Imagery Interview [a largely qualitative tool]).
- Computerized imagery training packages are being developed to improve positive imagery for people with depression. This area is likely to evolve rapidly for assessing patients' use of imagery and developing training tools.

FOR STUDENTS AND EDUCATORS

- Cognitions can take the forms of verbal thoughts and mental images. Verbal thoughts consist of words and sentences—for example, in social anxiety, "They will notice me shaking." In contrast, a mental image is a sensory representation, so in social anxiety one might picture oneself from an observer's point of view shaking violently, and imagine the sounds of observers laughing.

- Experimental research has demonstrated that mental imagery has a greater impact on both negative and positive emotions than verbal thoughts.
- It is therefore important for both researchers and clinicians to continue to investigate the role of mental imagery in both clinical and nonclinical populations.

ACKNOWLEDGMENTS

Susie Hales was supported by a Wellcome Trust fellowship (WT088217) awarded to Emily A. Holmes. Simon E. Blackwell, Martina Di Simplicio, and Emily A. Holmes are supported by the Medical Research Council (United Kingdom) intramural programme (No. MC-A060-5PR50). Simon E. Blackwell and Emily A. Holmes were supported by a grant from the Lupina Foundation. Emily A. Holmes is supported by a Wellcome Trust Clinical Fellowship (No. WT088217) and the National Institute for Health Research (NIHR) Oxford Biomedical Research Centre based at Oxford University Hospitals National Health Service (NHS) Trust, Oxford University. Lalitha Iyadurai was supported by an NIHR Doctoral Research Fellowship (No. NIHR-DRF-2011-04-076). The views expressed are our own and not necessarily those of the NHS, the NIHR, or the Department of Health.

Thank you to our MAPP assistants Ian Clark, Aiysha Malik, and Sophie Wallace-Hadrill for their help with MAPP.

REFERENCES

Addis, D. R., Pan, L., Vu, M., Laiser, N., & Schacter, D. L. (2009). Constructive episodic simulation of the future and the past: Distinct subsystems of a core brain network mediate imagining and remembering. *Neuropsychologia, 47,* 2222–2238.

American Psychiatric Association. (2013). *Diagnostic and statistical manual of mental disorders* (5th ed.). Arlington, VA: Author.

Arntz, A. (2012). Imagery rescripting as a therapeutic technique: Review of clinical trials, basic studies, and research agenda. *Journal of Experimental Psychopathology, 3,* 121–126.

Beck, A. T. (1971). Cognitive patterns in dreams and day dreams. In J. H. Masserman (Ed.), *Dream dynamics: Science and psychoanalysis* (Vol. 19, pp. 2–7). New York: Grune & Stratton.

Beck, A. T., & Steer, R. A. (1993). *Beck Anxiety Inventory manual.* San Antonio, TX: Psychological Corporation.

Berna, C., Vincent, K., Moore, J., Tracey, I., Goodwin, G. M., & Holmes, E. A. (2011). Presence of mental imagery associated with chronic pelvic pain: A pilot study. *Pain Medicine, 12*(7), 1086–1093.

Blackwell, S. E., & Holmes, E. A. (2010). Modifying interpretation and imagination in clinical depression: A single case series using cognitive bias modification. *Applied Cognitive Psychology, 24*(3), 338–350.

Butler, G., & Mathews, A. (1983). Cognitive processes in anxiety. *Advances in Behaviour Research and Therapy, 5*(1), 51–62.

Clark, D. M., & Wells, A. (1995). A cognitive model of social phobia. In R. G. Heimberg, M. Liebowitz, D. Hope, & F. Schneier (Eds.), *Social phobia: Diagnosis, assessment, and treatment* (pp. 69–93). New York: Guilford Press.

Crisp, R. J., Birtel, M. D., & Meleady, R. (2011). Mental simulations of social thought and action: Trivial tasks or tools for transforming social policy? *Current Directions in Psychological Science, 20*(4), 261–264.

Cui, X., Jeter, C. B., Yang, D., Montague, P. R., & Eagleman, D. M. (2007). Vividness of mental imagery: Individual variability can be measured objectively. *Vision Research, 47*(4), 474–478.

Cummings, C., Olphin, T., & Law, M. (2007). Self-reported psychological states and physiological responses to types of motivational general imagery. *Journal of Sport and Exercise Psychology, 29*, 629–644.

D'Argembeau, A., Renaud, O., & Van der Linden, M. (2011). Frequency, characteristics, and functions of future-oriented thoughts in daily life. *Applied Cognitive Psychology, 25*(1), 96–103.

Day, S. J., Holmes, E. A., & Hackmann, A. (2004). Occurrence of imagery and its link with early memories in agoraphobia. *Memory, 12*(4), 416–427.

Deeprose, C., & Holmes, E. A. (2010). An exploration of prospective imagery: The Impact of Future Events Scale. *Behavioural and Cognitive Psychotherapy, 38*(2), 201–209.

Di Simplicio, M., McInerney, J. E., Goodwin, G. M., Attenburrow, M., & Holmes, E. A. (2012). Revealing the mind's eye: Bringing (mental) images into psychiatry. *American Journal of Psychiatry, 169*(12), 1245–1246.

Dror, I. E., & Kosslyn, S. M. (1994). Mental imagery and aging. *Psychology and Aging, 9*(1), 90–102.

Edwards, D. (2007). Restructuring implicational meaning through memory-based imagery: Some historical notes. *Journal of Behavior Therapy and Experimental Psychiatry, 38*(4), 306–316.

Ehlers, A., & Clark, D. M. (2000). A cognitive model of posttraumatic stress disorder. *Behaviour Research and Therapy, 38*(4), 319–345.

Engelhard, I. M., van den Hout, M. A., Janssen, W. C., & van der Beek, J. (2010). Eye movements reduce vividness and emotionality of "flashforwards." *Behaviour Research and Therapy, 48*(5), 442–447.

First, M. B., Spitzer, R. L., Gibbon, M., & Williams, J. B. W. (2002). *Structured Clinical Interview for DSM-IV-TR Axis I Disorders, Research Version, Patient Edition (SCID-I/P).* New York: Biometrics Research, New York State Psychiatric Institute.

Giesen-Bloo, J., van Dyck, R., Spinhoven, P., van Tilburg, W., Dirksen, C., van Asselt, T., et al. (2006). Outpatient psychotherapy for borderline personality disorder: A randomized clinical trial of schema-focused therapy versus transference-focused psychotherapy. *Archives of General Psychiatry, 63*(6), 649–658.

Goodman, W. K., Price, L. H., Rasmussen, S. A., Mazure, C., Fleischmann, R. L., Hill, C. L., et al. (1989). The Yale–Brown Obsessive Compulsive Scale:

I. Development, use and reliability. *Achives of General Psychiatry*, *46*(11), 1006–1011.

Hackmann, A., Bennett-Levy, J., & Holmes, E. A. (2011). *Oxford guide to imagery in cognitive therapy*. Oxford, UK: Oxford University Press.

Hagenaars, M. A., & Holmes, E. A. (2012). Mental imagery in psychopathology: Another step [Editorial for the special issue of *Journal of Experimental Psychopathology*]. *Journal of Experimental Psychopathology*, *3*(2), 121–126.

Hales, S. A., Deeprose, C., Goodwin, G. M., & Holmes, E. A. (2011). Cognitions in bipolar disorder versus unipolar depression: Imagining suicide. *Bipolar Disorders*, *13*(7–8), 651–661.

Holmes, E. A., Arntz, A., & Smucker, M. R. (2007). Imagery rescripting in cognitive-behavior therapy: Images, treatment techniques, and outcomes. *Journal of Behavior Therapy and Experimental Psychiatry*, *38*(4), 297–305.

Holmes, E. A., Coughtrey, A. E., & Connor, A. (2008). Looking at or through rose-tinted glasses?: Imagery perspective and positive mood. *Emotion*, *8*(6), 875–879.

Holmes, E. A., Crane, C., Fennell, M. J. V., & Williams, J. M. G. (2007). Imagery about suicide in depression—"Flash-forwards"? *Journal of Behavior Therapy and Experimental Psychiatry*, *38*(4), 423–434.

Holmes, E. A., Geddes, J. R., Colom, F., & Goodwin, G. M. (2008). Mental imagery as an emotional amplifier: Application to bipolar disorder. *Behaviour Research and Therapy*, *46*(12), 1251–1258.

Holmes, E. A., & Hackmann, A. (2004). Mental imagery and memory in psychopathology [Special issue]. *Memory*, *12*(4).

Holmes, E. A., James, E. L., Blackwell, S. E., & Hales, S. (2011). "They flash upon that inward eye." *The Psychologist*, *24*(5), 2–5.

Holmes, E. A., James, E. L., Coode-Bate, T., & Deeprose, C. (2009). Can playing the computer game "Tetris" reduce the build-up of flashbacks for trauma?: A proposal from cognitive science. *PLoS ONE*, *4*(1), e4153.

Holmes, E. A., Lang, T. J., Moulds, M. L., & Steele, A. M. (2008). Prospective and positive mental imagery deficits in dysphoria. *Behaviour Research and Therapy*, *46*(8), 976–981.

Holmes, E. A., Lang, T. J., & Shah, D. M. (2009). Developing interpretation bias modification as a "cognitive vaccine" for depressed mood—Imagining positive events makes you feel better than thinking about them verbally. *Journal of Abnormal Psychology*, *118*(1), 76–88.

Holmes, E. A., & Mathews, A. (2010). Mental imagery in emotion and emotional disorders. *Clinical Psychology Review*, *30*(3), 349–362.

Holmes, E. A., Mathews, A., Mackintosh, B., & Dalgleish, T. (2008). The causal effect of mental imagery on emotion assessed using picture–word cues. *Emotion*, *8*(3), 395–409.

Insel, T., Cuthbert, B., Garvey, M., Heinssen, R., Pine, D. S., Quinn, K., et al. (2010). Research Domain Criteria (RDoC): Toward a new classification framework for research on mental disorders. *American Journal of Psychiatry*, *167*, 748–751.

Jacob, G. A., Arendt, J., Kolley, L., Scheel, C. N., Bader, K., Lieb, K., et al. (2011). Comparison of different strategies to decrease negative affect and increase positive affect in women with borderline personality disorder. *Behaviour Research and Therapy, 49*, 68–73.

Kosslyn, S. M., Ganis, G., & Thompson, W. L. (2001). Neural foundations of imagery. *Nature Reviews Neuroscience, 2*(9), 635–642.

Krans, J. (2011). Introduction to the special issue: Intrusive imagery in psychopathology: New research findings, implications for theory and treatment, and future directions. *International Journal of Cognitive Therapy, 4*, 117–121.

Kupfer, D. J., & Regier, D. A. (2011). Neuroscience, clinical evidence, and the future of psychiatric classification in DSM-5. *American Journal of Psychiatry, 168*, 172–174.

Kuyken, W., Padesky, C. A., & Dudley, A. (2009). *Collaborative case conceptualization: Working effectively with clients in cognitive-behavioral therapy.* New York: Guilford Press.

Lang, P. J. (1979). A bio-informational theory of emotional imagery. *Psychophysiology, 16*(6), 495–512.

Lang, T. J., Blackwell, S. E., Harmer, C. J., Davison, P., & Holmes, E. A. (2012). Cognitive bias modification using mental imagery for depression: Developing a novel computerized intervention to change negative thinking styles. *European Journal of Personality, 26*(2), 145–157.

Morina, N., Deeprose, C., Pusowski, C., Schmid, M., & Holmes, E. A. (2011). Prospective mental imagery in patients with major depressive disorder or anxiety disorders. *Journal of Anxiety Disorders, 25*(8), 1032–1037.

Morris, S. E., & Cuthbert, B. N. (2012). Research domain criteria: Cognitive systems, neural circuits, and dimensions of behavior. *Dialogues in Clinical Neuroscience, 14*(1), 29–37.

Moulds, M. L., & Holmes, E. A. (2011). Intrusive imagery in psychopathology: A commentary. *International Journal of Cognitive Therapy, 4*(2), 197–207.

Narrow, W. E., & Kuhl, E. A. (2011). Dimensional approaches to psychiatric diagnosis in DSM-5. *Journal of Mental Health Policy and Economics, 14*(4), 197–200.

Neisser, U. (1967). *Cognitive psychology.* New York: Appleton-Century-Crofts.

Pearson, D. G., Deeprose, C., Wallace-Hadrill, S. M. A., Burnett Heyes, S., & Holmes, E. A. (2013). Assessing mental imagery in clinical psychology: A review of imagery measures and a guiding framework. *Clinical Psychology Review, 33*(1), 1–23.

Perlis, R. H., Ostacher, M. J., Miklowitz, D. J., Hay, A., Nierenberg, A. A., Thase, M. E., et al. (2010). Clinical features associated with poor pharmacologic adherence in bipolar disorder: Results from the STEP-BD study. *Journal of Clinical Psychiatry, 71*(3), 296–303.

Pictet, A., Coughtrey, A. E., Mathews, A., & Holmes, E. A. (2011). Fishing for happiness: The effects of positive imagery on interpretation bias and a behavioral task. *Behaviour Research and Therapy, 49*(12), 885–891.

Rachman, S., & de Silva, P. (1978). Abnormal and normal obsessions. *Behaviour Research and Therapy, 16*, 233–238.

Reisberg, D., Pearson, D. G., & Kosslyn, S. M. (2003). Intuitions and introspections about imagery: The role of imagery experience in shaping an investigator's theoretical views. *Applied Cognitive Psychology, 17*(2), 147–160.

Rude, S. S., Wenzlaff, R. M., Gibbs, B., Vane, J., & Whitney, T. (2002). Negative processing biases predict subsequent depressive symptoms. *Cognition and Emotion, 16*(3), 423–440.

Rush, J., Trivedi, M., Ibrahim, H., Carmody, T., Arnow, B., Klein, D., et al. (2003). The 16-item Quick Inventory of Depressive Symptomatology (QIDS), clinician rating (QIDS-C), and self-report (QIDS-SR): A psychometric evaluation in patients with chronic major depression. *Biological Psychiatry, 54*(5), 573–583.

Schacter, D. L., Addis, D. R., & Buckner, R. L. (2008). Episodic simulation of future events: Concepts, data, and applications. *Annals of the New York Academy of Sciences, 1124*, 39–60.

Shepard, R. N., & Cooper, L. A. (1982). *Mental images and their transformations*. Cambridge, MA: MIT Press.

Simon, N. M., Zalta, A. K., Otto, M. W., Ostacher, M. J., Fischmann, D., Chow, C. W., et al. (2007). The association of comorbid anxiety disorders with suicide attempts and suicidal ideation in outpatients with bipolar disorder. *Journal of Psychiatric Research, 41*, 225–264.

Stöber, J. (2000). Prospective cognitions in anxiety and depression: Replication and methodological extension. *Cognition and Emotion, 14*(5), 725–729.

Weiss, D. S., & Marmer, C. R. (1997). The Impact of Event Scale—Revised. In J. P. Wilson & T. M. Keane (Eds.), *Assessing psychological trauma and PTSD: A handbook for practitioners* (pp. 399–411). New York: Guilford Press.

Wheatley, J., Brewin, C. R., Patel, T., Hackmann, A., Wells, A., Fisher, P., et al. (2007). "I'll believe it when I can see it": Imagery rescripting of intrusive sensory memories in depression. *Journal of Behavior Therapy and Experimental Psychiatry, 38*(4), 371–385.

5

Assessment of Cognitive Vulnerability to Psychopathology

Issues in Theory and Practice

Lyndsay E. Evraire, David J. A. Dozois,
and Elizabeth P. Hayden

Ingram and Price (2010) captured the centrality of concepts of vulnerability in the field when they noted that "efforts to understand vulnerability to psychopathology underlie virtually all efforts to understand psychopathology itself" (p. 3). By gaining a better understanding of vulnerability, researchers aim to both refine basic theory on the causes of disorder and to contribute to targeted preventative and intervention efforts. Although adversity is clearly linked to negative mental health outcomes, most individuals who experience stress do not develop disorder; this general observation has led to the search for vulnerability factors that differentiate between those most likely to show an adverse reaction to stress and those who will not (Ingram, Atchley, & Segal, 2011).

In cognitive models of vulnerability, individual differences in cognition are held to play a key explanatory role in accounting for why some individuals exhibit maladaptive emotional and behavioral outcomes in the context of adversity (Riskind & Alloy, 2006). Put differently, most cognitive theories follow a diathesis–stress framework, in that characteristic patterns of cognition are hypothesized to eventuate in disorder or symptoms only under specific environmental conditions. Numerous

94

influential models of how cognition interacts with the broader context to predict psychopathology and other behaviors have emerged. For example, research on social information processing has demonstrated that the way that children interpret specific situations predicts whether they will respond aggressively (Crick & Dodge, 1994; Dodge & Crick, 1990). Individuals high in anxiety sensitivity, a fear of physical symptoms of anxiety based on distorted beliefs about their potential harmfulness, are more prone to develop panic disorder in situations that elicit feared physical sensations (Reiss & McNally, 1985; Taylor, Koch, & McNally, 1992). In particular, multiple, highly influential models have emerged that aim to capture how cognition interacts with contextual events to predict depression. For example, Beck's (1967) cognitive model describes three levels of thinking involved in the development, maintenance, and exacerbation of depression: self-schemas, maladaptive beliefs and assumptions, and automatic thoughts (see Dozois & Beck, 2008). When latent negative self-schemas are activated by adversity, cognitive errors, information-processing biases, and negative automatic thoughts lead to an increase in depressive symptoms. Another important model by Bower (1981) emphasizes the activating role of emotions within broader sematic networks, and Teasdale and Barnard (1993) developed the multilevel Interacting Cognitive Subsystems framework, which speaks to the role of emotional experience in shaping belief systems. Other cognitive models of depression focus on the role of hopelessness and dysfunctional attributional styles, positing that individuals are more likely to experience depression when they attribute negative life events to stable and global causes, and believe that the occurrence of such events is attributable to their own actions (Abramson, Metalsky, & Alloy, 1989; Alloy, Abramson, Walshaw, & Neeren, 2006). Adopting a developmental perspective, Gotlib and Hammen (1992) advanced a cognitive-interpersonal model of vulnerability through which developmental experiences shape emerging cognitive, behavioral, and interpersonal vulnerabilities. Such vulnerabilities lead to the development of psychopathology when they become activated in response to stressful life events.

The process of assessing cognitive vulnerability involves making decisions about how vulnerability is to be conceptualized and operationalized, and therefore plays a central, yet often underappreciated role in research aimed at testing and refining these models. Thus, in our view, assessment and theory are intimately linked to one another in research on vulnerability; indeed, assessment methods constitute the backbone of etiological models of disorder. With this orientation in mind, the primary focus of this chapter is to address what we believe are the most critical conceptual and methodological issues surrounding the assessment of cognitive vulnerability to psychopathology, with a particular emphasis on the role of cognition in depression risk. We begin by providing an overview of the concept of vulnerability, and proceed to evaluate the adequacy of various assessment strategies in mapping this concept. Next, issues related to the measurement of cognitive vulnerability for the purposes of research and practice are addressed. We conclude with a review of the current status of the field of cognitive vulnerability assessment and a discussion of future directions.

COGNITIVE VULNERABILITY DEFINED

The conceptualization of vulnerability and its defining features have been described by various researchers (Hankin & Abela, 2005; Ingram & Price, 2010; Monroe & Simons, 1991). In this chapter, we focus on those features most consistently identified in accounts of cognitive vulnerability, drawing on Ingram and Price's (2010) excellent review of this topic, and discuss the extent to which research on the role of cognition supports the notion that negative cognition is indeed a vulnerability marker. More specifically, as most theorists hold that a vulnerability factor should evince some degree of stability over time, and that vulnerability itself is an endogenous characteristic that is possibly latent in nature (or at least, not always readily observable), we consider the extent to which research supports such characterizations of cognitive vulnerability.

Stability of Cognitive Vulnerability

In contrast to episodic disorders that wax and wane between states of relative severity and relative wellness, vulnerability factors are held to exhibit relative temporal stability. In other words, vulnerability factors are held to be trait-like and present before the onset of a disorder and remain present following its remission (Ingram et al., 2011). As such, an important step in theories of cognitive vulnerability is to determine whether a putative cognitive vulnerability possesses temporal stability, as opposed to simply covarying with the severity of the disorder. It is therefore surprising how little research has been conducted to address the stability of cognitive risk. A small body of work documents the moderate stability of cognitive vulnerability to depression in adulthood (e.g., Alloy et al., 2000; Dozois & Dobson, 2001a; Hankin, Fraley, & Abela, 2005). For example, Zuroff, Blatt, Sanislow, Bondi, and Pilkonis (1999) found that dysfunctional attitudes (measured using the Dyfunctional Attitude Scale [DAS]) in individuals with major depressive disorder showed both state- and trait-like components. More specifically, DAS scores decreased as a result of treatment, yet also demonstrated high levels of relative stability across the 18-month duration of the study. Unfortunately, most studies of the stability of cognitive vulnerability comprise only two waves of data collection and focus on short follow-up intervals. Furthermore, most examine the stability of self-reported cognition rather than laboratory measures, despite the widespread use of the latter paradigms in the field, as we discuss in subsequent sections.

Important, related work that speaks to the stability of childhood cognitive vulnerability is accruing (e.g., Cole et al., 2009), with evidence also supporting both stability and change (Hankin, 2008; Hankin et al., 2009; Hayden et al., 2013b). For example, in a sample of youth in early to middle adolescence, Hankin (2008) reported an average test–retest correlation of $r = .52$ for an array of self-reports of negative cognitive style across four waves of assessment separated by 5-week intervals. Cole et al. (2009) found greater evidence for trait-like aspects of self-reported negative cognition in cohorts comprised of children in middle and later childhood, assessed across several grades (i.e., grades 4–7). Voelz, Walker, Pettit, Joiner, and Wagner (2003) reported a moderately high test–retest correlation of .40 and considerable mean-level stability of a self-reported measure of attributions in an inpatient sample of young adolescents, despite the occurrence of a decrease in depressive symptoms over the same time interval (which ranged from 2 to 24 days). Intriguingly, some very recent work (Hayden et al., 2013b) suggests that cognitive vulnerability may show modest evidence for stability even earlier in life than previously thought. Overall, the extant research supports at least moderate stability of cognitive vulnerability; however, further longitudinal work is needed to better characterize the stability of cognitive risk across multiple waves of assessment, lengthier follow-up periods, diverse measures of cognitive risk, and different developmental stages using developmentally sensitive indices of cognition.

Research on the stability of other trait-like constructs (e.g., personality/temperament; Durbin, Hayden, Klein, & Olino, 2007) suggests that evidence for change in cognitive vulnerability over time will also be found. Such change could be related to developmental processes, life events, or direct intervention or preventative efforts, among other processes. Cognitive vulnerability factors may also become less salient, or increasingly latent, as symptoms remit. Dozois et al. (2009), for example, found that individuals with depression who received cognitive therapy plus pharmacotherapy showed significant changes in cognitive organization following treatment. Conversely, exposure to negative life events, especially those that are consistent with preexisting negative self-views, may further consolidate negative views of the self, world, and the future (e.g., Seeds & Dozois, 2010). Further work that examines which factors contribute to the stability and change of cognitive vulnerability is badly needed; by necessity, such work will require multiwave, longitudinal approaches.

Endogenous, Latent Properties of Cognitive Vulnerability

While individual differences in cognitive vulnerability almost certainly develop through a combination of intrinsic characteristics, life experiences, and learning processes, the locus of vulnerability is endogenous, or within the individual. Evidence suggests that cognitive vulnerability is often the most salient during periods of clinically significant symptoms, diminishing during successful treatment or naturally occurring remission and becoming latent, or at least, less readily observed during periods of normal mood (Ingram, Miranda, & Segal, 1998; Ingram & Price, 2010). This phenomenon has important implications for increasing the likelihood that negative cognition is reliably tapped during assessment protocols, particularly in individuals who are not currently experiencing significant symptoms.

The finding that cognitive vulnerability waxes and wanes along with symptom fluctuations calls into question whether such markers are best conceptualized as trait-like vulnerabilities or simply epiphenomena of disorder. Early research on cognitive vulnerability to depression tended to support the conclusion that the cognitive factors being tested were merely correlates of the disorder, rather than preexisting vulnerabilities (e.g., Barnett & Gotlib, 1988), as these studies tended to assess cognition without regard to the context in which negative cognition is activated. However, work over the past couple of decades, which has capitalized on the use of priming techniques (e.g., negative mood inductions), supports the notion that cognitive vulnerability to depression is a clinically meaningful, trait-like factor that can be activated and assessed outside of depressive states (see Scher, Ingram, & Segal, 2005, for a review). As we discuss in the next section, studies indicate that negative cognition requires priming to activate and thus validly assess (see Ingram et al., 1998), with priming now commonly regarded as an essential element in the assessment of latent cognitive processes.

PRIMING AND VULNERABILITY

Consistent with diathesis–stress models of cognitive vulnerability, which posit that negative cognition is activated in contexts of stress, research indicates that a negative mood state facilitates the priming of negative cognition and increases the accessibility of cognitive vulnerabilities.

More specifically, based on the mood-congruency hypothesis (see Ingram et al., 1998; Segal, 1988), constructs with affective content are more likely to be activated, and thus amenable to assessment, when an individual is in the relevant mood state (e.g., negative mood states increase the extent to which negative self-concepts can be readily retrieved). Further, in the case of depression, negative mood primes are thought to create an affective state similar to that experienced in the context of life stressors, stressors that are important, proximal factors in the onset of disorder (Persons & Miranda, 1992). Thus, when a negative mood prime is used, vulnerable persons should display maladaptive cognitions and information-processing biases similar to those manifested during times of stress, whereas individuals without vulnerability should not exhibit cognitive risk, despite also experiencing a negative mood. Evidence generally supports this pattern of effects (for a review, see Scher et al., 2005).

Although more recent research indicates that some cognitive structures relevant to vulnerability can be validly assessed in the absence of priming (e.g., Dozois, 2007), priming is still recommended as it enhances the accessibility of cognitive structures, their processes, and products. Furthermore, the magnitude of cognitive reactivity following a sad mood prime has been shown to predict relapse/recurrence in individuals who were no longer depressed (Segal, Gemar, & Williams, 1999; Segal et al., 2006). Thus, although priming adds burden to experimental protocols, it often plays an important role in the ability to discriminate between those with and without cognitive vulnerability.

Priming Techniques

If priming is a critical feature of cognitive vulnerability assessment, then the relative effectiveness of various mood induction procedures becomes a major issue in the validity of cognitive vulnerability assessment. A wide range of techniques has been developed to induce an array of mood states in individuals, although negative mood states are most commonly the focus of investigations of psychopathology risk. The most recent meta-analytic review of such techniques examined the effectiveness and validity of a number of different mood induction procedures in adult, nonclinical samples (Westermann, Spies, Stahl, & Hesse, 1996). Mood induction procedures (MIPs) were grouped into various categories: imagination (i.e., participants imagine an affectively charged life event), Velten (i.e., individuals read self-referent mood statements), affective film clips or stories, music, positive or negative feedback on task performance, social interaction, facial expressions (i.e., participants generate a facial expression that maps onto the mood to be induced), and protocols that combine various induction approaches (see Westermann et al., 1996). Analyses indicated that film and/or story approaches and approaches that combined multiple techniques tended to produce the largest mood changes. Effect sizes for the remaining MIPs were relatively comparable and moderate, with the exception of the facial expression MIP, which produced a considerably weaker effect. Thus, film clips and/ or stories may be the single most effective technique for eliciting elated or depressed mood states. Interestingly, a review by Brenner (2000) suggested that films also tended to be effective MIPs for children, although this review was not a meta-analysis.

However, there remains a need in the field for additional, basic descriptive work on MIPs. Research that directly compares the effects of different induction approaches in children is needed, as is an examination of the effects of various MIPs above and beyond the use of participant self-reported mood change, which may be subject to demand characteristics. For example, incorporating facial affect coding to assess mood change in the context of MIPs would be a valuable complement to self-reported mood status. Additionally, a better understanding of the parameters of MIPs is required. For example, how long do their effects last? Does mood duration vary across the type of mood induced? Which procedures are most effective for negative mood reversal? Further, interactions with participant gender, age, clinical status, and other variables in predicting MIP effectiveness are not well understood.

ASSESSMENT OF COGNITIVE VULNERABILITY

There are many approaches to the assessment of cognitive vulnerability across different levels of cognitive taxonomy (Beck & Dozois, 2011; Ingram & Kendall, 1986; Ingram et al., 1998). By "taxonomy," we refer to the notion that a broad cognitive system relevant to psychopathology consists of different levels ranging from relatively surface-level thoughts (i.e., cognitive products) to deeper structures (i.e., cognitive structures). Through an array of mechanisms (i.e., cognitive operations/processes), structural aspects of cognition are thought to give rise to the aforementioned cognitive products (see also Dunkley, Blankstein, & Segal, 2010, for a further review of the assessment of these facets of cognition). Each aspect of the broader system is likely relevant to disorder risk, and it is not yet resolved which aspect has the greatest relevance to maladaptive outcomes, as we discuss in subsequent sections. Here we present examples of commonly used approaches to these different levels of cognition with the goal of illustrating critical issues in the measurement of vulnerability.

Products

Self-report measures constitute the primary means of assessing the products of cognitive vulnerability; indeed, it has been argued that self-report measures are solely capable of tapping cognitive products (as opposed to mechanisms or processes; Mineka, Rafaeli, & Yovel, 2003) and may thus be inappropriate for assessing other, relatively latent aspects of vulnerability. While this is an empirical question worthy of further study, it seems clear that self-report is limited with respect to directly assessing cognitive processes such as memory, attention, processing depth and speed, and other operational aspects that contribute to structure. Hence, while we focus on self-report methods in the next few paragraphs addressing assessment of cognitive products, the caveat remains that these methods may be less appropriate for other aspects of vulnerability.

The DAS (Weissman & Beck, 1978) is a 40-item self-report measure that has been widely used to assess cognitive vulnerability in numerous populations. Short forms (9 items each) of the DAS have been developed based on applications of item response theory to provide parallel versions for pre- and postpriming assessments (Beevers, Strong, Meyer, Pilkonis, & Miller, 2007). With respect to its validity, DAS scores are clearly associated with dysphoric mood (see Scher et al., 2005, for review), and they may be a marker of cognitive vulnerability to depression. For example, formerly depressed individuals have been found to show an increase in DAS scores following a negative mood prime, whereas the DAS scores of those without a depression history did not change (Lau, Haigh, Christensen, Segal, & Taube-Schiff, 2012). In contrast, Jarrett et al. (2012) found that DAS scores did not increase following a negative mood prime in individuals with recurrent major depressive disorder who had responded to cognitive therapy, possibly because these participants acquired skills over the course of therapy that diminished the effects of dysfunctional attitudes, even in the presence of low mood (see also Dozois et al., 2009). This possibility is supported by findings from Segal and colleagues (Segal et al., 1999, 2006) demonstrating that individuals who have recovered from depression following cognitive therapy displayed less cognitive reactivity than did individuals who recovered with pharmacotherapy.

Numerous studies support the predictive validity of the DAS for other important clinical outcomes. In high-risk studies, individuals with a negative cognitive style, as indexed by the DAS, are more vulnerable to developing an initial episode of depression, experience a greater number of depressive episodes, and have more severe symptomatology, and a more chronic course of depression than do low-risk participants (Alloy, Abramson, Whitehouse, et al., 2006; Iacoviello, Alloy, Abramson,

Whitehouse, & Hogan, 2006).[1] The DAS is also sensitive to changes as a result of psychotherapy, and has been used to evaluate attitude change and overall response to treatment (Beevers, Keitner, Ryan, & Miller, 2003; Jarrett et al., 2012; Jarrett, Vittengl, Doyle, & Clark, 2007).

Taken together, these findings suggest that self-reported dysfunctional attitudes, indexed using the DAS, are a valid index of cognitive vulnerability to depression. Although DAS scores differentiate between individuals with depression and psychiatric controls, individuals with panic disorder, generalized anxiety disorder, anorexia nervosa, bipolar disorder, schizophrenia, and dysthymia may also manifest abnormally high DAS scores (Dobson & Shaw, 1986; Horan et al., 2010; Reilly-Harrington et al., 2010). Thus, its specificity as an index of depression risk is questionable, although the same limitation likely applies to many indices of cognitive vulnerability.

Cognitive Operations/Information Processing

Laboratory measures of information processing have long been used to assess operations that putatively indicate cognitive risk for depression. Indeed, one of the strengths of cognitive clinical research is its long-standing history of objective laboratory measures of attention and memory bias of affective stimuli (e.g., Kuiper & Derry, 1982). In contrast to self-report measures, laboratory indices of attention and memory are thought to be more suitable for the purposes of assessing individual differences in information-processing biases. A complete review of such tasks would be beyond the scope of this chapter. Hence, we select a few widely used measures for more detailed discussion.

Various modifications of the basic Stroop Task are among the most widely used methods in psychopathology rescarch. As a measure of attentional bias, these procedures examine how particular emotional stimuli interfere with performance on a color-naming task and how such disruptions might be related to psychopathology (Williams, Mathews, & MacLeod, 1996). Delayed naming of relevant word stimuli (usually affectively-valenced words such as words with depressive content), compared to irrelevant words, is held to reflect an attentional bias that may hold etiological significance for disorder (Gotlib, Roberts, & Gilboa, 1996). Meta-analytic reviews can now be found for Stroop performance in various disorders (Bar-Haim, Lamy, Pergamin, Bakermans-Kranenburg, & van IJzendoorn, 2007; Cisler et al., 2011; Cox, Fadardi, & Pothos, 2006; Dobson & Dozois, 2004; Epp, Dobson, Dozois &

---

[1]Without negative mood induction procedures, associations between DAS scores and clinical outcomes are less consistent.

Frewen, 2012; Lansbergen, Kenemans, & van Engeland, 2007; Schwartz & Verhaeghen, 2008; Westerhausen, Kompus, & Hugdahl, 2011), with results indicating increased color-naming response latencies in the comparison of patients versus controls on the emotional Stroop paradigms. Moreover, disorder-specific content tends to yield longer latencies than matched control words across studies. However, the extent to which cognitive interference reflects the operation of stable vulnerability factors rather than state-like mood variations is less clear.

Dot-probe tasks are widely used computerized measures of information processing also intended to identify attentional biases in the processing of affective information (e.g., MacLeod, Mathews, & Tata, 1986). In this task, participants are presented with a series of picture pairs consisting of one affectively neutral image and one affectively valenced image (e.g., a fear-eliciting or threatening stimulus). At stimulus offset, one of the images is replaced with a probe stimulus, which participants have been instructed to identify as quickly as possible. Quicker responses to probes replacing affective images relative to neutral images are thought to reflect attentional biases for information of that affective valence (MacLeod et al., 1986). Meta-analyses using the dot-probe task exist for anxiety disorders, depression, and disordered eating behavior (Brooks, Prince, Stahl, Campbell, & Treasure, 2011; Frewen, Dozois, Joanisse, & Neufeld, 2008; Peckham, McHugh, & Otto, 2010). These studies indicate that stimulus exposure duration plays a critical role in relating to different forms of psychopathology. For example, in the depression literature, individuals diagnosed with depression and those exhibiting subclinical symptoms demonstrate a bias toward negative information at exposure durations of 1,000 ms or longer (Gotlib, Krasnoperova, Yue, & Joormann, 2004; Joormann & Gotlib, 2007). Anxious participants, on the other hand, have an attentional bias toward threatening information at the subliminal and supraliminal level, but avoid threatening stimuli at longer exposure durations (Mathews & MacLeod, 2005; Mogg & Bradley, 2005). This paradigm has been most widely used in depression and anxiety research. However, further research exploring the role of attention bias is needed with respect to other forms of psychopathology.

Despite their popularity in clinical experimental psychopathology, support for attentional biases as an index of cognitive vulnerability is mixed for some disorders (for a review, see Scher et al., 2005). In the depression literature, Ingram and Ritter (2000) found that previously depressed individuals were more attentive to negative stimuli than nonvulnerable individuals, but only when they experienced a negative mood state. In contrast, other studies using an emotional Stroop paradigm have not found evidence for an attentional bias following a mood or self-focused induction (Gilboa & Gotlib, 1997; Hedlund & Rude, 1995).

While some variability in the literature may be related to whether studies have used mood-priming procedures (Scher et al., 2005), even priming studies have not consistently yielded support for attentional biases as a vulnerability marker. Thus, further research is needed to determine which disorders are related to vulnerabilities in attentional biases, which methods of assessing attentional bias are most valid, and the extent to which aspects of stimulus presentation (e.g., exposure duration) impact findings.

Memory biases for affectively charged, self-descriptive stimuli are also considered to play a critical role in risk for certain disorders, such as depression. The Self-Referent Encoding Task (SRET; Kuiper & Derry, 1982) is a widely used information-processing task that assesses memory biases for positive and negative self-referent information. In this task, participants are presented with a series of positive and negative adjectives and are asked to indicate whether each adjective is self-descriptive. This task is followed by an unexpected free recall period in which participants recall as many of the presented adjectives as possible. Typically, two indices of memory processing relevant to depression are calculated: a positive schematic processing score (the proportion of positive words rated as self-descriptive and recalled relative to all words rated as self-descriptive) and a negative schematic processing score (the proportion of negative words self-described and recalled) (Gencoz, Voels, Gencoz, Pettit, & Joiner, 2000; Hammen & Zupan, 1984; Johnson, Joorman, & Gotlib, 2007; Taylor & Ingram, 1999). A meta-analysis of recall performance demonstrated that individuals with depression tended to recall more negative than positive self-referent information whereas the reverse was true for nondepressed adults (Matt, Vazquez, & Campbell, 1992). Children with depression (Garber & Kaminski, 2000) and children of depressed mothers (Taylor & Ingram, 1999) also exhibit biased performance on SRETs (see Scher et al., 2005, for a review). Furthermore, in two independent samples of young children, performance on a SRET showed moderate stability over multiple 1-year follow-ups and was significantly associated with self-reported depressive symptoms and attributional styles (Hayden et al., 2006, 2013b). Thus, some evidence supports the validity of this task as an index of cognitive vulnerability to depression, although further research examining its predictive validity for clinically significant episodes of depression is needed.

Cognitive Organization

Only a few approaches to indexing cognitive organization/structure are available (Dozois & Dobson, 2001b; Segal, Gemar, Truchon, Guirguis, & Horowitz, 1995; Segal & Vella, 1990). The Psychological Distance

Scaling Task (PDST; Dozois & Dobson, 2001a, 2001b) is a computerized task in which participants place self-referential adjectives in two-dimensional space based on valence and self-descriptiveness. The resulting clusters of adjectives are thought to reflect the degree of interconnectedness of self-referent content or schema consolidation with relevance to cognitive vulnerability to depression. First, depressed individuals have stronger associations among negative interpersonal self-referent content and less interconnectedness for positive content (Dozois & Dobson, 2001a). Also, negative self-referent content is found in remitted individuals with past major depression (Dozois & Dobson, 2001b), in support of its role as a vulnerability factor. Additionally, Lumley and Harkness (2009) found that a depressotypic schema organization, indexed using a version of the PDST, mediated the relation between childhood maltreatment and depression, indicating that it may play a role as a mediator between early adversity and depression. At this point, the construct of cognitive organization appears to be a promising index of cognitive vulnerability. However, additional research using developmentally appropriate adaptations of the PDST is needed to establish whether prospective, longitudinal associations exist between cognitive organization and the initial onset of disorder.

CONCEPTUAL AND MEASUREMENT ISSUES

Content Specificity

According to the content-specificity hypothesis, different forms of psychopathology are associated with relatively specific, characteristic cognitive risks (Beck, 1976; D. A. Clark & Beck with Alford, 1999). Anxiety, for example, is characterized by an orientation toward future threat of harm or danger. In contrast, the emphasis in depression is on past events, with cognitions characterized by themes of loss, deprivation, self-deprecation, and hopelessness (Beck, 1967; Beck, Rush, Shaw, & Emery, 1979). Although research has provided some support for the content-specificity hypothesis (see Baranoff & Oei, Chapter 8, this volume; Beck & Dozois, 2011), high rates of comorbidity of disorders are the rule rather than the exception (Cole, Truglio, & Peeke, 1997; Dobson, 1985a, 1985b; Feldman, 1993), suggesting the possibility of shared diatheses across disorders, some of which may be cognitive in nature. In recognition of the high likelihood of common vulnerabilities that span disorders, theoretical models, including the tripartite and hierarchical models (Barlow, 1991; Barlow, Chorpita, & Turovsky, 1996; L. A. Clark & Watson, 1991; L. A. Clark, Watson, & Mineka, 1994), have highlighted mechanisms common to multiple forms of psychopathology, including depression and anxiety. Additionally, transdiagnostic interventions—approaches that identify and target vulnerability factors that apply to multiple disorders—may inform basic etiological models and enhance the efficiency and efficacy of treatment and prevention efforts (Dozois, Seeds, & Collins, 2009; Suárez, Bennett, Goldstein, & Barlow, 2008; Smith, Ratcliff, & Norton, Chapter 9, this volume). There remains a greater need in the field for investigations of dimensions of cognitive vulnerability that cut across multiple forms of psychopathology, as such models are more likely to map more closely onto the shared etiological underpinnings of these comorbid conditions.

Assessment across Development

A case for the causal status of cognitive vulnerability can be better made when it is established that markers of cognitive risk precede the onset of disorder. Such efforts require the use of longitudinal designs, preferably ones using multiple waves of follow-up. Further, given that the disorders for which cognitive factors are most strongly implicated (e.g., depression) commonly onset in adolescence and early adulthood rather than childhood (Garber, Gallerani, & Frankel, 2009), such studies require developmentally sensitive assessment approaches to assessing cognitive vulnerability in youth. Such design features are also compatible with the goals of early intervention and preventative efforts (see Dozois & Dobson, 2004). As a result, the capacity to validly assess cognitive vulnerability across different developmental stages becomes an important consideration for theory and prevention.

A number of self-report scales originally developed for adults have been adapted for use with children and adolescents. For example, the Automatic Thoughts Questionnaire, which taps aspects of negative cognition, has been used with children and adolescents (Hollon & Kendall, 1980; Kazdin, 1990), demonstrated excellent internal consistency, and differentiates depressed from nondepressed children. There are also assessment approaches specifically for children and adolescents (e.g., Conley, Haines, Hilt, & Metalsky, 2001). However, measures designed to tap cognitive risks relevant to youth may be less relevant to adult manifestations of vulnerability. As noted in the previous section on stability of cognitive risk, relatively little longitudinal work has been done on the long-term stability of cognitive vulnerability across different developmental stages, as well as the extent to which early cognitive vulnerability predicts the development of depressive symptoms and disorders.

The lack of research on this topic may relate to questions in the field regarding when children's cognitive vulnerability for internalizing disorders can be reliably and validly assessed. Much of the work that addresses this issue has focused on self-reported cognitive risk in later childhood and early adolescence across relatively brief follow-ups, factors that may increase estimates of stability relative to work on younger samples using information-processing measures and longer follow-up intervals. There is ongoing debate regarding when meaningful, stable aspects of cognitive risk emerge (e.g., Abela & Hankin, 2011; Cole et al., 2008; Gibb & Coles, 2005), and evidence may vary depending on when it is measured. The developmental literature indicates that children develop a more stable yet differentiated sense of self in middle childhood (Abela & Hankin, 2008; Harter, 2012), suggesting that appropriate measures may yield meaningful information about depressive cognition in children this age. Further, increases in depression risk in middle childhood, as well as greater crystallization of risk, could account for the subsequent increase in depression prevalence found in adolescence. This latter point highlights the importance of longitudinal work on children's emerging cognitive risk addressing the possibility of sex differences in negative cognition as a mechanism that accounts for girls' heightened risk for depression in puberty.

CLINICAL APPLICATIONS
OF ASSESSING COGNITIVE VULNERABILITY

In addition to research focusing on cognitive factors that play an etiological role in psychopathology, research has also examined the role of such factors in relapse and recurrence. It is entirely possible the same cognitive variables that predict disorder course may also have causal significance and so have direct clinical implications for relapse prevention. Some of this research was recently summarized by Jarrett, Vittengl, and Clark (2008), who provided guidelines for clinicians on how to prevent relapse and recurrence in those who have received cognitive therapy for depression (see Hunsley & Elliott, Chapter 6, this volume). With respect to cognitive risk for relapse, Segal et al. (2006) demonstrated that remitted depressed clients who reported greater dysfunctional cognitions during a mood prime had significantly greater risk of relapse during the 18 months following treatment. Another potential predictor of relapse and recurrence is negative cognitive organization, as measured using the PDST, which has been shown to persist past an episode of depression and is a stable vulnerability marker for depression (Dozois, 2007; Dozois & Dobson, 2001a). Future work examining the predictive power of cognitive factors for relapse is needed. This work should focus on effect sizes with respect to clinical outcomes to better clarify which indices of cognitive vulnerability have the greatest relevance for preventive work, above and beyond the predictive value of previous episodes of depression, which are a known, powerful predictor of future risk. Meta-analyses would also be highly useful in this respect.

A more refined typological approach wherein the goal is to establish measurement scores that reliably identify those at greatest risk for psychopathology onset and relapse could be taken in order to more accurately determine which individuals should be prioritized for prevention and targeted interventions (Dozois, Covin, & Brinker, 2003). Dozois et al. published data on six measures of depressive cognition in adults that were selected because of their high clinical and research utility based on criteria established by Nezu, Ronan, Meadows, and McClure (2000). They suggested that the norms provided may be used to make normative comparisons in research, to assess clinically significant cognitive change in treatment outcome, to assist with case conceptualization and treatment planning, to decide when treatment may be terminated, and to evaluate clinical significance in psychotherapy outcome trials. Ingram, Nelson, Steidtmann, and Bistricky (2007) extended this work by collecting normative data on six child–adolescent measures of depression-related cognition. Although norms on cognitive vulnerability measures are becoming more readily available, additional research is needed to develop a comprehensive normative database for a broad range of relevant cognitive measures used in vulnerability and prevention work and to test their predictive validity and utility.

With respect to relationships between specific scores on measures of vulnerability and course and outcomes of disorder, greater knowledge has accrued regarding the predictive validity of self-reports, rather than laboratory indices, of cognitive vulnerability for depression onset and relapse. This is due to the fact that stimuli used in laboratory measures of vulnerability are not standardized, varying across studies in terms of stimuli used and other experimental procedures. Adoption of standardized stimuli that are normed for different ages, research initiatives (e.g., depression vulnerability), and processes (e.g., auditory attention) may help address this issue in the long term, although self-reports are likely to continue to play a more dominant role in predicting treatment response in vulnerable individuals because of their ease of integration into clinical practice.

CONCLUSIONS AND FUTURE DIRECTIONS

Understanding vulnerability processes lies at the heart of basic science as well as of prevention and intervention in psychopathology. While cognitive models of psychopathology vulnerability have assumed a central position in efforts to understand and treat many common disorders (e.g., depression, anxiety), a number of core issues remain unresolved. For example, basic descriptive work that characterizes the long-term stability of cognitive vulnerability across different development periods is needed. Such work is no small task, as it necessitates the formulation and use of developmentally sensitive indices of cognition that have comparable construct validity for participants at these different periods. Research such as this will benefit from the collaborative efforts of experts in depression and cognitive development and will also facilitate research that more conclusively establishes the causal role of cognition in disorder. It has long been clear that, while cognitive factors predict subsequent disorder, disorder also predicts later cognition (e.g., Stewart et al., 2004). Longitudinal studies that begin prior to the age of risk for disorder and include careful screening of participants for clinically significant levels of symptoms and past disorder are still needed to better establish the causal role of cognitive vulnerability factors.

Research on the assessment of cognitive vulnerability will also benefit from the development and testing of more refined models of diatheses and stressors. For example, Abela and Sarin (2002) found that it was adolescents' most depressive inferential style (which they deemed their "weakest link"), rather than their overall inferential style, that interacted with life stress to predict depressive symptomatology. Nuanced tests such as these may highlight which facets of cognitive risk hold the greatest predictive power for disorder onset, although such analyses will not be possible without a fine-grained assessment of cognitive vulnerability. Further, intriguing work suggests the possibility that cognitive vulnerability may show specific predictive power for more refined disorder subtypes (Struijs, Groenewold, Oude Voshaar, & de Jonge, 2013). This may have important implications for targeted interventions, although it also relies upon careful assessment of both cognitive risk *and* symptoms of disorder. Additionally, researchers have begun to test diathesis–stress interactions in more precise, fine-grained ways to better map the predictive value of cognitive vulnerability. Employing multiple assessments periods (e.g., using daily diary methodologies) and more sophisticated data-analytic techniques (e.g., hierarchical linear modeling), for instance, may better capture the dynamic nature of cognitive vulnerability-stress interactions as they unfold over time (cf. Abela & Skitch, 2007; Hankin et al., 2005). Finally, intriguing work on the neural and genetic correlates of cognitive vulnerability is beginning to accrue (e.g., Hayden et al., 2013a; Smoski, Keng, Schiller, Minkel, & Dichter, 2013). This research not only contributes to basic theory on the biological substrates of cognitive risk, it may also ultimately inform treatments that focus on reducing cognitive risk through combined medication and cognitive therapy, for example. Such work hinges on the selection and assessment of cognitive endophenotypes (Gottesman & Gould, 2003) that map well onto biological substrates of disorder.

Studies that address each of these suggested future directions will benefit from the use of multiple methods of assessing cognitive risk. Ideally, we could conclude this chapter with a set of recommendations for specific measures of negative cognition to be utilized in both research and applied settings; however, given that many studies have focused on a single method of assessing cognitive risk, it remains generally unclear which indices of vulnerability have the best predictive power for the development of disorder, and it is difficult to conclusively say which measures, if any, should be the "gold standard" for various indices of cognitive vulnerability. To address these issues, multitrait–multimethod approaches to the assessment of cognitive vulnerability using self-report and laboratory indices of relevant cognitive constructs are badly needed, particularly in longitudinal studies of emerging disorder risk over time. Such work will help resolve the question of which indices of negative cognition pose the greatest etiological significance for disorder.

Thus, while we strongly recommend the use of multiple methods of assessment of cognitive vulnerability that tap the domains of cognition previously reviewed (i.e., products, processes, structure) whenever possible, in the interim, researchers and clinicians will continue to rely on common sense and practical considerations in choosing measures of cognitive vulnerability. For example, while a self-report measure of attentional bias would be unlikely to pass muster as an index of cognitive process in research on basic cognition, it may not generally be feasible for clinicians to use state-of-the-art laboratory measures of attentional bias (e.g., eye-tracking equipment) as a part of routine practice. In this respect, collaborations between researchers and clinicians could be mutually beneficial if it means that clinicians can access laboratory data with putative predictive power for clinical outcomes, and researchers, in turn, can access patient samples. Practice Research Networks (e.g., Castonguay, Locke, & Hayes, 2011) may play a critical role in fostering such collaborative efforts.

In conclusion, cognitive models of psychopathology vulnerability have assumed a preeminent role in both etiological theories and treatments of many common, chronic disorders that impact individuals across the lifespan. While a large body of research has accrued in support of these models, an array of both fundamental and more nuanced questions remain unresolved, including issues concerning the long-term stability of cognitive vulnerability, the early predictive power of cognitive vulnerability for later disorder, and more fine-grained questions about how specific facets of cognitive risk relate to disorder onset, its course, and its clinical presentation. The assessment of cognitive vulnerability lies at the heart of these issues, as the answers to these questions may well differ depending on how vulnerability is operationalized. Answering the question of which specific aspects of vulnerability hold the greatest predictive power for clinical outcomes, including the critical goal of targeted preventions, will necessitate the collaborative efforts of experts in both applied and basic science.

KEY POINTS

FOR PRACTITIONERS

- Enhance collaborative efforts with researchers toward the goal of generating data from clinical samples on cognitive risk and preventative and intervention efforts.
- Choose assessment instruments based on the goals and targets of therapy.
- Incorporate developmentally sensitive paradigms that are suitable to the client.
- Use longitudinal approaches that track change in both cognitive vulnerability and symptoms across time and treatment (when relevant).
- Use the norms available on cognitive risk to interpret data.

FOR RESEARCHERS

- Use effective and developmentally sensitive priming techniques (e.g., films/stories).
- Select a battery of measures that fully maps the spectrum of cognitive vulnerability (e.g., products, processes, structures, in the case of depression).
- Incorporate developmentally sensitive paradigms that are suitable to the target population.
- Use longitudinal approaches that track change in both cognitive vulnerability and symptoms across time and treatment (when relevant).
- Use normative data available on cognitive risk to interpret data.
- Use multiple methods that provide a fine-grained assessment of cognitive vulnerability and a stringent test of links between cognitive risk and the criterion disorder.
- Enhance collaborative efforts with clinicians toward the goal of better assessing cognitive vulnerability in clinical samples and its predictive validity for important outcomes.
- Additional, rigorous studies of the long-term stability and causal significance of early-emerging cognitive vulnerability are needed.

FOR STUDENTS AND EDUCATORS

- Incorporate developmentally sensitive paradigms that are suitable to the client.
- Additional, rigorous studies of the long-term stability and causal significance of early-emerging cognitive vulnerability are needed.
- Train students in the identification and evaluation of both symptom-based indices and cognitive measures of risk and vulnerability.

REFERENCES

Abela, J. R. Z., & Hankin, B. L. (2008). Cognitive vulnerability to depression in children and adolescents: A developmental psychopathology perspective. In J. R. Z. Abela & B. L. Hankin (Eds.), *Handbook of depression in children and adolescents* (pp. 35–78). New York: Guilford Press.

Abela, J. R. Z., & Hankin, B. L. (2011). Rumination as a vulnerability factor to depression during the transition from early to middle adolescence: A multi-wave longitudinal study. *Journal of Abnormal Psychology, 120,* 259–271.

Abela, J. R. Z., & Sarin, S. (2002). Cognitive vulnerability to hopelessness depression: A chain is only as strong as its weakest link. *Cognitive Therapy and Research, 26,* 811–829.

Abela, J. R. Z., & Skitch, S. A. (2007). Dysfunctional attitudes, self-esteem, and hassles: Cognitive vulnerability to depression in children of affectively ill parents. *Behaviour Research and Therapy, 45,* 1127–1140.

Abramson, L. Y., Metalsky, G. I., & Alloy, L. B. (1989). Hopelessness depression: A theory-based subtype of depression. *Psychological Review, 96,* 358–372.

Alloy, L. B., Abramson, L. Y., Hogan, M. E., Whitehouse, W. G., Rose, D. T., Robinson, M. S., et al. (2000). The Temple–Wisconsin Cognitive Vulnerability to Depression project: Lifetime history of Axis I psychopathology in individuals at high and low cognitive risk for depression. *Journal of Abnormal Psychology, 109,* 403–418.

Alloy, L. B., Abramson, L. Y., Walshaw, P. D., & Neeren, A. M. (2006). Cognitive vulnerability to unipolar and bipolar mood disorders. *Journal of Social and Clinical Psychology, 25,* 726–754.

Alloy, L. B., Abramson, L. Y., Whitehouse, W. G., Hogan, M. E., Panzarella, C., & Rose, D. T. (2006). Prospective incidence of first onsets and recurrences of depression in individuals at high and low cognitive risk for depression. *Journal of Abnormal Psychology, 115,* 145–156.

Bar-Haim, Y., Lamy, D., Pergamin, L., Bakermans-Kranenburg, M. J., & van IJzendoorn, M. H. (2007). Threat-related attentional bias in anxious and nonanxious individuals: A meta-analytic study. *Psychological Bulletin, 133,* 1–24.

Barlow, D. H. (1991). Disorders of emotion. *Psychological Inquiry, 2,* 58–71.

Barlow, D. H., Chorpita, B. F., & Turovsky, J. (1996). Fear, panic, anxiety, and disorders of emotion. In D. A. Hope (Ed.), *Nebraska Symposium on Motivation, 1995: Perspectives on anxiety, panic, and fear* (pp. 251–328). Lincoln: University of Nebraska Press.

Barnett, P. A., & Gotlib, I. A. (1988). Psychosocial functioning and depression: Distinguishing among antecedents, concomitants, and consequences. *Psychological Bulletin, 104,* 97–126.

Beck, A. T. (1967). Development of depression. In *Depression: Clinical, experimental, and theoretical aspects* (pp. 275–290). New York: Harper & Row.

Beck, A. T. (1976). *Cognitive therapy and the emotional disorders.* New York: Basic Books.

Beck, A. T., & Dozois, D. J. A. (2011). Cognitive therapy: Current status and future directions. *Annual Review of Medicine, 62,* 397–409.

Beck, A. T., Rush, A. J., Shaw, B. F., & Emery, G. (1979). *Cognitive therapy of depression.* New York: Guilford Press.

Beevers, C. G., Keitner, G., Ryan, C., & Miller, I. W. (2003). Cognitive predictors of symptom return following depression treatment. *Journal of Abnormal Psychology, 112,* 488–496.

Beevers, C. G., Strong, D. R., Meyer, B., Pilkonis, P. A., & Miller, I. W. (2007). Efficiently assessing negative cognition in depression: An item response theory analysis of the Dysfunctional Attitude Scale. *Psychological Assessment, 19,* 199–209.

Bower, G. H. (1981). Mood and memory. *American Psychologist, 36,* 129–148.

Brenner, E. (2000). Mood induction in children: Methodological issues and clinical implications. *Review of General Psychology, 4,* 264–283.

Brooks, S., Prince, A., Stahl, D., Campbell, I. C., & Treasure, J. (2011). A systematic review and meta-analysis of cognitive bias to food stimuli in people with disordered eating behavior. *Clinical Psychology Review, 31,* 37–51.

Castonguay, L. G., Locke, B. D., & Hayes, J. A. (2011). The Center for Collegiate Mental Health: An example of a practice-research network in university counseling centers. *Journal of College Student Psychotherapy, 25,* 105–119.

Cisler, J. M., Wlitzky-Taylor, K. B., Adams, T. G., Babson, K. A., Badour, C. L., & Willems, J. L. (2011). The emotional Stroop task and posttraumatic stress disorder: A meta-analysis. *Clinical Psychology Review, 31,* 817–828.

Clark, D. A., & Beck, A. T., with Alford, B. A. (1999). *Scientific foundations of cognitive theory and therapy of depression.* New York: Wiley.

Clark, L. A., & Watson, D. (1991). Tripartite model of anxiety and depression: Psychometric evidence and taxonomic implications. *Journal of Abnormal Psychology, 100,* 316–336.

Clark, L. A., Watson, D., & Mineka, S. (1994). Temperament, personality, and the mood and anxiety disorders. *Journal of Abnormal Psychology, 103,* 103–116.

Cole, D. A., Ciesla, J. A., Dallaire, D. H., Jacquez, F. M., Pineda, A. Q., Lagrange, B., et al. (2008). Emergence of attributional style and its relation to depressive symptoms. *Journal of Abnormal Psychology, 117,* 16–31.

Cole, D. A., Jacquez, F. M., Truss, A. E., Pineda, A. Q., Weitlauf, A. S., Tilghman-Osborne, C. E., et al. (2009). Gender differences in the longitudinal structure of cognitive diatheses for depression in children and adolescents. *Journal of Clinical Psychology, 65,* 1312–1326.

Cole, D. A., Truglio, R., & Peeke, L. (1997). Relation between symptoms of anxiety and depression in children: A multitrait–multimethod–multigroup assessment. *Journal of Consulting and Clinical Psychology, 65,* 110–119.

Conley, C. S., Haines, B. A., Hilt, L. M., & Metalsky, G. I. (2001). The Children's Attributional Style Interview: Developmental tests of cognitive diathesis–stress theories of depression. *Journal of Abnormal Child Psychology, 29,* 445–463.

Cox, W. M., Fadardi, J. S., & Pothos, E. M. (2006). The addiction-Stroop test: Theoretical considerations and procedural recommendations. *Psychological Bulletin, 132,* 443–476.

Crick, N. R., & Dodge, K. A. (1994). A review and formulation of social information-processing mechanisms in children's social adjustment. *Psychological Bulletin, 115,* 74–101.

Dobson, K. S. (1985a). An analysis of anxiety and depression scales. *Journal of Personality Assessment, 49,* 522–527.

Dobson, K. S. (1985b). The relationship between anxiety and depression. *Clinical Psychology Review, 5,* 307–324.

Dobson, K. S., & Dozois, D. J. A. (2004). Attentional biases in eating disorders: A meta-analytic review of Stroop performance. *Clinical Psychology Review, 23,* 1001–1022.

Dobson, K. S., & Shaw, B. F. (1986). Cognitive assessment with major depressive disorders. *Cognitive Therapy and Research, 10,* 13–29.

Dodge, K. A., & Crick, N. R. (1990). Social information-processing bases of aggressive behavior in children. *Personality and Social Psychology Bulletin, 16,* 8–22.

Dozois, D. J. A. (2007). Stability of negative self-structures: A longitudinal comparison of depressed, remitted, and nonpsychiatric controls. *Journal of Clinical Psychology, 63,* 319–338.

Dozois, D. J. A., & Beck, A. T. (2008). Cognitive schemas, beliefs, and assumptions. In K. S. Dobson & D. J. A. Dozois (Eds.), *Risk factors in depression* (pp. 121–144). Oxford, UK: Elsevier.

Dozois, D. J. A., Bieling, P. J., Patelis-Siotis, I., Hoar, L., Chudzik, S., McCabe, K., et al. (2009). Changes in self-schema structure in cognitive therapy for major depressive disorder: A randomized clinical trial. *Journal of Consulting and Clinical Psychology, 77,* 1078–1088.

Dozois, D. J. A., Covin, R., & Brinker, J. K. (2003). Normative data on cognitive measures of depression. *Journal of Consulting and Clinical Psychology, 71,* 71–80.

Dozois, D. J. A., & Dobson, K. S. (2001a). A longitudinal investigation of information processing and cognitive organization in clinical depression: Stability of schematic interconectedness. *Journal of Consulting and Clinical Psychology, 69,* 914–925.

Dozois, D. J. A., & Dobson, K. S. (2001b). Information processing and cognitive organization in unipolar depression: Specificity and comorbidity issues. *Journal of Abnormal Psychology, 110,* 236–246.

Dozois, D. J. A., & Dobson, K. S. (2004). The prevention of anxiety and depression: Promises and prospects. In K. S. Dobson & D. J. A. Dozois (Eds.), *The prevention of anxiety and depression: Theory, research, and practice* (pp. 283–295). Washington, DC: American Psychological Association.

Dozois, D. J. A., Seeds, P. M., & Collins, K. A. (2009). Transdiagnostic approaches to the prevention of depression and anxiety. *Journal of Cognitive Psychotherapy: An International Quarterly, 23*, 44–59.

Dunkley, D. M., Blankstein, K. R., & Segal, Z. V. (2010). Cognitive assessment: Issues and methods. In K. S. Dobson (Ed.), *Handbook of cognitive-behavioral therapies* (3rd ed., pp. 133–171). New York: Guilford Press.

Durbin, E. C., Hayden, E. P., Klein, D. N., & Olino, T. M. (2007). Stability of laboratory-assessed emotionality traits from ages 3 to 7. *Emotion, 7*, 388–399.

Epp, A. M., Dobson, K. S., Dozois, D. J. A., & Frewen, P. A. (2012). A systematic meta-analysis of the Stroop task in depression. *Clinical Psychology Review, 32*, 316–328.

Feldman, L. A. (1993). Distinguishing depression and anxiety in self report: Evidence from confirmatory factor analysis on nonclinical and clinical samples. *Journal of Consulting and Clinical Psychology, 61*, 631–638.

Frewen, P. A., Dozois, D. J. A., Joanisse, M. F., & Neufeld, R. W. J. (2008). Selective attention to threat versus reward: Meta-analysis and neural-network modeling of the dot-probe task. *Clinical Psychology Review, 28*, 307–337.

Garber, J., Gallerani, C. M., & Frankel, S. A. (2009). Depression in children. In I. H. Gotlib & C. L. Hammen (Eds.), *Handbook of depression* (2nd ed., pp. 405–443). New York: Guilford Press.

Garber, J., & Kaminski, K. M. (2000). Laboratory and performance-based measures of depression in children and adolescents. *Journal of Clinical Child Psychology, 29*, 509–525.

Gencoz, T., Voels, Z. R., Gencoz, F., Pettit, J. W., & Joiner Jr., T. E. (2000). Specificity of information-processing styles to depressive symptoms in youth psychiatric inpatients. *Journal of Abnormal Child Psychology, 29*, 255–262.

Gibb, B. E., & Coles, M. E. (2005). Cognitive vulnerability-stress models of psychopathology: A developmental perspective. In B. E. Gibb & M. E. Coles (Eds.), *Development of psychopathology: A vulnerability–stress perspective* (pp. 104–135). Thousand Oaks, CA: Sage.

Gilboa, E., & Gotlib, I. H. (1997). Cognitive biases and affect persistence in previously dysphoric and never-dysphoric individuals. *Cognition and Emotion, 11*, 517–538.

Gotlib, I. H., & Hammen, C. L. (1992). *Psychological aspects of depression: Toward a cognitive-interpersonal integration.* Chichester, UK: Wiley.

Gotlib, I. H., Krasnoperova, E., Yue, D. N., & Joormann, J. (2004). Attentional biases for negative interpersonal stimuli in clinical depression. *Journal of Abnormal Psychology, 113*, 127–135.

Gotlib, I. H., Roberts, J. E., & Gilboa, E. (1996). Cognitive interference in depression. In I. G. Sarason, G. R. Pierce, & B. R. Sarason (Eds.), *Cognitive interference: Theories, methods, and findings* (pp. 347–377). Mahwah, NJ: Erlbaum.

Gottesman, I. I., & Gould, T. D. (2003). The endophenotype concept in psychiatry: Etymology and strategic intentions. *American Journal of Psychiatry, 160,* 636–645.

Hammen, C., & Zupan, B. A. (1984). Self-schemas, depression, and the processing of personal information in children. *Journal of Experimental Child Psychology, 37,* 598–608.

Hankin, B. L. (2008). Stability of cognitive vulnerabilities to depression: A short-term prospective multiwave study. *Journal of Abnormal Psychology, 117,* 324–333.

Hankin, B. L., & Abela, J. R. Z. (2005). Depression from childhood through adolescence and adulthood: A developmental vulnerability and stress perspective. In B. L. Hankin & J. R. Z. Abela (Eds.), *Development of psychopathology: A vulnerability–stress perspective* (pp. 245–288). Thousand Oaks, CA: Sage.

Hankin, B. L., Fraley, C. R., & Abela, J. R. Z. (2005). Daily depression and cognitions about stress: Evidence for a trait-like depressogenic cognitive style and the prediction of depressive symptoms in a prospective daily diary study. *Journal of Personality and Social Psychology, 88,* 673–685.

Hankin, B. L., Oppenheimer, C., Jenness, J., Barrocas, A., Shapero, B. G., & Goldband, J. (2009). Developmental origins of cognitive vulnerabilities to depression: Review of processes contributing to stability and change across time. *Journal of Clinical Psychology, 65,* 1327–1338.

Harter, S. (2012). Emerging self-processes during childhood and adolescence. In M. R. Leary & J. P. Tangney (Ed.), *Handbook of self and identity* (2nd ed., pp. 680–715). New York: Guilford Press.

Hayden, E. P., Klein, D. N., Durbin, C. E., & Olino, T. M. (2006). Positive emotionality at age three predicts cognitive styles in seven-year-old children. *Development and Psychopathology, 18,* 409–423.

Hayden, E. P., Olino, T. M., Bufferd, S. J., Miller, A., Dougherty, L. R., Sheikh, H. I., et al. (2013a). The serotonin transporter linked polymorphic region and brain-derived neurotrophic factor valine to methionine at position 66 polymorphisms and maternal history of depression: Associations with cognitive vulnerability to depression in childhood. *Development and Psychopathology, 25,* 587–598.

Hayden, E. P., Olino, T. M., Mackrell, S. V. M., Jordan, P. J., Desjardins, J., & Katsiroumbas, P. (2013b). Cognitive vulnerability to depression during middle childhood: Stability and associations with maternal affective styles and parental depression. *Personality and Individual Differences, 55,* 892–897.

Hedlund, S., & Rude, S. S. (1995). Evidence of latent depressive schemas in formerly depressed individuals. *Journal of Abnormal Psychology, 104,* 517–525.

Hollon, S. D., & Kendall, P. C. (1980). Cognitive self-statements in depression: Development of an Automatic Thoughts Questionnaire. *Cognitive Therapy and Research, 4,* 383–395.

Horan, W. P., Rassovsky, Y., Kern, R. S., Lee, J., Wynn, J. K., & Green, M. F. (2010). Further support for the role of dysfunctional attitudes in models of real-world functioning in schizophrenia. *Journal of Psychiatric Research*, 44, 499–505.

Iacoviello, B. M., Alloy, L. B., Abramson, L. Y., Whitehouse, W. G., & Hogan, M. E. (2006). The course of depression in individuals at high and low cognitive risk for depression: A prospective study. *Journal of Affective Disorders*, 93, 61–69.

Ingram, R. E., Atchley, R. A., & Segal, Z. V. (2011). *Vulnerability to depression: From cognitive neuroscience to prevention and treatment*. New York: Guilford Press.

Ingram, R. E., & Kendall, P. C. (1986). Cognitive clinical psychology: Implications of an information processing perspective. In R. E. Ingram (Ed.), *Information processing approaches to clinical psychology* (pp. 3–21). Orlando, FL: Academic Press.

Ingram, R. E., Miranda, J., & Segal, Z. V. (1998). *Cognitive vulnerability to depression*. New York: Guilford Press.

Ingram, R. E., Nelson, T., Steidtmann, D. K., & Bistricky, S. L. (2007). Comparative data on child and adolescent cognitive measures associated with depression. *Journal of Consulting and Clinical Psychology*, 75, 390–403.

Ingram, R. E., & Price, J. M. (2010). Understanding psychopathology: The role of vulnerability. In R. E. Ingram & J. M. Price (Eds.), *Vulnerability to psychopathology: Risk across the lifespan* (pp. 3–17). New York: Guilford Press.

Ingram, R. E., & Ritter, J. (2000). Vulnerability to depression: Cognitive reactivity and parental bonding in high-risk individuals. *Journal of Abnormal Psychology*, 109, 588–596.

Jarrett, R. B., Minhajuddin, A., Borman, P. D., Dunlap, L., Segal, Z. V., Kidner, C. L., et al. (2012). Cognitive reactivity, dysfunctional attitudes, and depressive relapse and recurrence in cognitive therapy responders. *Behaviour Research and Therapy*, 50, 280–286.

Jarrett, R. B., Vittengl, J. R., & Clark, L. A. (2008). How much cognitive therapy, for which patients, will prevent depressive relapse. *Journal of Affective Disorders*, 111, 185–192.

Jarrett, R. B., Vittengl, J. R., Doyle, K., & Clark, L. A. (2007). Changes in cognitive content during and following cognitive therapy for recurrent depression: Substantial and enduring, but not predictive of change in depressive symptoms. *Journal of Consulting and Clinical Psychology*, 75, 432–446.

Johnson, S. L., Joorman, J., & Gotlib, I. H. (2007). Does processing of emotional stimuli predict symptomatic improvement and diagnostic recovery from major depression? *Emotion*, 7, 201–206.

Joormann, J., & Gotlib, I. H. (2007). Selective attention to emotional faces following recovery from depression. *Journal of Abnormal Psychology*, 116, 80–85.

Kazdin, A. E. (1990). Evaluation of the Automatic Thoughts Questionnaire: Negative cognitive processes and depression among children. *Psychological Assessment: A Journal of Consulting and Clinical Psychology*, 2, 73–79.

Kuiper, N. A., & Derry, P. A. (1982). Depressed and nondepressed content self-reference in mild depressives. *Journal of Personality, 50,* 67–80.

Lansbergen, M. M., Kenemans, J. L., & van Engeland, H. (2007). Stroop interference and attention-deficit/hyperactivity disorder: A review and meta-analysis. *Neuropsychology, 21,* 251–262.

Lau, M. A., Haigh, E. A. P., Christensen, B. K., Segal, Z. V., & Taube-Schiff, M. (2012). Evaluating the mood state dependence of automatic thoughts and dysfunctional attitudes in remitted versus never-depressed individuals. *Journal of Cognitive Psychotherapy: An International Quarterly, 26,* 381–389.

Lumley, M. N., & Harkness, K. L. (2009). Childhood maltreatment and depressotypic cognitive organization. *Cognitive Therapy and Research, 33,* 511–522.

MacLeod, C., Mathews, A., & Tata, P. (1986). Attentional bias in emotional disorders. *Journal of Abnormal Psychology, 95,* 15–20.

Mathews, A., & MacLeod, C. (2005). Cognitive vulnerability to emotional disorders. *Annual Review of Clinical Psychology, 1,* 167–195.

Matt, G. E., Vazquez, C., & Campbell, W. K. (1992). Mood-congruent recall of affectively toned stimuli: A meta-analytic review. *Clinical Psychology Review, 12,* 227–255.

Mineka, S., Rafaeli, E., & Yovel, I. (2003). Cognitive biases in emotional disorders: Information processing and social cognitive perspectives. In S. Mineka, E. Rafaeli, & I. Yovel (Eds.), *Handbook of affective sciences* (pp. 976–1009). New York: Oxford University Press.

Mogg, K., & Bradley, B. P. (2005). Attentional bias in generalized anxiety disorder versus depressive disorder. *Cognitive Therapy and Research, 29,* 29–45.

Monroe, S. M., & Simons, A. D. (1991). Diathesis-stress theories in the context of life stress research: Implications for the depressive disorders. *Psychological Bulletin, 110,* 406–425.

Nezu, A. M., Ronan, G. F., Meadows, E. A., & McClure, K. S. (2000). *Practitioner's guide to empirically based measures of depression.* New York: Kluwer Academic/Plenum.

Peckham, A. D., McHugh, K. R., & Otto, M. W. (2010). A meta-analysis of the magnitude of biased attention in depression. *Depression and Anxiety, 27,* 1135–1142.

Persons, J. B., & Miranda, J. (1992). Cognitive theories of vulnerability to depression: Reconciling negative evidence. *Cognitive Therapy and Research, 16,* 485–502.

Reilly-Harrington, N. A., Miklowitz, D. J., Otto, M. W., Frank, E., Wisniewski, S. R., Thase, M. E., et al. (2010). Dysfunctional attitudes, attributional styles, and phase of illness in bipolar disorder. *Cognitive Therapy and Research, 34,* 24–34.

Reiss, S., & McNally, R. J. (1985). The expectancy model of fear. In S. Reiss & R. R. Bootzin (Eds.), *Theoretical issues in behavior therapy* (pp. 107–122). New York: Academic Press.

Riskind, J. H., & Alloy, L. B. (2006). Cognitive vulnerability to emotional disorders: Theory and research design/methodology. In L. B. Alloy & J. H. Riskind (Eds.), *Cognitive vulnerability to emotional disorders* (pp. 1–32). Mahwah, NJ: Erlbaum.

Scher, C. D., Ingram, R. E., & Segal, Z. V. (2005). Cognitive reactivity and vulnerability: Empirical evaluation of construct activation and cognitive diatheses in unipolar depression. *Clinical Psychology Review, 25*, 487–510.

Schwartz, K., & Verhaeghen, P. (2008). ADHD and Stroop interference from age 9 to 41 years: A meta-analysis of developmental effects. *Psychology Medicine, 38*, 1607–1616.

Seeds, P. M., & Dozois, D. J. A. (2010). Prospective evaluation of a cognitive vulnerability–stress model for depression: The interaction of schema self-structure and negative life events. *Journal of Clinical Psychology, 66*, 1307–1323.

Segal, Z. V. (1988). Appraisal of the self-schema construct in cognitive models of depression. *Psychological Bulletin, 103*, 147–162.

Segal, Z. V., Gemar, M., Truchon, C., Guirguis, M., & Horowitz, L. M. (1995). A priming methodology for studying self-representation in major depressive disorder. *Journal of Abnormal Psychology, 104*, 205–213.

Segal, Z. V., Gemar, M., & Williams, S. (1999). Differential cognitive response to a mood challenge following successful cognitive therapy or pharmacotherapy for unipolar depression. *Journal of Abnormal Psychology, 108*, 3–10.

Segal, Z. V., Kennedy, S., Gemar, M., Hood, K., Pedersen, R., & Buis, T. (2006). Cognitive reactivity to sad mood provocation and the prediction of depressive relapse. *Archives of General Psychiatry, 63*, 749–755.

Segal, Z. V., & Vella, D. D. (1990). Self-schema in major depression: Replication and extension of a priming methodology. *Cognitive Therapy and Research, 14*, 161–176.

Smoski, M. J., Keng, S. L., Schiller, C. E., Minkel, J., & Dichter, G. S. (2013). Neural mechanisms of cognitive reappraisal in remitted major depressive disorder. *Journal of Affective Disorders, 151*(1), 171–177.

Stewart, S. M., Kennard, B. D., Lee, P. W. H., Hughes, C. W., Mayes, T. L., Emslie, G. J., et al. (2004). A cross-cultural investigation of cognitions and depressive symptoms in adolescents. *Journal of Abnormal Psychology, 113*, 248–257.

Struijs, S. Y., Groenewold, N. A., Oude Voshaar, R. C., & de Jonge, P. (2013). Cognitive vulnerability differentially predicts symptom dimensions of depression. *Journal of Affective Disorders, 151*(1), 92–99.

Suárez, L., Bennett, S., Goldstein, C., & Barlow, D. H. (2008). Understanding anxiety disorders from a "triple vulnerabilities" framework. In M. M. Antony & M. B. Stein (Eds.), *Oxford handbook of anxiety and related disorders* (pp. 153–172). New York: Oxford University Press.

Taylor, L., & Ingram, R. E. (1999). Cognitive reactivity and depressotypic information processing in children of depressed mothers. *Journal of Abnormal Psychology, 108*, 202–210.

Taylor, S., Koch, W. J., & McNally, R. J. (1992). How does anxiety sensitivity vary across the anxiety disorders? *Journal of Anxiety Disorders, 6,* 249–259.

Teasdale, J. D., & Barnard, P. J. (1993). *Affect, cognition, and change: Remodelling depressive thought.* Hove, UK: Erlbaum.

Voelz, Z. R., Walker, R. L., Pettit, J. W., Joiner, T. E., & Wagner, K. D. (2003). Depressogenic attributional style: Evidence of trait-like nature in youth psychiatric inpatients. *Personality and Individual Differences, 34,* 1129–1140.

Weissman, A. N., & Beck, A. T. (1978). *Development and validation of the Dysfunctional Attitude Scale: A preliminary investigation.* Paper presented at the 86th annual meeting of the American Educational Research Association, Toronto, Ontario, Canada.

Westerhausen, R., Kompus, K., & Hugdahl, K. (2011). Impaired cognitive inhibition in schizophrenia: A meta-analysis of the Stroop interference effect. *Schizophrenia Research, 133,* 172–181.

Westermann, R., Spies, K., Stahl, G., & Hesse, F. W. (1996). Relative effectiveness and validity of mood induction procedures: A meta-analysis. *European Journal of Social Psychology, 26,* 557–580.

Williams, J. M. G., Mathews, A., & MacLeod, C. (1996). The Emotional Stroop task and psychopathology. *Psychological Bulletin, 120,* 3–24.

Zuroff, D. C., Blatt, S. J., Sanislow, C. A., III, Bondi, C. M., & Pilkonis, P. A. (1999). Vulnerability to depression: Reexamining state dependence and relative stability. *Journal of Abnormal Psychology, 108,* 76–89.

6

Implementing an Evidence-Based Approach to Cognitive-Behavioral Assessment

John Hunsley and Katherine Elliott

Attention to the critical role that assessment plays in interventions for all client age groups has long been a hallmark of the cognitive-behavioral family of treatment approaches (Kendall & Korgeski, 1979; Mash & Hunsley, 1990, 2004). Since their initial development, behavior therapies, cognitive therapies, and cognitive-behavioral therapies (hereafter referred to collectively as CBT) have all emphasized the importance of accurately assessing clients before commencing treatment, closely monitoring the impact of treatment, and evaluating treatment outcome. Because of this, clinicians providing these treatments are particularly well placed to engage in evidence-based practices, including evidence-based assessment activities. In this chapter, we begin by briefly describing the nature of evidence-based psychological practice and, especially, evidence-based assessment (EBA). After examining the current state of EBA, we focus specifically on EBA within the context of CBT and, in particular, on the assessment of cognitive variables assumed to mediate the effects of treatment. Some of these issues are illustrated in a presentation of a theoretically driven, evidence-based approach to assessment in the treatment of generalized anxiety disorder. We conclude the chapter by considering the current challenges and barriers associated with being truly evidence-based in assessment activities associated with treatment provision.

EVIDENCE-BASED PSYCHOLOGICAL PRACTICE

In an attempt to reduce the time between the publication of replicated research findings and their incorporation into daily practice, many efforts were made in the United States during the 1980s and 1990s to develop medical practice guidelines. The purpose of these guidelines was to provide both practitioners and, to some extent, patients with statements about the most appropriate treatment for a particular condition (Institute of Medicine, 1992). Around this time, in Canada and the United Kingdom, the evidence-based medicine movement was developed on the premise that applying empirical knowledge to medical services would improve patient care (Sackett, Rosenberg, Gray, Haynes, & Richardson, 1996). This movement subsequently spread to the United States (e.g., Institute of Medicine, 2001) and many other countries.

The term "evidence-based" refers to a concept that is increasingly applied to many forms of work in a diverse number of fields. It involves the examination and synthesis of information drawn from a wide array of sources in order to guide the practitioner to consider the best available treatment option for a particular patient (Institute of Medicine, 2001). The sources of information that are typically considered include systematically collected data, clinical expertise, and patient preference. The goal is for the practitioner to be able to offer a patient the best options for treatment, according to the current state of research, for the particular problem being addressed (Hunsley, 2007a). Although this may seem to be a fairly straightforward process, the development of evidence-based practice has encountered many obstacles. Translating research findings into practice guidelines, and then disseminating these guidelines in a comprehensive and timely manner has proven to be more challenging than anticipated.

It might seem self-evident that providing CBT to clients ensures, almost by definition, that clients are receiving evidence-based services. Unfortunately, this is not a safe assumption to make. For example, in their survey of psychologists who provided interventions for eating disorders, Mussell et al. (2000) found that although 70% of respondents reported using evidence-based treatments (EBTs), three-quarters of these psychologists had not been trained in the provision of these treatments. Similarly, Becker, Zayfert, and Anderson (2004) surveyed psychologists who provided treatments for posttraumatic stress disorder (PTSD) and found that only one in four had received training in the use of exposure and that only 17% reported using any form of exposure in their treatment of clients with PTSD. In other words, "doing CBT" is not necessarily the same as "doing CBT properly."

Because it can be difficult for practitioners to keep up with research developments, there is a need for summaries of evidence provided by expert reviews (Chambless & Ollendick, 2001). Several databases have been developed that provide this information, such as the Cochrane Collaboration. Similarly, nongovernmental organizations, such as the National Institute for Health and Care Excellence (NICE) in England and Wales, provide both policy directives and clinician-friendly clinical guidelines. These guidelines are based on the best available evidence and are refined through extensive consultation procedures. Although problems and concerns exist regarding the use and accuracy of these types of data sources (cf. Chambless & Ollendick, 2001; Hunsley, 2007b), there is little doubt that the evidence-based movement has established itself within the field of medicine and is growing within professional psychology.

Psychology's initial efforts in this regard focused on identifying "empirically validated" or "empirically supported" treatments based on specific criteria mainly focused on methodological issues (Chambless & Ollendick, 2001). A great deal of debate ensued following these efforts, involving questions about the nature and suitability of the research base used to identify treatments and the exclusive focus on treatment outcome studies. More recently, national psychology organizations, such as the American Psychological Association, have adopted evidence-based practice as a key strategy for promoting effective psychological services (American Psychological Association Presidential Task Force on Evidence-Based Practice, 2006). It is now generally accepted that evidence-based practice must include all relevant research evidence, not just the results of clinical trials (cf. Norcross, 2011). For much of the research literature, evidence hierarchies can be used to indicate the best available research evidence. In general, all health care professions (including psychology) typically consider expert opinion to be at the bottom of the hierarchy. Above this are case studies, followed by controlled case studies, group research designs with threats to internal validity, then group research designs with strong internal validity (including the gold standard, randomized controlled trials). At the top of this research hierarchy are systematic reviews and meta-analyses of studies with the most rigorous methodologies (Hunsley, 2007a).

EVIDENCE-BASED ASSESSMENT

Consistent with the principles of evidence-based psychological practice, EBA is an approach to psychological assessment that emphasizes the use of research and theory to guide decisions related to assessment activities and the interpretation of data obtained from these activities. This entails (1) the selection of constructs to be assessed for a specific assessment purpose, (2) the methods and measures to be used in the assessment, and (3) the manner in which the assessment process proceeds (Hunsley & Mash, 2007; Mash & Hunsley, 2005; McLeod, Jensen-Doss, & Ollendick, 2013). Whether the assessment is being conducted as a stand-alone service (such as with forensic or psychoeducational evaluations) or as part of the delivery of treatment services, the assessment process is inherently a decision-making task that requires hypotheses to be itera-tively formulated and tested. The resulting data, even when collected with psychometrically strong measures, are likely to be incomplete or have inconsistencies, and the clinician must strive to make sense of these data. As a result, an evidence-based approach to assessment must involve attention to this complex decision-making task in light of (1) potential errors and biases in data synthesis and interpretation, (2) the need to balance the costs of the assessment process with a desire for additional clinical data, and (3) the potential impact of the assessment data on treatment-related clinical outcomes such as the provision, alteration, and termination of treatment.

As we mentioned, whenever possible, psychometrically strong measures—those that have consistent evidence of reliability, validity, and, ideally, clinical utility—should be used to assess the constructs targeted in the assessment (for guidelines, see Hunsley & Mash, 2008b). Because assessment instruments can be used for a wide range of purposes, including screening, diagnosis, case conceptualization, treatment monitoring, and treatment evaluation, and because the psychometric properties of these instruments are conditional on the assessment purpose and the population assessed (Haynes, Smith, & Hunsley, 2011), clinicians and researchers face a considerable challenge in selecting measures that are scientifically sound. They must decide, for example, what evidence is most relevant for the assessment task at hand. Although indices of validity such as specificity, sensitivity, positive predictive power, and negative predictive power are crucial in determining whether a measure will be appropriate for screening pur-poses (Hsu, 2002), sensitivity to change is likely to be the most relevant aspect of validity when using measures to monitor and evaluate the impact of treatment. Moreover, as required by the *Standards for Edu-cational and Psychological Testing* (American Educational Research Association, American Psychological Association, & National Coun-cil on Measurement in Education, 1999), assessment measures must have appropriate norms (for norm-referenced interpretation) and/or replicated supporting evidence for the accuracy of cutoff scores (for criterion-referenced interpretation; see also Achenbach, 2005). When evaluating the relevance of norms and/or cutoff scores, the clinician must determine whether the instrument is appropriate for use with the client being assessed. This, in turn, means that attention must be paid to the characteristics of the samples (including age, gender, and ethnicity) on which the supporting scientific evidence was derived.

Considerable progress has been made in identifying EBA instruments (Hunsley & Mash, 2011) for many assessment purposes across a wide range of client ages and conditions (e.g., Antony, Orsillo, & Roemer, 2001; Cohen et al., 2008; Hunsley & Mash, 2008a; Nezu, Ronan, Meadows, & McClure, 2000). These sources provide clinicians with invaluable guides for selecting instruments to be included in EBAs. However, EBA involves much more than the data collected from psychometrically strong measures. Data from psychological measures are typically combined with other sources of information, including life history information, observations of client behavior, collateral information, and, frequently, assessments by other health care professionals. An evidence-based approach to assessment must involve steps to minimize the many ways that error and misinterpretation can occur when integrating and synthesizing these assessment data. Although clear, evidence-based guidelines on how best to assess common disorders and problems are not yet widely available, considerable effort is now focused on how assessment data can be used in an evidence-based manner in routine clinical practice (e.g., Ebesutani, Bernstein, Chorpita, & Weisz, 2012; Jenkins, Youngstrom, Youngstrom, Feeny, & Findling, 2012).

Consistent with how most assessment and treatment research is conducted, EBA encourages a problem-specific approach to assessment, allowing EBA to be seamlessly integrated into EBTs; many examples of this can be found in Hunsley and Mash (2008a) and Antony and Barlow (2010). Although diagnostic systems provide one common alternative for framing the range of disorders and problems to be considered in assessment and treatment, commonly experienced emotional and relational problems (e.g., excessive anger, social skills deficits) that occur in the absence of a diagnosable disorder may also be the focus of EBAs and EBTs (e.g., Chorpita & Daleiden, 2009). Additionally, there are generic assessment strategies or tools that have considerable research support for a range of client problems, such as functional analytic assessments (Haynes, Leisen, & Blaine, 1997; Haynes, O'Brien, & Kaholokula, 2011) and treatment-monitoring systems (Lambert & Shimokawa, 2011). We have much more to stay about treatment monitoring in subsequent sections of the chapter.

On first glance, it might seem that there is little in EBA that goes beyond good assessment practices. In some ways, this is correct, as EBA guides the clinician and researcher to follow scientific evidence and scientific principles throughout the assessment process, and this should be what all are trained to do. Unfortunately, it appears that, for many reasons, standard psychological assessment practices often fall well short of EBA recommendations. For example, (1) many of the psychological instruments most commonly used in clinical settings have little or no supporting scientific evidence of their reliability and validity (e.g., Hunsley, Lee, Wood, & Taylor, 2015); (2) measures are commonly used for populations for which they were neither developed nor normed (e.g., Therrien & Hunsley, 2012); (3) evidence for the clinical utility of most psychological measures and clinical decision-making processes is almost nonexistent (Youngstrom, 2013); and (4) the majority of researchers publishing in psychology journals fail to address or report the reliability values of the scores obtained with the measures used in their studies (e.g., Vacha-Haase & Thompson, 2011). Clearly, all is not well with respect to the attention to science evident in current psychological assessment practices.

Assessment practices associated with CBT practices are not immune to these problems. For example, all clinicians and researchers should know the basic fact that reliability is a property of the scores obtained with a measure in a given sample, not an immutable property of the measure itself. Nevertheless, a meta-analysis of the reliability values obtained with the Beck Depression Inventory (BDI) found that only 7.5% of published articles in which the BDI was used reported meaningful reliability estimates for the samples used in the research (Yin & Fan, 2000). To obtain a sense of how widespread the failure to report sample reliability values is in the current CBT literature, we reviewed the most recent issue of *Cognitive Therapy and Research* at the time of writing of this chapter (Volume 36, Issue 6). This journal was selected because of its CBT focus and the high quality of the research it publishes. Of the 20 articles published in the issue, 11 (55%) reported sample reliability values for all or almost all of the measures used in the study. Of the other 9 articles, 5 provided reliability values found in other studies (i.e., reliability induction) and 4 failed to even mention reliability. Among the 11 articles reporting sample reliability values, a total of 83 different measures were used for which internal consistency values were relevant (i.e., total scores, scales, subscales, etc.). For 64% of these measures, the reported sample reliability value was above .70; for 17% of the measures, the reported sample reliability value was below .70, and for 19%, no value was reported (usually this was in the context of giving a range of sample reliability values for a multiscale instrument). Our point is not intended to be a criticism of the journal or of the quality of other aspects of the articles we examined. Nevertheless, assuming the representativeness of these findings, attention is most definitely lacking to the basic psycho-metric construct of reliability in much CBT-relevant research.

The lack of evidence for the clinical utility of assessment tools and procedures also affects the provision of CBT services. Many cognitive-behavioral EBTs involve the repeated use of a recommended set of instruments at several points before, during, and after treatment. These instruments are aimed at providing the clinician or researcher with a wide range of cognitive, affective, behavioral, and interpersonal data deemed to be relevant to the provision of treatment and the evaluation of its impact on the client. However, it is common to hear in clinical settings that there is insufficient time to administer an extensive battery of measures, and only one or two very brief measures may be consid-ered for routine clinical use. Although the downplaying of the need for assessment data may well be a cause for concern, it is next to impos-sible to mount an empirically based argument against such practices, as there is very little evidence that using the instruments recommended in treatment manuals is necessary for treatment success. What assessment data are necessary to enhance the likelihood of a positive outcome for clients? At this point in time, we simply do not know this for any form of cognitive-behavioral intervention.

EVIDENCE-BASED ASSESSMENT IN CBT

Despite these gaps in our knowledge, there is a natural fit between EBA and cognitive-behavioral interventions. Many of the assumptions and principles of EBA are consistent with cognitive-behavioral assessment practices, and an emphasis on diagnosis, research-informed case formu-lations, and the monitoring of treatment effects throughout the dura-tion of services are all common components of most CBT approaches. Moreover, many of the evidence-based instruments available to assess clients of all ages measure constructs central to CBT approaches (e.g., symptom classes and profiles, interpersonal and social functioning, and, of course, cognitive phenomena). In the following sections we outline some of the issues to be considered when striving to conduct EBAs as part of CBT treatments.

Diagnostic Assessment

EBA relies on scientific evidence from research on psychopathology, assessment, and intervention, among other areas, to aid clinicians in selecting relevant constructs to assess. Given that much of this litera-ture is based on research participants who were diagnosed with specific mental disorders, the results of a diagnostic evaluation allow the clinician to search the psychological literature for key constructs to assess as part of the case formulation and for treatment options to offer the client. Within a CBT framework this could involve consideration of client health issues (e.g., common comorbid conditions and chronic health problems), social/interpersonal characteristics (e.g., conflictual intimate and work relationships, work functioning, and health care utilization), and cognitive characteristics (e.g., dysfunctional beliefs, rumination tendencies, and counterproductive self-statements) that warrant further evaluation. Even the most casual observer of the psychological treatment literature knows that, notwithstanding recent efforts to develop transdiagnostic treatments, most CBT treatment research focuses on the treatment of a specific diagnostic category, usually from the American Psychiatric Association's *Diagnostic and Statistical Manual of Mental Disorders* (DSM). Indeed, this tendency is so ingrained in the treatment research literature that most attempts to identify and disseminate psychological EBTs explicitly organize such treatments by diagnostic categories (e.g., Nathan & Gorman, 2007). This means that, at a very basic level, diagnosis has utility in determining which treatments are most likely to be beneficial for a diagnosed client.[1]

Of course, many practitioners with a behavioral orientation are skeptical about the clinical utility of diagnosis. This is not the appropriate venue to examine the merits or limitations of such a perspective. We would simply note that, based on the extent to which diagnostic categories inform the content and organization of most CBT handbooks and texts, diagnostic considerations are important for most professionals working within a CBT framework. Additionally, although hardly a scientific consideration, the reality for many clinicians is that the extent of reimbursement for their services is dependent, in large part, on the diagnoses received by clients. Accurate diagnosis, therefore, can be critically important in order to obtain access to appropriate services.

The first assessment challenge confronting the CBT clinician who

---

[1]The gold standard in evaluating such treatments is, of course, the use of randomized controlled trials in which participants diagnosed with a specific disorder are randomly assigned to various treatment conditions. For numerous conceptual and ethical reasons, there is no research in which a range of psychological treatments are randomly assigned to participants with differing diagnoses (e.g., how well does cognitive therapy for depression fare with those diagnosed with specific phobias as compared to participants diagnosed with major depressive disorder?). Without intentionally "mismatching" treatments to clients and evaluating the resulting treatment effects, it is probably more accurate to say that diagnosis has pseudo-utility with respect to the identification of treatments likely to be of benefit (Nelson-Gray, 2003).

wishes to implement an appropriate EBT is to accurately diagnose the client for whom a treatment plan is being developed. Depending on the client's age and general presenting problems, there are a range of psychometrically sound assessment options to consider, most of which are semistructured interviews (Hunsley & Mash, 2008a). The importance of accurately diagnosing a client's problems cannot be understated. Diagnostic inaccuracies can result in the use of potentially suboptimal, inappropriate, or irrelevant treatment strategies. A study of community-based treatments for adolescents by Jensen-Doss and Weisz (2008) nicely illustrates this point. Disagreement between clinician-generated and research-based diagnoses were associated with treatment implementation problems, including an increased number of client "no-shows," cancelled treatment appointments, and treatment dropouts. Not surprisingly, compared to situations in which there was diagnostic agreement, inaccurate clinician-generated diagnoses were also associated with smaller treatment gains. So, does accurate diagnosis necessarily improve CBT outcomes? Given the dearth of evidence on the clinical utility of most assessment tools and practices, there is no direct evidence that answers this question. We suggest, however, that the Jensen-Doss and Weisz (2008) findings should be seriously considered by all CBT practitioners.

In addition to the need to accurately assess a primary diagnosis, the clinician must consider additional diagnoses, as comorbidity is typically the rule in most clinical settings. In a large-scale epidemiology study, Kessler, Chiu, Demler, and Walters (2005) evaluated the extent of comorbidity in adults meeting diagnostic criteria for a mental disorder during the preceding 12-month period. Almost half of diagnosable respondents met criteria for two or more disorders. Furthermore, it is common in studies of comorbidity for individuals to present with three or more disorders (Krueger & Markon, 2006)! Only when a clinician is aware of the presence of comorbidity can a treatment plan be devised to address the full range of clinically significant problems experienced by the client. Our knowledge of the nature and course of comorbid conditions has grown dramatically in recent years (e.g., Kessler et al., 2011; Links & Eynan, 2013). Nevertheless, there is little in the way of evidence-based guidelines for determining how best to assess or treat comorbid conditions (Youngstrom, 2013), thus requiring the clinician to exercise good judgment (informed by relevant research and clinical experience) in determining how to prioritize a client's treatment needs and/or when to consider treatment options based on transdiagnostic principles. Knowing what disorders the client has is, in most instances, the best way for clinicians to consult the research literature in order to make these decisions.

Case Formulation

For many mental health professionals, the term "diagnosis" has a meaning that encompasses, but is more than, a narrow focus on a taxonomy of mental disorders. Terms such as "diagnostic formulation," "case conceptualization," or "case formulation" are probably more accurate reflections of what the term means. For those operating within a CBT framework, the taxonomic diagnosis provides an organizing structure around which an idiographic formulation is developed. This formulation identifies the nature of the client's problems, the factors that are hypothesized to cause and/or maintain the problems, treatment options to address the problems, and predictions about the eventual outcome of the problems if left untreated (Haynes, O'Brien, et al., 2011; Mash & Hunsley, 2007). In the early days of CBT there was often tension regarding the incorporation of nomothetic information (e.g., empirically based models of mental disorders, data from standardized psychological instruments) into case formulations (Mash & Hunsley, 1990). Many concerns were raised about the relevance of generalized self-report measures, trait measures, and unsystematic observations for conducting functional analyses of behavior. With an increased focus on developing and using appropriate assessment measures and processes, most current CBT assessment and case formulation approaches routinely include such nomothetically based data (e.g., McLeod et al., 2013; Persons, 2005). Indeed, most CBT treatment manuals explicitly encourage the clinician to begin with a scientifically sound model of psychopathology and then individually tailor the treatment to optimally fit a client's needs. Kendall and colleagues have aptly termed this approach "flexibility within fidelity" (Kendall & Beidas, 2007; Kendall, Gosch, Furr, & Sood, 2008). At the risk of stating the obvious, the assessments underlying the tailoring of treatments must be accurate and should include data obtained with evidence-based instruments.

Case formulations are presumed to have clinical value because they guide the clinician to develop a treatment focused on modifiable hypothesized causal and/or maintaining factors, thus potentially permitting the greatest possible changes in client functioning (cf. Haynes, O'Brien, et al., 2011). Despite the almost ubiquitous reliance on case formulations to guide treatment provision in CBT and other theoretical orientations, the evidence base for the reliability and validity of these procedures is remarkably limited (Beiling & Kuyken, 2003). Moreover, with the exception of functional analytic case formulations (Haynes et al., 1997), there is virtually no evidence addressing the clinical utility of case formulations. For example, compared to providing treatment based solely on taxonomic diagnoses, we do not know whether individually tailored case formulations result in treatment that is more effective, of shorter duration, or less costly.

Most clinicians take it as an article of faith that case formulations are critical for providing professionally responsible treatments. In order to develop formulations that are truly informed by evidence, what is required is an extensive scientific literature on the environmental, interpersonal, and intrapersonal factors that consistently serve to moderate the effects of treatment. With this information in hand, clinicians and researchers could turn their attention to developing and using assessment tools and procedures designed specifically to assess these factors. Thus there is much work to be done before one can safely conclude that case formulations, including CBT case formulations, are truly evidence-based and essential in ensuring high-quality services.

Treatment Monitoring and Outcome Evaluation

The relation between EBA and EBT involves much more than simply formulating an accurate diagnosis and then selecting and tailoring a designated EBT for this disorder. In the broader realm of psychological service provision, Weisz, Chu, and Polo (2004) have noted how the dialectic of assess → treat → reassess → adjust treatment → reassess is not well articulated in relation to current clinical practice. With respect to CBT, however, the situation is entirely different. Since its inception, CBT has been predicated on the importance of having assessment data guide treatment efforts throughout the course of services. Clinicians working within a CBT framework are likely to be very well versed in monitoring the impact of treatment as it unfolds, and then using these data to adjust treatment strategies and directions as needed. Indeed, almost every CBT manual or book explicitly recommends variables that might need to be assessed throughout treatment and, usually, offer suggestions on the use of specific instruments and the frequency with which they should be used. Indeed many of the guides currently available for monitoring the impact of treatment have been based on cognitive-behavioral assessment principles (e.g., Woody, Detweiler-Bedell, Teachman, & O'Hearn, 2003).

Surprisingly, much of the evidence on the impact of treatment monitoring on treatment outcome has been conducted by researchers who are outside of the CBT tradition, and recent reviews of this work (e.g., Duncan, 2012; Overington & Ionita, 2012) fail to mention that, for several decades, it was only CBT practitioners who routinely tracked client progress in a systematic manner. This is rather ironic, as it has been contended that much of the clinical success of EBTs, most of which are CBT interventions, stems from the use of treatment-monitoring strategies (Hunsley & Mash, 2010). After all, in the clinical trials that provide the evidence supporting EBTs, some form of session-by-session evaluation and/or evaluation at selected treatment points always occurs, and the outcome of treatment is always evaluated against pretreatment levels of functioning.

The bottom line is that there is now compelling evidence of the value of using client progress data in treatment provision. In a recent meta-analysis, data were summarized from several large-scale randomized trials involving the tracking of treatment effects for thousands of adult clients, across a range of treatment approaches (Lambert & Shimokawa, 2011). Tracking client progress influenced both treatment successes and failures: Compared to the clients of therapists who did not receive treatment progress data, the clients of therapists who received these data had 3.5 times higher odds of achieving reliable clinical change and less than half the odds of experiencing deterioration during treatment. Clearly, CBT practitioners should continue the practice of closely monitoring clients' responses to treatment. They may also want to consider incorporating one of the progress-monitoring tools reviewed by Overington and Ionita (2012) into their practices. One of the main advantages of such tools, compared to the use of a self-report measure such as the Beck Depression Inventory–II, is that session-by-session norms have been developed to indicate whether a client's treatment progress is consistent with likely treatment success or failure.

AN EVIDENCE-BASED APPROACH TO ASSESSING COGNITIVE CONSTRUCTS

As demonstrated by the extensive research presented in other chapters in this volume, considerable progress has been made in the development of tools to evaluate cognitive phenomena, and the range of standardized approaches available for these purposes is impressive. In addition to commonly used self-report methods that employ endorsement, recall, or production instructions, there are now a number of performance-based approaches to measuring cognitive variables (e.g., implicit association tasks, eye tracking). There is growing evidence that many of these instruments and procedures have strong psychometric properties. For example, using the tripartite classification system of cognitive structures, cognitive processes, and cognitive content, Dunkley, Blankstein, and Segal (2010) presented summary information on literally scores of measures available for the cognitive assessment of anxiety and depression. For many CBT interventions it is highly likely that cognitive constructs will play a central role, both in clinicians' case formulations and in the variables targeted for change as part of a comprehensive treatment plan. As a result, select cognitive variables will undoubtedly be measured at multiple points throughout the treatment process.

As we have already highlighted, the question of the clinical utility of assessment tools and strategies is one that has been largely neglected in clinical psychology (Hunsley & Mash, 2007; Youngstrom, 2013) and, unfortunately, this is also true in the realm of cognitive assessment. Evaluations of cognitive measures for research purposes have not been matched by efforts to establish their value in clinical contexts. As has been the case for observational coding systems, assessment tools that have repeatedly shown their value for research purposes do not necessarily have a significant role to play in typical clinical practice (Mash & Foster, 2001).

Many assessment issues fundamental to a clinician's decision to use a cognitive measure with clients have simply not been explored. Is one measure better than another for assessing the same cognitive construct across clients with the same diagnosis? Does the assessment of cognitive structures, processing, and/or content predict psychological functioning or diagnostic status above and beyond other readily available life history data or other psychological measures? Do data from cognitive measures result in more complete or more useful case formulations, and are such formulations reasonably consistent across time and clinicians? Is there any clinical value in assessing clients with cognitive performance tasks (such as Stroop procedures and methodologies described in other chapters), and is there value beyond what can be gained with more commonly used and readily available endorsement or production measures of cognitive content? Given the relatively limited time available for obtaining assessment data throughout treatment, what level of specificity is best in assessing cognitive phenomena, and does this conclusion hold for cognitive structures, processes, and content? Does the monitoring of cognitive phenomena, in addition to the tracking of symptoms and psychological functioning, result in treatment that is more efficient, more powerful, or more cost-effective? Cognitive assessment researchers (and psychological assessment researchers in general, for that matter) have much work to do in order to adequately consider the applied value of instruments and procedures frequently used in research studies.

Keeping in mind that the development of EBA tools and strategies, much like construct validity, is always a "work in progress," what would an evidence-based approach to cognitive assessment look like? As described earlier in this chapter, the constructs to be included as part of case formulation and treatment-monitoring efforts would have solid, replicated empirical evidence for these assessment purposes. The best standardized tools to assess these constructs (i.e., extensive evidence of reliability and validity, availability of appropriate norms or cutoff scores) would be chosen. As evident in this volume, there are a number of instruments and procedures that may be potentially relevant, at least based on reliability and validity data. To accurately interpret the data yielded by these measures, appropriate norms are required and, although some encouraging steps have also been taken in establishing normative data for cognitive measures (e.g., Dozois, Covin, & Brinker, 2003), this is an aspect that definitely needs more attention if the measures are to have clinical utility. Ideally, the synthesis and interpretation of these data, incorporating other cognitive and noncognitive psychological measures, would be guided by empirically derived rules. In the absence of these rules, awareness of the potential impact of decision-making biases and heuristics is important, and steps would be taken to reduce the occurrence and impact of assessment errors stemming from these factors. All in all, this is a rather tall order, but it is certainly possible within the foreseeable future for some well-established cognitive measures.

As we indicated previously in the chapter, suggestions such as these may seem obvious to many clinicians and researchers and may appear to add little to what is assumed to be good assessment practices. EBA principles do serve as reminders about the importance of science in psychological assessment. Although for some clinicians such reminders may not be necessary, it is important to remember that, as we have described, surveys have found that many clinicians offering CBT services have not actually received much training to provide these services. For many, therefore, attention to EBA principles may enhance the quality of the services they provide.

EBA AND CBT: AN ILLUSTRATION IN THE ASSESSMENT OF GENERALIZED ANXIETY DISORDER

Dugas, Gagnon, Ladouceur, and Freeston (1998) developed a theoretical model for understanding and treating generalized anxiety disorder (GAD) that has direct clinical implications. Their model provides a fine example of how instruments can be developed and validated for both research and clinical purposes. It involves four key constructs: intolerance of uncertainty, beliefs about worry, negative problem orientation, and cognitive avoidance. The researchers proposed that if one possesses a general intolerance of uncertainty, ambiguous situations can activate beliefs held about worry. This, in turn, leads to anxiety, at which point, as a coping mechanism, one will engage in either cognitive avoidance or poor problem orientation, which further fuels the anxiety within the ambiguous situation.

Intolerance of uncertainty is the central component of the model. The assumption is that this dispositional characteristic is developed based on negative beliefs and attitudes toward uncertainty (e.g., uncertainty is unfair, stressful, interferes with functioning, and should be avoided). In turn, this characteristic is hypothesized to affect the way one attends to, appraises, and retains ambiguous information in the environment, thereby directly affecting information processing that leads to increased worry about the outcome of uncertain events (Sexton, Francis, & Dugas, 2007).

The second key construct in the model involves beliefs about worry, which can be both positive and negative (Sexton et al., 2007). Positive beliefs about worry refer to the frequent reports of those who suffer from GAD that worry is a positive personality trait and serves a beneficial purpose (e.g., it is motivating, facilitates problem solving, and can even alter events). However, beliefs about worry can also include negative themes. For example, commonly reported negative beliefs include the belief that worry can disrupt performance, increase a problem, as well as cause emotional discomfort. Finally, a distinguishing feature of worry associated with GAD has been the worry about the negative consequences of worrying itself.

The third construct in Dugas's model is negative problem orientation. This is the belief that one is unable to solve a problem, or that the process of solving a problem is very difficult and challenging. This is distinct from a person's actual ability to solve a problem that appears to be unrelated to GAD (Dugas, Freeston, & Ladouceur, 1997).

The final construct in the model is cognitive avoidance. In the model, worry is treated as a predominantly verbal–linguistic experience that allows one to avoid the physiological arousal associated with negative images and, therefore, the emotional processing of the feared, negative outcomes (Sexton et al., 2007). Cognitive avoidance includes strategies such as thought suppression, thought substitution, the transformation of images to verbal thoughts, distraction, and the avoidance of threatening stimuli.

Most relevant for our purposes, extensive efforts by Dugas and colleagues have been made to develop measures designed to assess the constructs of this model. These include the Intolerance of Uncertainty Scale (IUS), the Why Worry–II (WW-II), the Negative Problem Orientation Questionnaire (NPOQ), and the Cognitive Avoidance Questionnaire (CAQ). The IUS is a 27-item measure that assesses the key uncertainty construct in Dugas's model (Buhr & Dugas, 2002). To date, the scale shows excellent internal consistency in a sample of French-speaking (N = 216) and English-speaking university students (N = 276) (alpha = .91 and .94, respectively). Test–retest reliability over a 5-week period has been demonstrated with the French version of the scale in a sample (N = 78) of French-speaking university students (r = .78) (Dugas et al., 1997). The scale further shows excellent convergent, criterion, and discriminant validity. Although prior studies have demonstrated five- and four-factor structures, a recent examination of the English translation has shown a two-factor structure which provides a good fit to the data (Sexton & Dugas, 2009).

The WW-II is a 25-item measure that assesses five possible beliefs about the usefulness of worry: It (1) aids in problem solving, (2) motivates, (3) protects against negative emotions, (4) can alter actual events (thought–action fusion), and (5) is a positive personality trait (Holowka, Dugas, Francis, & Laugesen, 2000). Based on results found in a study using undergraduate university students (N = 165), the measure showed excellent internal consistency (alpha = .93) overall as well as for each of the above-mentioned subscales (alpha = .81, .84, .81, .75, and .71, respectively). It further showed good test–retest reliability over a 6-week period (r = .80).

The NPOQ is a 12-item measure of negative attitudes toward problems as well as the ability to solve them (Robichaud & Dugas, 2005a). Based on results found in a study using a sample of university students (N = 201), this Likert-type scale demonstrated excellent internal consistency (alpha = .92) as well as good test–retest reliability over 5 weeks (r = .80). This measure further demonstrated both convergent and divergent validity in a second study using a sample of university students (N = 148) with other measures of negative and positive problem orientation and showed strong correlations with measures of worry, anxiety, and depression (Robichaud & Dugas, 2005b).

The CAQ is a 25-item measure of five cognitive strategies: thought substitution, transformation of images into thoughts, distraction, avoidance of threatening stimuli, and thought suppression (Sexton & Dugas, 2008). Based on results found in a study of university students (N = 456) the English translation showed excellent overall internal consistency (alpha = .95) as well as good internal consistency for each of the above-mentioned subscales (alpha = .86, .73, .89, .87, and .87, respectively). The CAQ demonstrated good test–retest reliability (N = 130) over a 4- to 6-week period (r = .85). There is support, based on confirmatory factor analysis, for the proposed subscales as well as evidence for convergent and divergent validity for the measures of worry, thought suppression, and dispositional coping styles (Sexton & Dugas, 2008).

Overall, the model is showing considerable promise in both improving our understanding of GAD and providing more accurate diagnoses of adults suffering from GAD. For example, Dugas, Marchand, and

Ladouceur (2005) found that the model (as measured by the CAQ, IUS, WW-II, and the Social Problem-Solving Inventory—Abridged) was related to explaining worry (an important component of GAD) and not to the fear of physiological symptoms of anxiety, agoraphobic cognitions, or behavioral avoidance (as seen in panic disorder with agoraphobia). They further found that intolerance of uncertainty (the key feature within the model) was specific to participants suffering from GAD. Although there is a need for research using the measures with clinical samples, the psychometric evidence gathered to date is very encouraging.

The model provides an excellent example of how attention to accurate assessment of cognitive variables is essential for an increased understanding of what is unique about GAD and what is shared in common with other anxiety disorders. This, is turn, should lead to new and/or improved options for CBT approaches to GAD. In light of a number of our comments in this chapter, a central concern from a clinician's standpoint is whether the use of these instruments is likely to lead to shorter, better, or more cost-effective treatment. Evidence for the clinical utility of these measures is likely to have a critical effect on the extent to which these measures are adopted by clinicians providing services to clients with GAD.

IMPLEMENTING EBA WITHIN CBT SERVICES

Cognitive-behavioral practitioners are more likely to be open to evidence-based practices than are clinicians espousing other theoretical orientations (e.g., Stewart, Chambless, & Baron, 2012). Moreover, because the value of assessment has long been recognized within CBT approaches to psychological services, there is a tradition of developing assessment tools and then using these measures to evaluate treatment progress and outcome (Mash & Hunsley, 1990, 2004). That being said, for quite some time many authors have commented on the limited attention paid to the utility of widely used assessment instruments and methods with respect to treatment process and outcome (e.g., Hayes, Nelson, & Jarrett, 1987). Without clear evidence of treatment utility, it is reasonable to question whether the considerable time necessary for accurate and repeated client assessment is truly cost-effective. As a case in point, Lima et al. (2005) found that the information available from clients' pretreatment Minnesota Multiphasic Personality Inventory–2 (MMPI-2) results did not meaningfully enhance the delivery or outcome of evidence-based interventions provided to the clients. Thus, evidence of reliability, content validity, criterion validity, and the like does not guarantee that a measure is useful for clinical purposes, and data on the treatment utility of many instruments are sorely needed.

However, as we described earlier, evidence shows that the availability of accurate diagnostic information and the use of treatment monitoring data can improve treatment outcomes for clients. For CBT practitioners, this result should be heartening, as the assessment tasks of diagnosis and ongoing treatment evaluation are integral components of most CBT approaches. Thus, these assessment activities should continue to be central to the delivery of cognitive-behavioral interventions, but clinicians need to ensure that the diagnostic and treatment monitoring data are obtained with psychometrically strong assessment procedures and measures. This necessitates that professionals make good decisions in their selection of assessment tools, decisions that are informed by the scientific evidence and that involve considering the match between the supporting evidence and the characteristics of the client to be assessed. As described previously, there are many resources available to aid in these tasks.

With the growing emphasis on quality assurance in health care services, there is an important role for assessment data in documenting treatment outcome. Again, clinicians working within a CBT framework are likely well-versed in conducting such evaluations. In selecting benchmarks against which services will be judged, the clinician must ensure that the treatment outcome results are relevant to their clients and that the benchmarks are based on measures shown to yield reliable and valid data across a range of samples. Furthermore, to employ these benchmarks in routine practice, CBT practitioners must then use assessment tools that have strong scientific support and are appropriate for the task at hand. For a number of psychological disorders and conditions, research-derived treatment benchmarks are now available to serve as aids in the evaluation of clinical services (e.g., Hunsley & Lee, 2007; Lee, Horvath, & Hunsley, 2013; Minami et al., 2008; Weersing, 2005).

Of course, all clinicians face considerable challenges in balancing the competing demands on their time. The time required for direct service provision must be balanced with the time needed for administrative tasks, supervisory work, continuing education efforts, and myriad other tasks. Within the context of direct service provision, the time devoted to assessment activities usually means that less time can be devoted to intervention activities. In some clinical settings, ensuring that adequate time is available for assessment before and during treatment may be extremely difficult, especially if assessment time is treated as nonbillable or nonreimbursable work. Thus the contingencies operating in many clinical settings may make it difficult to adequately assess clients and to stay informed about developments in clinical assessment.

CONCLUSIONS

Based on their training, cognitive-behavioral researchers and clinicians should be well-versed in the use of a variety of assessment methods and strategies and should have considerable experience in turning to empirical evidence to guide their assessment activities. However, both critical reviews of the psychological research and surveys of clinicians' assessment practices indicate that more effort must be made to ensure that the selection and use of assessment instruments is informed by scientific evidence and scientific thinking. Thorough diagnostic evaluations and the consistent tracking of treatment progress have been shown to yield considerable benefits to clients receiving psychological treatments. Assessment activities such as these are critical for the efficient and effective delivery of intervention services, and cognitive-behavioral clinicians should be routinely incorporating them into their clinical services. Likewise, we encourage cognitive-behavioral researchers to continue to develop and validate assessment tools that both explicate important psychological processes and aid clinicians in their efforts to enhance client psychosocial functioning and well-being.

KEY POINTS

FOR PRACTITIONERS

- Select and use psychometrically strong assessment measures, with appropriate norms and clinical cutoffs.
- Actively collaborate with clients in all assessment activities, ensuring that they understand the reasons for the assessments.
- Provide clients with timely feedback based on the assessment data.
- Ensure the accuracy of diagnostic evaluations, taking into account diversity considerations and the likely presence of comorbid disorders.
- Monitor client symptoms, treatment goals, and other relevant variables on a consistent and regular basis.
- Use these monitoring data to inform decisions to modify or discontinue treatment strategies.

FOR RESEARCHERS

- Calculate and report in publications the reliability values of all measures used in a study (including structured interviews, self-report measures, and performance measures).
- Be sensitive to age and diversity considerations: Ensure that items and norms are appropriate for the study sample.

- If developing a measure, follow current guidelines for scale development and validation.

FOR STUDENTS AND EDUCATORS

- Have solid knowledge of psychometrics and scientifically informed measurement practices.
- View client assessment as an iterative, hypothesis-testing task.
- Learn about assessment strategies and instruments directly relevant to conducting diagnostic evaluations, developing cognitive-behavioral case formulations, and monitoring treatment progress.
- Recognize the potential impact of cognitive heuristics and biases on all assessment activities, and learn how to take steps to counteract or minimize their effects.
- Stay informed about scientific developments in clinical assessment.

REFERENCES

Achenbach, T. M. (2005). Advancing assessment of children and adolescents: Commentary on evidence-based assessment of child and adolescent disorders. *Journal of Clinical Child and Adolescent Psychology, 34,* 541–547.

American Educational Research Association, American Psychological Association, & National Council on Measurement in Education. (1999). *Standards for educational and psychological testing.* Washington, DC: American Educational Research Association.

American Psychological Association Presidential Task Force on Evidence-Based Practice. (2006). Evidence-based practice in psychology. *American Psychologist, 61,* 271–285.

Antony, M. M., & Barlow, D. H. (Eds.). (2010). *Handbook of assessment and treatment planning for psychological disorders* (2nd ed.). New York: Guilford Press.

Antony, M. M., Orsillo, S. M., & Roemer, L. (Eds.). (2001). *Practitioner's guide to empirically based measures of anxiety.* New York: Plenum Press.

Becker, C. B., Zayfert, C., & Anderson, E. (2004). A survey of psychologists' attitudes towards and utilization of exposure therapy for PTSD. *Behaviour Research and Therapy, 42,* 277–292.

Beiling, P. J., & Kuyken, W. (2003). Is cognitive case formulation science or science fiction? *Clinical Psychology: Science and Practice, 10* 52–69.

Buhr, K., & Dugas, M. J. (2002). The Intolerance of Uncertainty Scale: Psychometric properties of the English version. *Behaviour Research and Therapy, 40,* 931–945.

Chambless, D. L., & Ollendick, T. H. (2001). Empirically supported psychological interventions: Controversies and evidence. *Annual Review of Psychology, 52,* 685–716.

Chorpita, B. F., & Daleiden, E. L. (2009). Mapping evidence-based treatments for children and adolescents: Application of the distillation and matching model to 615 treatments for 322 randomized trials. *Journal of Consulting and Clinical Psychology, 77, 566–579.*

Cohen, L. L., La Greca, A. M., Blount, R. L., Kazak, A. E., Holmbeck, G. N., & Lemanek, K. L. (2008). Introduction to the special issue: Evidence-based assessment in pediatric psychology. *Journal of Pediatric Psychology, 33, 911–915.*

Dozois, D. J. A., Covin, R., & Brinker, J. K. (2003). Normative data on cognitive measures of depression. *Journal of Consulting and Clinical Psychology, 71, 71–80.*

Dugas, M. J., Freeston, M. H., & Ladouceur, R. (1997). Intolerance of uncertainty and problem orientation in worry. *Cognitive Therapy and Research, 21, 593–606.*

Dugas, M. J., Gagnon, F., Ladouceur, R., & Freeston, M. H. (1998). Generalized anxiety disorder: A preliminary test of a conceptual model. *Behaviour Research and Therapy, 36, 215–226.*

Dugas, M. J., Marchand, A., & Ladouceur, R. (2005). Further validation of a cognitive-behavioral model of generalized anxiety disorder: Diagnostic and symptom specificity. *Journal of Anxiety Disorders, 19, 329–343.*

Duncan, B. L. (2012). The Partners for Change Outcome Management System (PCOMS): The Heart and Soul of Change Project. *Canadian Psychology, 53, 93–104.*

Dunkley, D. M., Blankstein, K. R., & Segal, Z. V. (2010). Cognitive assessment: Issues and methods. In K. S. Dobson (Ed.), *Handbook of cognitive-behavioral therapies* (3rd ed., pp. 148–186). New York: Guilford Press.

Ebesutani, C., Bernstein, A., Chorpita, B. F., & Weisz, J. R. (2012). A transportable assessment protocol for prescribing youth psychosocial treatments in real-world settings: Reducing assessment burden via self-report scales. *Psychological Assessment, 24, 141–155.*

Hayes, S. C., Nelson, R. O., & Jarrett, R. B. (1987). The treatment utility of assessment: A functional approach to evaluating assessment quality. *American Psychologist, 42, 963–974.*

Haynes, S. N., Leisen, M. B., & Blaine, D. D. (1997). Design of individualized behavioral treatment programs using functional analytic clinical case methods. *Psychological Assessment, 9, 334–348.*

Haynes, S. N., O'Brien, W. H., & Kaholokula, J. K. (2011). *Behavioral assessment and case formulation.* Hoboken, NJ: Wiley.

Haynes, S. N., Smith, G., & Hunsley, J. (2011). *Scientific foundations of clinical assessment.* New York: Taylor & Francis.

Holowka, D. W., Dugas, M. J., Francis, K., & Laugesen, N. (2000, November). *Measuring beliefs about worry: A psychometric evaluation of the Why Worry–II Questionnaire.* Poster presented at the annual meeting of the Association for Advancement of Behavior Therapy, New Orleans, LA.

Hunsley, J. (2007a). Training psychologists for evidence-based practice. *Canadian Psychology, 48, 32–42.*

Hunsley, J. (2007b). Addressing key challenges in evidence-based practice in psychology. *Professional Psychology: Research and Practice, 38, 113–121.*

Hunsley, J., & Lee, C. M. (2007). Research-informed benchmarks for psychological treatments: Efficacy studies, effectiveness studies, and beyond. *Professional Psychology: Research and Practice, 38,* 21–33.

Hunsley, J., Lee, C. M., Wood, J. M., & Taylor, W. (2015). Controversial and questionable assessment techniques. In S. O. Lilienfeld, S. J. Lynn, & J. Lohr (Eds.), *Science and pseudoscience in clinical psychology* (2nd ed., pp. 42–82). New York: Guilford Press.

Hunsley, J., & Mash, E. J. (2007). Evidence-based assessment. *Annual Review of Clinical Psychology, 3,* 29–51.

Hunsley, J., & Mash, E. J. (Eds.). (2008a). *A guide to assessments that work.* New York: Oxford University Press.

Hunsley, J., & Mash, E. J. (2008b). Developing criteria for evidence-based assessment: An introduction to assessments that work. In J. Hunsley & E. J. Mash (Eds.), *A guide to assessments that work* (pp. 3–14). New York: Oxford University Press.

Hunsley, J., & Mash, E. J. (2010). Role of assessment in evidence-based practice. In M. M. Antony & D. H. Barlow (Eds.), *Handbook of assessment and treatment planning for psychological disorders* (2nd ed., pp. 3–22). New York: Guilford Press.

Hunsley, J., & Mash, E. J. (2011). Evidence-based assessment. In D. H. Barlow (Ed.), *Oxford handbook of clinical psychology* (pp. 76–97). New York: Oxford University Press.

Hsu, L. M. (2002). Diagnostic validity statistics and the MCMI-III. *Psychological Assessment, 14,* 410–422.

Institute of Medicine. (1992). *Guidelines for clinical practice.* Washington, DC: National Academy Press.

Institute of Medicine. (2001). *Crossing the quality chasm: A new health system for the 21st century.* Washington, DC: National Academy Press.

Jenkins, M. M., Youngstrom, E. A., Youngstrom, J. K., Feeny, N. C., & Findling, R. L. (2012). Generalizability of evidence-based assessment recommendations for pediatric bipolar disorder. *Psychological Assessment, 24,* 269–281.

Jensen-Doss, A., & Weisz, J. R. (2008). Diagnostic agreement predicts treatment process and outcomes in youth mental health clinics. *Journal of Consulting and Clinical Psychology, 76,* 711–722.

Kendall, P. C., & Beidas, R. S. (2007). Smoothing the trail for dissemination of evidence-based practices for youth: Flexibility within fidelity. *Professional Psychology: Research and Practice, 38,* 13–20.

Kendall, P. C., Gosch, E., Furr, J. M., & Sood, E. (2008). Flexibility within fidelity. *Journal of the American Academy of Child and Adolescent Psychiatry, 47,* 987–993.

Kendall, P. C., & Korgeski, G. P. (1979). Assessment and cognitive-behavioral interventions. *Cognitive Therapy and Research, 3,* 1–21.

Kessler, R. C., Chiu, W. T., Demler, O., & Walters, E. E. (2005). Prevalence, severity, and comorbidity of 12-month DSM-IV disorders in the National Comorbidity Survey Replication. *Archives of General Psychiatry, 62,* 617–627.

Kessler, R. C., Ormel, J., Petukhova, M., McLaughlin, K. A., Green, J. G., Russo, L. J., et al. (2011). Development of lifetime comorbidity in the World Health Organization World Mental Health Surveys. *Archives of General Psychiatry*, *68*, 90–100.

Krueger, R. F., & Markon, K. E. (2006). A model-based approach to understanding and classifying psychopathology. *Annual Review of Clinical Psychology*, *2*, 111–133.

Lambert, M. J., & Shimokawa, K. (2011). Collecting client feedback. In J. C. Norcross (Ed.), *Psychotherapy relationships that work: Evidence-based responsiveness* (2nd ed., pp. 203–223). New York: Oxford University Press.

Lee, C. M., Horvath, C., & Hunsley, J. (2013). Does it work in the real world?: The effectiveness of treatments for psychological problems in children and adolescents. *Professional Psychology: Research and Practice*, *44*, 81–88.

Lima, E. N., Stanley, S., Kaboski, B., Reitzel, L. R., Richey, J. A., Castro, Y., et al. (2005). The incremental validity of the MMPI-2: When does therapist access not enhance treatment outcome? *Psychological Assessment*, *17*, 462–468.

Links, P. S., & Eynan, R. (2013). The relationship between personality disorders and Axis I psychopathology: Deconstructing comorbidity. *Annual Review of Clinical Psychology*, *9*, 529–534.

Mash, E. J., & Foster, S. L. (2001). Exporting analogue behavioral observation from research to clinical practice: Useful or cost-defective? *Psychological Assessment*, *13*, 86–98.

Mash, E. J., & Hunsley, J. (1990). Behavioral assessment: A contemporary approach. In A. S. Bellack, M. Hersen, & A. E. Kazdin (Eds.), *International handbook of behavior modification and therapy* (2nd ed., pp. 87–106). New York: Plenum.

Mash, E. J., & Hunsley, J. (2004). Behavioral assessment: Sometimes you get what you need. In M. Hersen (Series Ed.) & S. N. Haynes & E. M. Heiby (Vol. Eds.), *Comprehensive handbook of psychological assessment: Vol. 3. Behavioral assessment* (pp. 489–501). Hoboken, NJ: Wiley.

Mash, E. J., & Hunsley, J. (2005). Evidence-based assessment of child and adolescent disorders: Issues and challenges. *Journal of Clinical Child and Adolescent Psychology*, *34*, 362–379.

Mash, E. J., & Hunsley, J. (2007). Assessment of child and family disturbance: A developmental–systems approach. In E. J. Mash & R. A. Barkley (Eds.), *Assessment of childhood disorders* (4th ed., pp. 3–50). New York: Guilford Press.

McLeod, B. D., Jensen-Doss, A., & Ollendick, T. H. (Eds.). (2013). *Handbook of child and adolescent diagnostic and behavioral assessment*. New York: Guilford Press.

Minami, T., Wampold, B. E., Serlin, R. C., Hamilton, E. G., Brown, G. S., & Kircher, J. C. (2008). Benchmarking the effectiveness of psychotherapy treatment for adult depression in a managed care environment: A preliminary study. *Journal of Consulting and Clinical Psychology*, *76*, 116–124.

Mussell, M. P., Crosby, R. D., Crow, S. J., Knopke, A. J., Peterson, C. B.,

Wonderlich, S. A., et al. (2000). Utilization of empirically supported psychotherapy treatments for individuals with eating disorders: A survey of psychologists. *International Journal of Eating Disorders, 27*, 230–237.

Nathan, P. E., & Gorman, J. M. (Eds.). (2007). *A guide to treatments that work* (3rd ed.). New York: Oxford University Press.

Nelson-Gray, R. O. (2003). Treatment utility of psychological assessment. *Psychological Assessment, 15*, 521–531.

Nezu, A. M., Ronan, G. F., Meadows, E. A., & McClure, K. S. (Eds.). (2000). *Practitioner's guide to empirically based measures of depression.* New York: Kluwer Academic/Plenum.

Norcross, J. C. (Ed.). (2011). *Psychotherapy relationships that work: Evidence-based responsiveness* (2nd ed.). New York: Oxford University Press.

Overington, L., & Ionita, G. (2010). Progress monitoring measures: A brief guide. *Canadian Psychology, 53*, 82–92.

Persons, J. B. (2005). Empiricism, mechanism, and the practice of cognitive-behavior therapy. *Behavior Therapy, 36*, 107–118.

Robichaud, M., & Dugas, M. J. (2005a). Negative problem orientation: Part 1. Psychometric properties of a new measure. *Behaviour Research and Therapy, 43*, 391–401.

Robichaud, M., & Dugas, M. J. (2005b). Negative problem orientation: Part 2. Construct validity and specificity to worry. *Behaviour Research and Therapy, 43*, 403–412.

Sackett, D. L., Rosenberg, W. M. C., Gray, J. A. M., Haynes, R. B., & Richardson, W. S. (1996). Evidence based medicine: What it is and what it isn't. *British Medical Journal, 312*, 71–72.

Sexton, K. A., & Dugas, M. J. (2008). The Cognitive Avoidance Questionnaire: Validation of the English translation. *Journal of Anxiety Disorders, 22*, 355–370.

Sexton, K. A., & Dugas, M. J. (2009). Defining distinct negative beliefs about uncertainty: Validating the factor structure of the Intolerance of Uncertainty Scale. *Psychological Assessment, 21*, 176–186.

Sexton, K. A., Francis, K., & Dugas, M. J. (2007). Generalized anxiety disorder. In M. Hersen (Series Ed.) & M. Hersen & J. Rosqvist (Vol. Eds.), *Handbook of psychological assessment, case conceptualization, and treatment: Vol. 1. Adults* (pp. 291–319). Hoboken, NJ: Wiley.

Stewart, R. E., Chambless, D. L., & Baron, J. (2012). Theoretical and practical barriers to practitioners' willingness to see training in empirically supported treatments. *Journal of Clinical Psychology, 68*, 8–23.

Therrien, Z., & Hunsley, J. (2012). Assessment of anxiety in older adults: A systematic review of commonly used measures. *Aging and Mental Health, 16*, 1–16.

Vacha-Haase, T., & Thompson, B. (2011). Score reliability: A retrospective look back at 12 years of reliability generalization studies. *Measurement and Evaluation in Counseling and Development, 44*, 159–168.

Weersing, V. R. (2005). Benchmarking the effectiveness of psychotherapy: Program evaluation as a component of evidence-based practice. *Journal of the American Academy of Child and Adolescent Psychiatry, 44*, 1058–1062.

Weisz, J. R., Chu, B. C., & Polo, A. J. (2004). Treatment dissemination and evidence-based practice: Strengthening intervention through clinician–researcher collaboration. *Clinical Psychology: Science and Practice, 11,* 300–307.

Woody, S. R., Detweiler-Bedell, J., Teachman, B., & O'Hearn, T. (2003). *Treatment planning in psychotherapy: Taking the guesswork out of clinical care.* New York: Guilford Press.

Yin, P., & Fan, X. (2000). Assessing the reliability of Beck Depression Inventory scores: Reliability generalization across studies. *Educational and Psychological Measurement, 60,* 201–223.

Youngstrom, E. (2013). Future directions in psychological assessment: Combining evidence-based medicine innovations with psychology's historical strengths to enhance utility. *Journal of Clinical Child and Adolescent Psychology, 42,* 139–159.

PART II

COGNITIVE ASSESSMENT AND DIAGNOSIS

7

Dimensionality in Cognitive-Behavioral Assessment

Amanda A. Uliaszek, Alison Alden,
and Richard E. Zinbarg

Diagnosis and assessment are intertwined concepts when exploring the topic of dimensionality in psychology and psychiatry assessment practice and research. We begin by noting that not only behavioral, but also cognitive aspects are found in nearly every diagnosis in the fourth edition, text revision of the *Diagnostic and Statistical Manual of Mental Disorders* (DSM-IV-TR; American Psychiatric Association, 2000). Thus, the ability to assess behavioral and cognitive symptoms is integral to the ability to diagnose many disorders. Examples include avoidance behavior in various anxiety disorders, suicide attempts in major depression, substance use in situations in which it is physically hazardous in substance use disorders, worry in generalized anxiety disorder, dissociation in borderline personality disorder, and delusions in schizophrenia. The ongoing debate between dimensional versus categorical models of diagnosis and assessment should therefore be of interest to all those interested in cognitive-behavioral assessment, diagnosis, and case formulation. This chapter outlines the pros and cons of continuous versus categorical assessment, the importance of taxometric research, the role of comorbidity, as well as implications from DSM-5 (American Psychiatric Association, 2013). The goal is to educate readers on both sides of the dimensionality debate and provide recommendations based on current taxometric research and changes in the most recent edition of DSM.

THE DEBATE BETWEEN CONTINUOUS VERSUS CATEGORICAL DIAGNOSIS AND ASSESSMENT

The debate regarding the superiority of continuous versus categorical diagnosis and assessment has been going on for decades, with dozens of books and articles outlining disparate views on the topic (e.g., Haslam, 2003; Kraemer, Noda, & O'Hara, 2004; Kraemer, 2007; Widiger, 1992). Over the previous 20 years, little has changed with regard to the arguments posed by each side. However, only recently has the traditionally categorical DSM attempted to integrate the two sides. The intention is to bring the main document driving clinical diagnosis and research more in line with strong opinions heralding the pros of continuous assessment. Here we present a brief history of the traditionally categorical DSM, as well as a detailed description of the pros and cons of categorical versus continuous diagnosis and assessment. A summary can be found in Table 7.1.

Categorical Diagnosis and Assessment

The diagnostic system utilized by both DSM-5 (American Psychiatric Association, 2013) and the *International Classification of Diseases and Related Health Problems, 10th Revision* (ICD-10; World Health Organization, 2004) is based largely on the structure of the nomenclature of the late 19th and early 20th centuries, often referred to as the "Kraepelinian approach" (e.g., Kraepelin, 1919, 1921). In this approach, disorders are classified after a careful observation of signs, symptoms, and course. This is in contrast to many medical diseases, which are classified based on underlying pathological abnormalities (Compton & Guze, 1995).

The first DSM was published (American Psychiatric Association, 1952) as a way to find consistency between the psychiatric conditions seen by military doctors after WWII and the diagnoses typically reported in psychiatric hospitals. The second edition, DSM-II (American Psychiatric Association, 1968), expanded on this approach with the goal of maximizing ease of communication among professionals. However, the first two editions of the DSM were both characterized by vague, imprecise categories. DSM-III (American Psychiatric Association, 1980) marked a major shift with the goal of operationalizing disorders more clearly by providing a description of symptoms, associated features, age of onset, course, impairment, prevalence estimates, gender ratio, familial pattern, and differential diagnosis (Compton & Guze, 1995). In many ways, this was similar to the Kraepelinian approach utilized over 50 years before. This approach to diagnosis stayed consistent throughout the most recent

TABLE 7.1. A Summary of the Pros and Cons of Categorical and Continuous Diagnosis and Assessment

Categorical	Continuous
Pros	
• Concise, parsimonious, clear	• Face validity for some disorders
• Common language	• Tracking treatment outcome
• Intervention and psychopharmacological selection	• Predicts clinical needs
• Outcome in etiological research	• Can provide normative data
• Inclusion criteria in randomized controlled trials	• Statistical benefits
	• Clarity of research results
Cons	
• Imperfect indicator of a disorder	• Availability
• Arbitrary lines of demarcation	• Difficulties in interpretability
• Does not provide a complete clinical picture	• Barriers to communication
• High rates of comorbidity	
• Reduce power (need to increase sample size)	
• Cutpoints may cause conflicting results	

DSM edition, DSM-5, although DSM-5 has made further gains toward the inclusion of dimensions. The categorical approach to classification has many benefits, but also has inherent problems.

Pros

This categorical assessment of symptoms and disorders has many bene-fits that speak to its stability as an approach for 100 years. Most notably, the system might be evaluated as a clear and concise representation of the various disorders. The disorders and associated diagnoses are opera-tionalized clearly with direct language. The criteria for various disorders frequently specify the number of symptoms that must be present (e.g., five out of nine symptoms must be present), the duration that the symp-toms must persist (e.g., 2 weeks or 6 months), and the frequency with which the symptoms must be experienced (e.g., the symptoms must be present more than 50% of the time, or the symptoms must last for at least 1 hour per day). This aids in ease of diagnosing, as well as improves interrater reliability. The resulting categorical diagnoses provide ease in communication between professionals. For example, when someone has a diagnosis of generalized anxiety disorder, we know chronic and uncontrollable worry is a primary symptom. Likewise, we have a common understanding of what defines a panic attack, a binge, or a compulsion. Categorical assessment is therefore useful for "quick and dirty" common language among professionals. Clinically, it can also be a useful starting point in terms of the selection of psychotherapy interventions and drug selection (Kraemer, 2007). For example, diagnostic categories can serve as a heuristic for selecting between exposure therapy (for specific phobia) and cognitive therapy (for unipolar depression or perhaps generalized anxiety disorder). Likewise, categorical diagnoses can guide a clinician in deciding whether to prescribe mood stabilizers (for bipolar disorder) or antipsychotic medication (for schizophrenia).

In addition to the clinical benefits of categorical diagnosis, there are many research benefits. Clinical researchers require a common language of psychopathology when completing literature reviews, replicating previous studies, or drawing hypotheses from a series of studies. In addition, categorical diagnoses may be preferred in certain types of research studies, such as examination of etiology. It is arguably easier to definitively identify causal risk factors or potential diatheses by relating variables to a categorical outcome as opposed to elevations on particular dimensions. Although a researcher could seek to predict a particular cutpoint on a dimensional measure, it is unclear whether this cutpoint has clinical relevance across populations; clinical relevance in a categorical diagnosis is implicit. Categorical diagnoses also are often used as inclusion criteria for randomized controlled trials to ensure a homogeneous sample when testing the efficacy of an intervention (Helzer, van den Brink, & Guth, 2006; Kraemer, 2007). One might argue that this could be accomplished by the use of cutpoints on a continuous measure. However, this becomes unnecessarily subject to the particular parameters of the study, the study population, and the opinions of the researchers involved. The DSM system provides a system for diagnoses without much room for subjective opinion.

Cons

Despite the listed benefits of this method, as well as the long-standing tradition of categorical diagnosis, there are many drawbacks. First, diagnoses refer to a clinician's expert opinion on whether someone has a disorder. Symptoms are, by definition, imperfect indicators of a disorder (Kraemer, 2007). When one is assessing a symptom or making a diagnosis, there is human error in both the assessment method and the diagnostic criteria itself. While both categorical and continuous measures contain error, it may be that the impact of measurement error on categorical diagnoses (or the dichotomizing of continuous measures by utilizing a cutpoint) has a greater impact. Unlike error on a continuous measure, which may cause the rating of a patient's level on a certain dimension to be off by a degree, error in categorical diagnosis yields a diametrically opposed result. In other words, in making categorical diagnoses, a clinician must make a judgment call regarding whether someone has the requisite number and type of symptoms, and error can result in either a false positive or a false negative diagnosis. For example, a person may meet criteria for only three symptoms of dependent personality disorder. According to the categorical system, he has no diagnosis and is not differentiated from the normal population. However, when dimensional scoring rules are utilized, he might be quite elevated relative to the average person and likely differs in impairment, distress, historical factors, and a range of other correlates relative to the average person.

Second, lines of demarcation between symptom and disorder presence or absence are often arbitrary or based on cutpoints from a limited amount of research. For example, if three people report the same symptoms of depression, one person who is depressed for 1 week, one depressed for 2 weeks, and one depressed for 20 years, the latter two receive the same diagnosis of major depressive disorder, even though it would appear that the former two are more similar and would require more similar treatment. In other cases, the diagnostic system has applied categorical distinctions between disorders that, in actuality, appear to be manifestations of the same unidimensional construct and only differ in terms of severity.

A third problem in the clinical setting is that the exact nature or essence of the client is not fully communicated by the diagnosis. For example, to qualify for a diagnosis of borderline personality disorder, one must meet five out nine criteria. Thus two people with the same diagnosis may overlap in only one symptom of the disorder. This is a considerable problem in personality disorder diagnoses in which there is not a defining symptom of any disorder. However, this also is the case with Axis I disorders—two people may each have a diagnosis of major depressive disorder, and one of them may not even report depressed affect. While diagnoses may aid in communication, much information is often missing, and diagnostic labels can sometimes be misleading.

Finally, one of the biggest criticisms of the current diagnostic system is the high rates of comorbidity found across disorders. However, we should note that the problem of high rates of comorbidity are not a necessary consequence of using a categorical diagnostic system. In fact, a poorly constructed continuous system could result in extremely high rates of correlations between disorder dimensions, again making for a highly redundant system. The problem of comorbidity is discussed further in the following section.

There are additional problems when considering categorical diagnoses and clinical research. In fact, many researchers supplant or supplement categorical diagnoses with continuous measures or forgo the use of categories in statistical analyses (Hudziak, Achenbach, Althoff, & Pine, 2007). A primary reason is the low statistical power when using a categorical indicator such as a categorical diagnosis of psychopathology (Cohen, 1983). When power is reduced, the necessary sample size needed to adequately test a hypothesis may increase dramatically. Kraemer (2007) provides a stunning hypothetical example in which a sample size of 200 is needed when a dichotomous diagnosis is utilized compared to a sample size of less than 20 when a continuous measure is used. Finally, results from the same dataset can be drastically different depending on what cutpoints are used (Kraemer et al., 2004). This can cause misleading results in such important areas as effective treatment or disorder etiology.

Continuous Diagnosis and Assessment

Continuous assessment of psychological constructs has a history as long as psychology itself. Whether focused on reaction times, normal personality traits, or skin conductance, psychologists have long since utilized continuous measurement to make sense of psychological constructs. The continuous measurement of psychopathology has a long-standing tradition as well. Many widespread continuous measures of psychopathology have been around for decades: the Minnesota Multiphasic Personality Inventory (Hathaway & McKinley, 1940), the Beck Depression Inventory (BDI; Beck, Ward, Mendelson, Mock, & Erbaugh, 1961), the Hare Psychopathy Checklist (Hare, 1980), and many more that could be added to this list. Thus, clinicians and researchers alike have felt the need for continuous measures of symptoms despite the availability of a categorical diagnostic system that is in widespread use. Next, we highlight the benefits of continuous assessment, as well as the potential drawbacks.

Pros

Consistent with the widespread use of continuous measures, there are a number of benefits to their use. In general, such measures may come across as having more face validity than a dichotomous diagnostic label. Clinicians often need and expect more than a diagnostic label in order to feel as though they have a complete clinical picture. It is unlikely that one would attend a case conference or a grand rounds and hear only a diagnostic label presented; instead, an indication of disorder severity, frequency of various problematic behaviors, and a general description of ancillary symptoms accompanies the diagnosis. Second, continuous measures are better predictors of treatment outcome and clinical needs (e.g., Van Os et al., 1999), as well as current and prospective dysfunction (Gunderson et al., 2000). Most would agree that comparing diagnostic status pre- and posttreatment is not an adequate assessment of treatment gains. Often, continuous measures of symptoms and behaviors are necessary to assess the full clinical picture. Concerning clinical needs, imagine a person presenting for therapy with a specific phobia of driving. This suggests a straightforward treatment of exposure therapy. Now imagine that the person also scores in the clinical range on the Penn State Worry Questionnaire (PSWQ; Meyer, Miller, Metzger, & Borkovec, 1990) and on the Beck Depression Inventory (BDI); it is likely that this person would also benefit from cognitive therapy and behavioral activation to target the worry and depressive symptoms.

Continuous measurement provides benefits to both the clinician and clinical researcher in terms of statistical sophistication. First, the utilization of continuous measures provides the opportunity to assess normative data in the general population and for specific groupings, such as by age, gender, or race (Hudziak et al., 2007). Clients and research participants alike can be assessed according to their specific demographic variables, and level of severity can be determined. In terms of statistical analyses, as described above, continuous measurement allows for an increase in power and lessens the likelihood that a ballooning sample size is needed. Finally, continuous measurement may aid in the clarity of research results. An exclusive focus on categorical findings results in a loss of information, with many of the nuances of the data being overlooked. For example, it is possible for participants to experience a significant decrease in symptoms or a significant increase adaptive coping, but this figure may not be large enough to result in a category jump (i.e., from diagnosis to remission or from low functioning to high functioning). Continuous measurement provides this numerical variation. In addition, the use of continuous measurement allows one to examine the shape of associations; assessing a linear versus curvilinear relationship can provide valuable information regarding the exact nature of the association between variables (e.g., Preacher, Rucker, MacCallum, & Nicewander, 2005).

Cons

First, the availability of some continuous measures may be limited. One must locate and often purchase these measures, as well as access a scoring key and normative data to ease interpretation. This also may be true of certain diagnostic interviews, although many clinical settings may use "in-house" standardized biopsychosocial interviews that are free and focus on the requirements of governmental and private billing agencies.

An additional point relates to ease of interpretation as some clinicians and clinical researchers may continue to have difficulty interpreting the results of such measures. There is little interpretation needed when one is presented with a diagnosis. However, a score of 23 on the BDI or a 47 on the PSWQ requires experience with the measure and knowledge about the related literature. Such interpretations can be somewhat facilitated by focusing on the average item score, as this gives a clinician or researcher some idea of where a person falls in reference to the range of the Likert scale of the measure's items (McDonald, 1999). Even using the average item score, however, it would not be clear whether a score fell in the clinical range.

Finally, communicating the results of continuous measures may be a barrier to treatment or to the dissemination of research findings. Other clinicians or researchers may not be familiar with the measure, the range of the scale, or the normative data and thus have trouble understanding the clinical or research picture. This problem also applies to third-party payment by insurance companies and other reimbursement agencies. Typically, third-party payment companies require categorical diagnoses to assess reimbursement requests. Before continuous measures could be utilized for third-party payments, either cutoffs would need to be established or else algorithms would have to be developed to relate amount of coverage to the severity of scores. Though neither of these tasks should be impossible, they would be challenging.

TAXOMETRIC RESEARCH

As should now be clear, determining whether disorders are better conceptualized as discrete categorical entities or phenomena represented by levels along one or more dimensions has important implications for assessment. However, attempting to distinguish whether something is categorical or dimensional is no easy undertaking. Depending on the sample of individuals that one examines, continuous phenomena can sometimes appear to be categorical and vice versa. For example, if one's sample of interest included only individuals who scored at the two extremes of an underlying dimension (such as detachment), one might mistakenly conclude that this phenomenon was categorical and that all individuals fell into one of two distinct types (e.g., pathologically detached and normal). Continuous phenomena can also appear to be categorical depending on the properties of the items in one's measure. Thus Grayson (1987) has pointed out that if the "difficulty level" (i.e., the point along the underlying latent trait at which an item is maximally discriminating) of most items of a continuous latent trait cluster around a similar level, the distribution of the resulting scale scores will be bimodal (or a cluster analysis would reveal distinct clusters), and one might mistakenly conclude that the phenomenon was categorical. Likewise, measurement error within distinct groups can sometimes make categorical phenomena appear continuous or even normally distributed.

Fortunately, powerful statistical techniques have been developed to test whether the underlying latent structures of constructs are categorical or continuous, and research utilizing such techniques is known as "taxometric research" (Meehl, 1995, 1999; Waller & Meehl, 1998). If a construct is categorical, or "taxonic," individuals are said to fall into nonarbitrary groups at the latent level. In cases in which there are only two latent groups, each individual is said to fall into either the taxon (e.g., disordered group) or its complement class (e.g., the nondisordered group).

An important principle behind taxometric research is that membership in latent classes (or taxa) or scores along latent dimensions influence, but do not completely determine, individuals' scores on manifest variables. The mathematical model underlying taxometric research breaks down the covariance between indicators of a presumptively taxonic phenomenon of interest into covariance within the taxon, covariance within the complement class, and the mean difference between the taxon and the complement class on each of the construct indicators. Each of these components of covariance is weighted in terms of the base rates of the taxon and complement classes within the population that one is studying (Meehl, 1992). Thus, if a phenomenon is truly categorical, two indicators of the taxon will not be associated at all within either the taxon class or the complement class, but will be differentially associated in the overall sample as the proportion of taxon and complement class members changes across subsamples. In contrast, two variables that are indicators of a latent dimension will covary in a fairly consistent manner across subsamples that have been ordered along a third indicator variable (Ruscio & Ruscio, 2004). This general model is the basis for a number of analytic procedures that attempt to determine whether phenomena are indeed taxonic (e.g., mean above minus below a cut [MAMBAC], Meehl & Yonce, 1994; maximum covariance [MAXCOV], Meehl & Yonce, 1996; and maximum eigenvalue [MAXEIG], Waller & Meehl, 1998).

Studies employing taxometric methods should be guided by our prior knowledge of assessment constructs. Both previous research and clinical experience assessing and treating different forms of psycho-pathology can suggest important targets for taxometric analysis. For example, clinicians and researchers alike have observed that there are individuals who appear to have features of personality disorders even if they don't strictly meet the criteria for a particular categorical diagnosis as defined by DSM-5 (American Psychiatric Association, 2013). This observation has prompted recent taxometric research on particularly personality disorders, especially borderline personality disorder (see discussion below). Further, prior assessment research can inform decisions about which indicators of constructs of interest to subject to taxometric analyses. Thus taxonic research has the potential to play an important part in research related to understanding the causes, correlates, and assessment of psychopathology, and the nature of comorbidity.

We would be remiss if we did not point out that Meehl's (e.g., Waller & Meehl, 1998) taxometric methods have some limitations. Thus the same condition that Grayson (1987) noted could lead an examination of bimodality or a cluster analysis to falsely conclude that a continu-ous trait was categorical—clustering of indicators around the same dif-ficulty level—can have similar effects on taxometric analyses (Ganges-tad & Snyder, 1985; Meehl, 1992). Although one may conduct "control analyses" to evaluate this possibility (e.g., Gangestad & Snyder, 1985), a more elegant alternative has been recently introduced. Thus Markon and Krueger (2006) have introduced an information-theoretic approach for distinguishing dimensional from categorical variables that involves comparing the fit of latent class versus latent trait models. As these mod-els explicitly incorporate indicator properties such as difficulty levels, they should be less vulnerable than Meehl's methods to problems such as clustering of difficulty levels.

A final point to make in this section is that as the taxometric litera-ture has matured, there has been growing recognition of the possibility that some phenomena may be neither purely taxonic nor purely dimen-sional (e.g., Bernstein et al., 2010). That is, it is logically possible that distinct classes (i.e., classes that differ qualitatively) might underlie a given observed variable but that there might be meaningful, dimensional variation within each class. Indeed, there is a form of quantitative struc-tural analysis, factor mixture modeling, that allows for modeling such phenomena (Bauer & Curran, 2004; Lubke & Muthen, 2005).

COMORBIDITY

Comorbidity is a phenomenon found across the psychopathology spec-trum. Many researchers consider comorbidity to be problematic and seek to "control" for its effects or exclude comorbid cases entirely. However, a growing body of research has found that comorbidity is a potential source of information regarding etiology, mechanisms, or underlying structure (e.g., L. A. Clark, 2007; Dolan-Sewell, Krueger, & Shea, 2001; Krueger, 2005). Much can be said about the implications for the current categorical diagnostic system on comorbidity. The high rates of comorbidity seen within and between Axis I and Axis II DSM-IV-TR disorders (see Cassin & von Ranson, 2005; Clark, 2005, 2007; Coid, Yang, Tyrer, Roberts, & Ullrich, 2006; Kessler, Chiu, Demler, & Walters, 2005; Skodol et al., 2011) is one of the largest criticisms of the pre-DSM-5 system.

High rates of comorbidity are problematic for a number of reasons. First, comorbidity will naturally increase as the number of diagnostic categories increase—as is the case with the progression from DSM-I to DSM-IV-TR. In this case, comorbidity increases in a spurious way; although it seems that more and more people have multiple diagnoses, this may be only the result of splitting a single syndrome into more and more syndromes. Second, as a result of this "splitting" of disorders, the "Use of This Manual" section in DSM-IV-TR encourages the assignment of multiple diagnoses. This becomes a problem because many clinicians have a limited capacity for actually capturing these additional diagnoses (Zimmerman & Mattia, 2000). Thus comorbid diagnoses are not always assessed, potentially misinforming treatment recommendations. Third, some third-party agencies and health information systems only allow for the coding of a single diagnosis. Analyses of these data then result in erroneous assumptions regarding base rates and treatment utilization (Pincus, Tew, & First, 2004).

There are many potential explanations for the high rates of comorbidity found across disorders. First, symptoms tend to reappear across the criterion for different disorders. Thus a person who meets criteria for one disorder is likely to meet criteria for another (Helzer, Bucholz, & Gossop, 2007). This can be seen in a symptom like restlessness/agitation (which appears across major depression, generalized anxiety disorder, and posttraumatic stress) or physical displays of anger (which appear in both borderline and antisocial personality disorders). Like these two examples, many symptoms are nonspecific and can be applied to a range of disorders, as well as states of normal functioning (Shuckit, 2006). Second, two (or more) disorders may have been inappropriately split when they actually represent a single dimension with inaccurately superimposed categories. This possibility is highlighted by the fact that some disorders have such high rates of comorbidity that they rarely appear in the absence of one another. This is especially true for the DSM-IV-TR Axis II disorders (Skodol et al., 2011); many Axis II disorders appear almost exclusively in the presence of DSM-IV-TR Axis I disorders (e.g., borderline personality disorder and major depressive disorder) and other Axis II disorders (e.g., histrionic and narcissistic personality disorders). In these cases, the explanation for comorbidity may be less about redundant symptoms and more about underlying continuous vulnerability factors that are common to various forms of psychopathology. This liability-spectrum approach is based on the understanding of psychiatric disorders as manifestations of a limited number of underlying liability factors shared by several disorders (Krueger & Markon, 2006).

Taxometric analyses can help clarify whether nominally different diagnoses that exhibit a high degree of diagnostic crossover or comorbidity are actually qualitatively distinct phenomena or lie on a continuum with each other. For example, Gleaves and colleagues conducted multiple taxometric analyses examining eating disorders and concluded that, while bulimia nervosa appears to be qualitatively distinct from normality, it may lie on a continuum with the binge-eating and purging subtype of anorexia nervosa (Gleaves, Lowe, Green, Corove, & Williams, 2000). Should these findings be replicated, it would suggest that we should change the way we assess eating disorders (Gleaves et al., 2000). Whether such changes should consist of adjusting the diagnostic boundaries between disorders or adding dimensional measures of relevant symptoms to our current assessment system is also a matter for future research. Given that, as in the case of anorexia nervosa and bulimia nervosa, seemingly similar disorders are sometimes differentially affected by cognitive therapy treatment packages (Pike, Walsh, Vitousek, Wilson, & Bauer, 2003; Wilson & Fairburn, 1998), using taxometric methods to clarify disorder boundaries and refine assessment measures accordingly is of paramount importance.

IMPLICATIONS FOR COGNITIVE ASSESSMENT AND COGNITIVE-BEHAVIORAL THERAPY

Findings from research examining the dimensionality debate, as well as research on comorbidity and taxometric methods, have important implications for the assessment, treatment, and research of psychopathology. More specifically, employing taxometric methods can enable researchers to answer a number of questions relevant to the debate over how to best assess psychological problems. First, taxometric methods can be used to determine whether a disorder represents a qualitatively distinct phenomenon or lies on the continuum with normal functioning. For example, taxometric methods have been employed in the study of borderline personality disorder. The fact that such methods have failed to find evidence of a latent borderline personality disorder taxon lent support to the proposal to incorporate dimensional measures in assessing this disorder in DSM-5 (Ayers, 2000; Edens, Marcus, & Ruiz, 2008; Rothschild, Cleland, Haslam, & Zimmerman, 2003; Simpson, 1994; Trull, Widiger, & Guthrie, 1990). Although this proposal remains in Section III of the DSM-5, current and future researchers are likely to continue to explore the dimensional conceptualization of personality disorder.

Using taxometric methods to determine whether a disorder, such as borderline personality disorder, is best conceptualized as categorical or dimensional allows clinicians and researchers to maximize the validity and reliability of their assessments (Ruscio & Ruscio, 2004). For example, by incorporating a dimensional measure in diagnosing borderline personality disorder, clinicians will have an organized means of retaining and communicating about clinically valuable information that would not have been captured by a simple categorical diagnosis.

Likewise, clear evidence that a disorder is taxonic can also increase the validity of assessment. Mistakenly conceptualizing categorical diagnoses as continuous can make it more difficult to distinguish the boundary between illness and health and can lead to the selection of nonoptimal cutoff scores on assessment measures (Ruscio & Ruscio, 2004). In other words, establishing that a psychological problem is taxonic can facilitate the development of more accurate standards for assessing it and subsequently determining which individuals could benefit from treatment. If a taxon is found, researchers can examine how closely it corresponds to diagnoses made upon the basis of current diagnostic criteria, and consider adjustments to these criteria that would better enable them to characterize the underlying construct (Meehl, 1986).

Taxometric analyses can clarify whether subtypes of different diagnoses represent qualitatively distinct phenomena or dimensions along which all cases of the disorder vary by degrees. For example, Haslam and colleagues conducted a series of taxometric analyses evaluating whether various cognitive and behavioral symptoms that can occur in the context of obsessive–compulsive disorder represent distinct subtypes of this disorder (Haslam, Williams, Kyrios, McKay, & Taylor, 2005). They found little support for this idea, instead finding that these symptoms appeared to represent different dimensions along which people varied. These findings were largely replicated by subsequent taxometric research that suggested that the only proposed subtype of obsessive–compulsive disorder that seemed to represent a discrete taxometric entity was hoarding (Olatunji, Williams, Haslam, Abramowitz, & Tolin, 2008). Such research suggests that, rather than assessing obsessive–compulsive disorder subtypes, it might be useful to develop some form of profile analysis in which individuals are allowed to vary along cognitive and behavioral symptom dimensions (D. A. Clark, 2005).

Identifying distinct categorical subtypes of disorders such as obsessive–compulsive disorder is important, given that such subtypes can also predict distinct patterns of temporal stability, comorbidity, and treatment response (Leckman et al., 2010). Therefore, assessment of well-validated subtypes of disorders can and should guide initial treatment decisions. However, when taxometric research suggests that "subtypes" are better conceptualized as dimensions, incorporating dimensional measures and profile analyses can help us appreciate the variations in symptom presentation across patients and adjust treatments accordingly (Leckman et al., 2010).

In general, taxometric research has significant implications for how we view psychopathology; more specifically, it builds a strong foundation supporting the benefits of continuous assessment in many circumstances. Because it elucidates the underlying structure of psychopathology and the nature of covariance among disorders, it has significant treatment implications as well. If we know that two disorders are differing points on the same continuum, only differing in severity, than this affects treatment planning and anticipating treatment course and outcome (Bender, Morey, & Skodol, 2011). In addition, if the evidence supporting a categorical distinction between two disorders is weak, then we might assume that an effective treatment for one disorder will be an effective treatment for another. In general, taxometric research has the potential to increase the usefulness and validity of treatment recommendations compared to a traditional system where diagnosis drives the entire treatment plan.

Thus taxometric research has the potential to greatly improve cognitive therapy assessment and treatment. It can be used to determine the fundamental nature of psychological problems, assess the validity of disorder boundaries, and clarify whether it is more relevant to talk about subtypes of a disorder or symptom dimensions. This can facilitate the development of better cognitive therapy assessment measures, which can, in turn, improve treatment decisions.

A PARTIAL SOLUTION: DSM-5

DSM was originally intended as a handbook to aid in clinician assessment and treatment. As described by Kraemer (2007), "diagnostic" or "diagnosis" refers to a clinician's expert opinion as to whether someone has an underlying disorder. "Statistical" refers to the act of counting cases in institutional settings and represents the epidemiological nature of the early DSM. Historically, DSM is categorical and seeks to epitomize and reinforce all of the above mentioned benefits of categorical diagnosis and assessment.

However, the purpose of DSM is no longer to represent a common language for psychiatrists treating a small number of vaguely defined disorders. With each revision, DSM has become more complex and comprehensive, and its purpose and its ramifications now reach a larger number of professionals (psychiatrists, psychologists, child psychologists, psychiatric nurses, etc.) with goals that expand on psychotherapy or psychopharmacological recommendations. DSM is now used as the basis for research, policy change, and pedagogy. The progression of the various versions of DSM have been characterized by the empirical and clinical flavor of the time, with DSM-I and DSM-II focused on clinical utility, DSM-III focused on reliability, and DSM-IV and DSM-IV-TR focused on evidence-based approaches to diagnosis (Kraemer, 2007). DSM-5 has been taxed with the burden of combining all: providing a clinically useful, empirically based tool used in both the clinical and research settings that provides reliable and valid diagnoses. Thus, preparations for DSM-5 spanned many years, involved many outstanding professionals in psychiatry and psychology, and involved the expenditure of thousands (probably millions) of dollars in epidemiological and psychopathology research. The result is several modifications with specific ramifications directly related to the continuous versus categorical debate. Below, we discuss a substantial change in DSM-5 directly related to the integration of continuous measurement into the categorical diagnosis framework. In addition, we discuss the implications for clinical research and clinical assessment.

Hybrid Diagnoses: Categorical plus Continuous

DSM-IV-TR predominantly employs the use of a binary system for diagnoses—someone has a disorder or they do not. However, there are some ways in which DSM-IV-TR has already included the integration of dimensional scoring to provide additional helpful information to a diagnosing clinician or researcher. This is most frequently seen when a binary diagnosis is given and there is an attached unit of severity—mild, moderate, severe—to provide the reader with additional important information. This can currently be seen in the diagnostic categories of alcohol and other substance use disorders, as well as the mood episodes. Dimensional add-ons such as these help increase the reliability and validity of the diagnosis (Helzer et al., 2007; Kraemer, 2007). Although these specifiers exist for a limited number of disorders in DSM-IV-TR, DSM-5 has made continuous methods of diagnosis more ubiquitous.

To this effect, DSM-5 includes several "emerging measures" in Section III. Currently, field trials are testing the reliability, validity, and clinical utility of several measures to use in place of or in tandem with the current diagnostic system. These include cross-cutting symptom measures, disorder-specific severity measures, and personality inventories (see the American Psychiatric Association website for more detail). An example of one such measure includes a measure of severity of illness rating that is applied to the previous week. A clinician using this measure would then answer the following question: "Considering your total clinical experience with this particular population, how mentally ill is the patient at this time?" Then the clinician would rate the client on a 0–7 Likert scale. Including continuous measures of the severity of each symptom and of the disorder as a whole allows for the benefits of categorical diagnoses to be augmented by those of continuous measurement.

A second example involves the anxiety disorders, in which a continuous measure of general severity is being tested to supplement the individual categorical diagnoses. This is different from the symptom-by-symptom or general severity continuous measures described previously. In this case, emotional (e.g., felt anxious, worried, or nervous), cognitive (e.g., thoughts of bad things happening), physiological (e.g., racing heart, sweaty, trouble breathing, faint, or shaky), and behavioral (e.g., avoidance, escape) symptoms common across anxiety disorders are rated by the clinician on a 5-point Likert scale to provide a total score for anxiety severity across all anxiety disorders.

The implementation of a continuous assessment of general anxiety holds benefits for both clinicians and clinical researchers. For clinicians, it provides the opportunity to (1) have a single assessment of anxiety severity, despite the likelihood of a single client's having multiple anxiety diagnoses (Kessler et al., 2005); or (2) assess the severity for each comorbid anxiety diagnosis and then determine the principal diagnosis as the one with the highest severity. In addition to the benefits in assessment, these measures also would be helpful for tracking treatment progress.

In the first approach, clients A and B may each present for cognitive-behavioral therapy for panic disorder with agoraphobia, each meeting full criteria. However, a closer look at the severity measure shows that client A is most distressed and impaired by the physiological symptoms of anxiety (e.g., racing heart, muscle tension, feeling faint), while client B strongly endorses cognitive symptoms (e.g., distracting self, worrying). Thus the treatment recommendations for each client would differ based on the severity measure. It might be best to start client A with progressive muscle relaxation, diaphragmatic breathing, and interoceptive exposures, whereas client B might start with cognitive restructuring and worry diaries.

The second approach would help drive treatment recommendations, sequencing of topics in psychotherapy, and medication selection. For example, imagine a man presenting for cognitive-behavioral therapy and meeting criteria for posttraumatic stress disorder, panic disorder, and specific phobia (spiders), with scores on the continuous severity measure for each individual diagnosis of 42, 30, and 12, respectively. The client arrives in the first session appearing nervous and states that he would like to focus on his fear of spiders, although the assessment shows that this is the least severe problem and the client is likely avoiding the difficult task of exposures to both trauma triggers and panic attack symptoms. The severity measure then helps the clinician collaborate with the client on the most effective means of treatment course.

As mentioned above, researchers often prefer continuous measures because of the increase in statistical power and added benefit of working with data that approaches a normal distribution. The continuous severity assessment provides an increase in options for those completing randomized control trials or research in psychopathology. For example, the severity measure might be used as a moderating factor to further elucidate the benefits of particular treatments on particular populations. A researcher may come to the conclusion that there is no evidence for the effectiveness of a treatment based on the absence of a significant main effect for the treatment. When a severity dimension is introduced as a moderator, results might show that the treatment is effective, but only for those at some particular level of severity. In terms of clinical research, we know that those who share a DSM diagnosis most likely share a series of symptoms or an underlying latent vulnerability. However, it is likely that different people differ in age of onset, impairment, distress, resistance to treatment, and a variety of other disorder characteristics (Kraemer et al., 2004). A continuous measure of severity paired with the diagnosis may help explain causes and concomitants of various other important explanatory variables. This might mean linking an early age of onset to high severity or low levels of resistance to treatment to low severity. Finally, while many researchers do apply continuous measures of psychopathology with the use of self-report questionnaires, symptom counts, and clinician severity ratings (Di Nardo & Barlow, 1988), a DSM-derived system will introduce uniformity across clinical and research settings in much the same way that it does for categorical diagnoses.

CONCLUSION

This chapter demonstrates that the question of "categorical or continuous?" does not have a correct or incorrect answer. As with many similar questions (e.g., "nature or nurture?"), the answer is sometimes one, sometimes the other, and often both. Through an examination of the benefits and drawbacks of the current diagnostic system, as well as the importance of taxometric research, we can state that there is a time and place for both categorical diagnoses and continuous measures in both research and clinical settings. We have the statistical tools available—namely, taxometric analyses, comparing the fit of latent class versus latent trait models, and factor mixture modeling—to determine if a particular set of symptoms best represents discrete taxons, continuous dimensions, or a combination of the two; researchers and clinicians alike should pay particular attention to the research available for their disorders of focus. If we look at the changes in DSM-5, particularly in Section III, we see movement toward a hybrid diagnostic system for many disorders. Thus, we can determine that what we will need is not a "one size fits all" diagnostic system that assumes all problems fit the same structure, but rather a system that distinguishes which problems belong to which of each of the three kinds of structures.

KEY POINTS

FOR PRACTITIONERS

- Attempts should be made to utilize both categorical and continuous measures of psychopathology.
- Categorical diagnoses are best used as a starting point for treatment and psychopharmacology selections.
- Continuous measures are best used to enhance the clinical picture, determine severity, and track treatment outcome.
- DSM-5 provides new information on the importance of continuous assessment.

FOR RESEARCHERS

- Attempts should be made to utilize both categorical and continuous measures of psychopathology.
- Categorical diagnoses are best used as inclusion criteria for highly controlled studies (e.g., randomized controlled trials) or as one of multiple outcome variables in longitudinal studies of etiology or diatheses.
- Continuous measures should be a part of nearly every research study, as they increase power, improve interpretation of results, and decrease required sample size for hypothesis testing.
- Pay close attention to recent developments in taxometric, latent class versus latent trait, and factor mixture modeling research to understand

the underlying structure of psychopathology. Changes from DSM-5 should be incorporated into research hypotheses and assessments.

FOR STUDENTS AND EDUCATORS

- Developments in taxometric, latent class versus latent trait, and factor mixture modeling provide important insight into the underlying structure of psychopathology.
- Be aware of the recent changes in DSM-5 that include additional continuous measures of severity, as well as a dimensional–categorical hybrid model of personality disorders.

REFERENCES

American Psychiatric Association. (1952). *Diagnostic and statistical manual of mental disorders*. Washington, DC: Author.

American Psychiatric Association. (1968). *Diagnostic and statistical manual of mental disorders* (2nd ed.). Washington, DC: Author.

American Psychiatric Association. (1980). *Diagnostic and statistical manual of mental disorders* (3rd ed.). Washington, DC: Author.

American Psychiatric Association. (2000). *Diagnostic and statistical manual of mental disorders* (4th ed., text rev.). Washington, DC: Author.

American Psychiatric Association. (2013). *Diagnostic and statistical manual of mental disorders* (5th ed.). Arlington, VA: Author.

Ayers, W. (2000). *Taxometric analysis of borderline and antisocial personality disorders in a drug and alcohol dependent population.* Unpublished doctoral dissertation, Fordham University.

Bauer, D. J., & Curran, P. J. (2004). The integration of continuous and discrete latent variable models: Potential problems and promising opportunities. *Psychological Methods, 9*, 3–29.

Beck A. T., Ward, C. H., Mendelson, M., Mock, J., & Erbaugh, J. (1961). An inventory for measuring depression. *Archives of General Psychiatry, 4*, 561–571.

Bender, D. S., Morey, L. C., & Skodol, A. E. (2011). Toward a model for assessing level of personality functioning in *DSM–5*: Part I. A review of theory and methods. *Journal of Personality Assessment, 93*, 332–346.

Bernstein, A., Stickle, T. R., Zvolensky, M. J., Taylor, S., Abramowitz, J., & Stewart, S. (2010). Dimensional, categorical, or dimensional-categories: Testing the latent structure of anxiety sensitivity among adults using factor-mixture modeling. *Behavior Therapy, 41*, 515–529.

Cassin, S. E., & von Ranson, K. M. (2005). Personality and eating disorders: A decade in review. *Clinical Psychology Review, 25*, 895–916.

Clark, D. A. (2005). Lumping versus splitting: A commentary on subtyping in OCD. *Behavior Therapy, 36*, 401–404.

Clark, L. A. (2007). Assessment and diagnosis of personality disorder: Perennial issues and an emerging reconceptualization. *Annual Review of Psychology, 58,* 227–257.

Cohen, J. (1983). The cost of dichotomization. *Applied Psychological Measurement, 7,* 249–253.

Coid, J., Yang, M., Tyrer, P., Roberts, A., & Ullrich, S. (2006). Prevalence and correlates of personality disorder in Great Britain. *British Journal of Psychiatry, 188,* 423–431.

Compton, W. M., & Guze, S. B. (1995). The neo-Kraepelinian revolution in psychiatric diagnosis. *European Archives of Psychiatry and Clinical Neuroscience, 245,* 196–201.

Di Nardo, P. A., & Barlow, D. H. (1988). *Anxiety Disorders Interview Schedule—Revised (ADIS-R).* Albany: Phobia and Anxiety Disorders Clinic, State University of New York.

Dolan-Sewell, R. G., Krueger, R. F., & Shea, M. T. (2001). Co-occurrence with syndrome disorders. In W. J. Livesley (Ed.), *Handbook of personality disorders: Theory, research, and treatment* (pp. 84–106). New York: Guilford Press.

Edens, J. F., Marcus, D. K., & Ruiz, M. A. (2008). Taxometric analyses of borderline personality features in a large-scale male and female offender sample. *Journal of Abnormal Psychology, 117*(3), 705–711.

Gangestad, S., & Snyder, M. (1985). "To carve nature at its joints": On the existence of discrete classes in personality. *Psychological Review, 92,* 317–349.

Gleaves, D. H., Lowe, M. R., Green, B. A., Corove, M. B., & Williams, T. L. (2000). Do anorexia and bulimia nervosa occur on a continuum?: A taxometric analysis. *Behavior Therapy, 31,* 195–219.

Grayson, D. A. (1987). Can categorical and dimensional views of psychiatric illness be distinguished? *British Journal of Psychiatry, 151,* 355–361.

Gunderson, J. G., Shea, M. T., Skodol, A. E., McGlashan, T. H., Morey, L. C., Stout, R. L., et al. (2000). The Collaborative Longitudinal Personality Disorders Study: Development, aims, design, and sample characteristics. *Journal of Personality Disorders, 14,* 300–315.

Hare, R. D. (1980). A research scale for the assessment of psychopathy in criminal populations. *Personality and Individual Differences, 1,* 111–120.

Haslam, N. (2003). Categorical versus dimensional models of mental disorders: The taxometric evidence. *Australian and New Zealand Journal of Psychiatry, 37,* 696–704.

Haslam, N., Williams, B. J., Kyrios, M., McKay, D., & Taylor, S. (2005). Subtyping obsessive–compulsive disorder: A taxometric analysis. *Behavior Therapy, 36,* 381–391.

Hathaway, S. R., & McKinley, J. C. (1940). A multiphasic personality schedule (Minnesota): I. Construction of the schedule. *Journal of Psychology, 10,* 249–254.

Helzer, J. E., Bucholz, K. K., & Gossop, M. (2007). A dimensional option for the diagnosis of substance dependence in DSM-IV. *International Journal of Methods in Psychiatric Research, 16,* S24–S33.

Helzer, J. E., van den Brink, W., & Guth, S. E. (2006). Should there be both categorical and dimensional criteria for the substance use disorders in DSM-V? *Addiction, 101*, 17–22.

Hudziak, J. J., Achenbach, T. M., Althoff, R. R., & Pine, D. S. (2007). A dimensional approach to developmental psychopathology. *International Journal of Methods in Psychiatric Research, 16*, S16–S23.

Kessler, R. C., Chiu, W. T., Demler, O., & Walters, E. E. (2005). Prevalence, severity, and comorbidity of 12-month DSM-IV disorders in the National Comorbidity Survey Replication. *Archives of General Psychiatry, 62*, 617–627.

Kraemer, H. C. (2007). DSM categories and dimensions in clinical and research contexts. *International Journal of Methods in Psychiatric Research, 16*, S8–S15.

Kraemer, H. C., Noda, A., & O'Hara, R. (2004). Categorical versus dimensional approaches to diagnosis: Methodological challenges. *Journal of Psychiatric Research, 38*, 17–25.

Kraepelin, E. (1919). *Dementia praecox and paraphrenia*. Edinburgh, Scotland: E. & S. Livingstone.

Kraepelin, E. (1921). *Manic-depressive insanity and paranoia*. Edinburgh, Scotland: E. & S. Livingstone.

Krueger, R. F. (2005). Continuity of Axes I and II: Toward a unified model of personality, personality disorders, and clinical disorders. *Journal of Personality Disorders, 19*(3), 233–261.

Krueger, R. F., & Markon, K. E. (2006). Reinterpreting comorbidity: A model-based approach to understanding and classifying psychopathology. *Annual Review of Clinical Psychology, 2*, 111–133.

Leckman, J. F., Denys, D., Simpson, H. B., Mataix-Cols, D., Hollander, E., Saxena, S., et al. (2010). Obsessive–compulsive disorder: A review of the diagnostic criteria and possible subtypes and dimensional specifiers for DSM-V. *Depression and Anxiety, 27*, 507–527.

Lubke, J. H., & Muthen, B. (2005). Investigating population heterogeneity with factor mixture models. *Psychological Methods, 10*, 21–39.

Markon, K. E., & Krueger, R. F. (2006). Information-theoretic latent distribution modeling: Distinguishing discrete and continuous latent variable models. *Psychological Methods, 11*(3), 228–243.

McDonald, R. P. (1999). *Test theory: A unified treatment*. Mahwah, NJ: Erlbaum.

Meehl, P. E. (1986). Diagnostic taxa as open concepts: Metatheoretical and statistical questions about reliability and construct validity in the grand strategy of nosological revision. In T. Millon & G. L. Klerman (Eds.), *Contemporary directions in psychopathology: Toward the DSM-IV* (pp. 215–231). New York: Guilford Press.

Meehl, P. E. (1992). Factors and taxa, traits, and types, differences in degree and differences in kind. *Journal of Personality, 60*, 117–174.

Meehl, P. E. (1995). Bootstraps taxometrics: Solving the classification problem in psychopathology. *American Psychologist, 50*, 266–274.

Meehl, P. E. (1999). Clarifications about taxometric method. *Applied and Preventive Psychology, 8*, 165–174.

Meehl, P. E., & Yonce, L. J. (1994). Taxometric analysis: I. Detecting taxonicity with two quantitative indicators using means above and below a sliding cut (MAMBAC procedure). *Psychological Reports, 74*, 1059–1274.

Meehl, P. E., & Yonce, L. J. (1996). Taxometric analysis: II. Detecting taxonicity using covariance of two quantitative indicators in successive intervals of a third indicator (MAXCOV procedure). *Psychological Reports, 78*, 1091–1227.

Meyer, T. J., Miller, M. L., Metzger, R. L., & Borkovec, T. D. (1990). Development and validation of the Penn State Worry Questionnaire. *Behaviour Research and Therapy, 28*, 487–495.

Olatunji, B. O., Williams, B. J., Haslam, N., Abramowitz, J. S., & Tolin, D. F. (2008). The latent structure of obsessive–compulsive symptoms: A taxometric study. *Depression and Anxiety, 25*, 956–968.

Pike, K. M., Walsh, B. T., Vitousek, K., Wilson, G. T., & Bauer, J. (2003). Cognitive behavioral therapy in the posthospitalization treatment of anorexia nervosa. *American Journal of Psychiatry, 160*(11), 2046–2049.

Pincus, H. A., Tew, J. D., & First, M. B. (2004). Psychiatric comorbidity: Is more less? *World Psychiatry, 3*, 18–23.

Preacher, K. J., Rucker, D. D., MacCallum, R. C., & Nicewander, W. A. (2005). Use of the Extreme Groups Approach: A critical reexamination and new recommendations. *Psychological Methods, 10*(2), 178–192.

Rothschild, L., Cleland, C., Haslam, N., & Zimmerman, M. (2003). A taxometric study of borderline personality disorder. *Journal of Abnormal Psychology, 112*(4), 657–666.

Ruscio, J., & Ruscio, A. M. (2004). Clarifying boundary issues in psychopathology: The role of taxometrics in a comprehensive program of structured research. *Journal of Abnormal Psychology, 113*(1), 24–38.

Shuckit, M. A. (2006). Comorbidity between substance use conditions and comorbidity. *Addiction, 101*, 76–88.

Simpson, W. B. (1994). *Borderline personality disorder: Dimension or category? A maximum covariance analysis.* Unpublished doctoral dissertation, Boston University.

Skodol, A. E., Bender, D. S., Morey, L. C., Clark, L. A., Oldham, J. M., Alarcon, R. D., et al. (2011). Personality disorder types proposed for DSM-5. *Journal of Personality Disorders, 25*, 136–169.

Trull, T. J., Widiger, T. A., & Guthrie, P. (1990). Categorical versus dimensional status of borderline personality disorder. *Journal of Abnormal Psychology, 99*, 40–48.

Van Os, J., Gilvarry, C., Bale, R., Van Horn, E., Tattan, T., White, I., et al. (1999). A comparison of the utility of dimensional and categorical representations of psychosis. *Psychological Medicine, 29*, 595–606.

Waller, N. G., & Meehl, P. E. (1998). *Multivariate taxometric procedures: Distinguishing types from continua.* Thousand Oaks, CA: Sage.

Widiger, T. A. (1992). Categorical versus dimensional classification: Implications from and for research. *Journal of Personality Disorders, 6*, 287–300.

Wilson, G. T., & Fairburn, C. G. (1998). Treatments for eating disorders. In

P. E. Nathan & J. M. Gorman (Eds.), *A guide to treatments that work* (3rd ed., pp. 579–609). New York: Oxford University Press.

World Health Organization. (2004). *International statistical classification of diseases and health related problems* (10th rev.). Geneva, Switzerland: Author.

Zimmerman, M., & Mattia, J. I. (2000). Principal and additional DSM-IV disorders for which outpatients seek treatment. *Psychiatric Services, 51,* 1299–1304.

8

The Cognitive Content-Specificity Hypothesis

Contributions to Diagnosis and Assessment

John Baranoff and Tian Po S. Oei

Cognitive theory has brought attention to the role of cognitions in the initiation and maintenance of emotional disorders (Beck, 1967, 1976, 2008). The "cognitive content-specificity hypothesis" (CCSH) is a key component of cognitive theory; it states that emotional disorders can be defined by cognitive content and cognitive profiles (Beck, 1976; see Figure 8.1, solid lines). Beck (1976) outlined eight domains of thought content linked to separate emotional disorders. For example, depression was defined by the presence of past-oriented negative automatic thoughts relating to self-criticism, hopelessness, and loss (Beck, 1967, 1976, 2008). More specifically, Beck (1976) described depression as characterized by a triad of negative thoughts about the self, the world, and the future. By contrast, thoughts related to anxiety were considered to be future-oriented and focused on danger (Beck, 1976; Beck, Emery, & Greenberg, 1985), while mania related to inflated self-evaluations and unrealistic expectations of abilities (Beck, 1976).

In the 40 years since the CCSH was proposed, research has highlighted a number of complexities. While the link between specific cognitive content and a given emotional response has gained empirical support, there is less research that supports the concept of a cognitive-affective relationship *unique* to each emotional response. Specifically, for a unique relationship between cognition and affective state, there should be no effect or at least a weak effect for the crossover of anxious thoughts to depression (R. Beck & Perkins, 2001; Lamberton & Oei, 2008; Smith & Mumma, 2008; see Figure 8.1, dashed lines). Although the evidence for a unique relationship is mixed, the CCSH has had a significant impact on the cognitive assessment of emotional disorders, case conceptualization, and selection of treatment targets in clinical practice.

THE AIMS OF THIS CHAPTER

The aims of this chapter are to provide an overview of the CCSH and outline conceptual and methodological challenges in testing the hypothesis. The current status of the CCSH in relation to anxiety and depression is assessed, and implications for assessment and diagnosis are discussed. According to R. Beck and Perkins (2001), the terms "cognitive specificity" and "cognitive content-specificity" have been used interchangeably. In this chapter, "cognition" and "cognitive content" denote the surface level of cognition referred to as "cognitive products" (Kendall & Ingram, 1987), "automatic thoughts" (Beck, 1967), and "self-statements" (Meichenbaum, 1977). The affective component has been

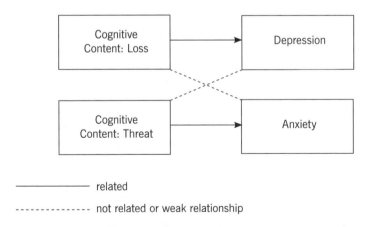

————————— related

-------------- not related or weak relationship

FIGURE 8.1. The cognitive content-specificity hypothesis. Solid line indicates strong positive relationship between cognitions and emotional disorder. Dashed line shows weak relationship or unrelated. Modified from Lamberton and Oei (2008) with permission from Elsevier.

considered as either an emotional response or an emotional disorder in the literature. The validity of diagnostic systems such as the *Diagnostic and Statistical Manual of Mental Disorders* (DSM; American Psychiatric Association, 2013) has been discussed by authors such as Pilgrim and Bentall (1999) and is beyond the scope of this chapter.

THE COGNITIVE CONTENT-SPECIFICITY HYPOTHESIS

Since the development of the cognitive model of depression (Beck, 1967, 1987, 2008; D. A. Clark & Beck, with Alford, 1999) and later of anxiety (Beck et al., 1985), cognitive models have been proposed for a diverse range of presentations including somatic problems, panic disorder, pain disorder, bipolar affective disorder, and personality disorders (Beck, Freeman, & Davis, 2004; Butler, Chapman, Forman, & Beck, 2006; Epp, Dobson, & Cottraux, 2009). The CCSH is a component of the cognitive model that can be empirically tested (e.g., Lamberton & Oei, 2008). The majority of studies that test the CCSH are focused on depression and anxiety. In the past decade, a small number of studies examining the differences in cognitive profiles between depression and states such as anger and mania have been published (e.g., Beck, Colis, Steer, Madrak, & Goldberg, 2006; Schniering & Rapee, 2004; Smith & Mumma, 2008).

Conceptual Issues

Beck's (1976) statement of the CCSH emphasized that each disorder is characterized by particular cognitive content, but did not clarify how the uniqueness aspect of a cognitive-affective relationship should be defined. Beck (1976, p. 83) stated that "on the basis of the clinical observations and systematic studies, I was able to distinguish among the common neurotic disorders according to differences in the content of ideation." The CCSH can be interpreted in a number of ways (R. Beck & Perkins, 2001). A strict interpretation of the CCSH would suggest no crossover between cognitive content and another emotional state (see Figure 8.1). The CCSH has been interpreted in a relative sense and analyzed accordingly (D. A. Clark, Beck, & Brown, 1989; Smith & Mumma, 2008). In this respect, a high frequency of failure cognitions is hypothesized to relate to depressed states to a greater extent than to anxiety states. Conversely, a high frequency of threat cognitions is hypothesized to relate to anxiety states more than to depressed states.

It may be useful to conceptualize the CCSH as consisting of two parts. The first part is the relationship between cognitive content and a specific emotional response. This part can be conceptualized as the "sensitivity" component or a "cognitive content hypothesis" (CCH). In a CCH, the focus is on determining the strength of the cognitive-affective relationship, and a distinction is not made between cognitive content that is common across affective states and unique content. The second conceptual part of the CCSH concerns the uniqueness of the relationship between cognitive content and a specific emotional response; it can be conceptualized as the "specificity" component of the CCSH. In contrast to the definition of the CCH, it may be helpful to refer to the uniqueness requirement as being a defining feature of the CCSH. At present, evidence for the CCSH is mixed, and the level of specificity in the model under consideration is often not clearly identified in the literature. Therefore, making the distinction between the CCH and CCSH will assist in the evaluation of the empirical evidence.

The two components of the CCSH have not received equal empirical support. A large number of studies support a positive relationship between particular cognitive content and emotional responses (i.e., the CCH; e.g., R. Beck & Perkins, 2001; D. A. Clark et al., 1999). By contrast, the evidence is mixed for a *unique* relationship between specific cognitions and specific emotional responses (e.g., R. Beck & Perkins, 2001; Lamberton & Oei, 2008). The evidence appears to be more inconsistent for anxiety than depression, and hence the CCSH may vary in how it applies to different affective states (R. Beck & Perkins, 2001). Even if conceptual precision is reached, methodological issues may limit the accuracy to which the CCSH can be tested.

Methodological Issues

Assessment of Cognitions by Questionnaires

In studies that test the CCSH, cognitions are primarily assessed by questionnaire. An awareness of the psychometric properties is required in order to distinguish between the various measures. We have selected three well-validated self-report measures that assess cognition at the level of automatic thoughts: the Catastrophic Cognitions Questionnaire—Modified (Khawaja, Oei, & Baglioni, 1994), Automatic Thoughts Questionnaire (Hollon & Kendall, 1980) and Cognition Checklist (Beck, Brown, Steer, Eidelson, & Riskind, 1987). The Catastrophic Cognitions Questionnaire—Modified and Automatic Thoughts Questionnaire are questionnaires developed to measure specific cognitive content relevant to panic disorder and depression, respectively. By contrast, the Cognition Checklist was developed to distinguish between anxiety-related and depressive cognitive content (Beck et al., 1987). We provide a brief overview of the development and validation of these measures of cognitive content.

Catastrophic Cognitions Questionnaire—Modified. The Catastrophic Cognitions Questionnaire—Modified (CCQ-M) consists of 21 items that assess catastrophic cognitions related to danger (Khawaja & Oei, 1992; Khawaja et al., 1994) and comprises three subscales: misperception of affective responses as danger (emotional catastrophe); sensitivity to physical symptoms (physical catastrophe); and the interpretation of strained cognitive capacity as dangerous (mental catastrophe). Exploratory and confirmatory factor analyses showed that the CCQ-M had a sound factor structure in clinical and nonclinical samples (Khawaja et al., 1994). Further, the CCQ-M showed statistically significant correlations with measures of anxiety (Beck, Epstein, Brown, & Steer, 1988). The emotional and mental catastrophes subscales discriminated between an anxiety disorder sample and a student sample (Khawaja et al., 1994). Nevertheless, the CCQ-M was not sufficiently sensitive to discriminate between different diagnostic categories of anxiety. In clinical practice, the CCQ-M may be useful for confirming the presence of anxious cognitions and identifying treatment targets, but may not be sufficient to differentiate specific anxiety disorders.

Automatic Thoughts Questionnaire. The Automatic Thoughts Questionnaire (ATQ; Hollon & Kendall, 1980) is a widely used measure of depressive cognitions. There are several versions of the ATQ. The ATQ—Revised (ATQ-R) was developed to measure positive and neutral cognitive content (10 statements) as well as negative cognitive content (30 statements; Kendall, Howard, & Hays, 1989); both subscales have been shown to have good internal reliability and discriminant validity (Hollon & Kendall, 1980; Kendall, Howard, & Hays, 1989). The ATQ-positive (ATQ-P; Ingram & Wisnicki, 1988) was developed to measure positive self-statements and has been shown to successfully discriminate between groups defined on the basis of depressive symptoms and negative affect (Ingram & Wisnicki, 1988). There is, however, evidence to suggest that the ATQ-P may not discriminate anxiety from depression. For example, Cho and Telch (2005) found the presence of ATQ negative cognitions was more important in discriminating depression from social anxiety than the absence of ATQ-P positive thoughts.

A modification to the ATQ, referred to as the ATQ-B, requires a rating of the degree of belief in the thought in addition to a rating of its frequency (Zettle & Hayes, 1986). This modification protects against a patient confusing the importance of a thought with the frequency of occurrence (Dunkley, Blankstein, & Segal, 2010). The ATQ-B has good internal reliability in both clinical and nonclinical samples and has good test–retest reliability (Zettle, 2010). Short forms of the ATQ have also been developed and have been shown to have sound psychometric properties (Netemeyer et al., 2002). Nevertheless, it is unclear to what extent these shortened measures are responsive to change across treatment.

Cognition Checklist. The Cognition Checklist (CCL; Beck et al., 1987) is the most frequently used measure in CCSH research (R. Beck & Perkins, 2001) and was developed to differentiate depression from anxiety (Beck et al., 1987). The CCL has two subscales: anxious cognitions (CCL-A) and depressive cognitions (CCL-D). The scale consists of 26 items (14 depressive content items and 12 anxious content items). Good internal reliability and adequate test–retest reliability have been reported for both subscales (Beck et al., 1987). The CCL-D has received more support than the CCL-A in the differentiation of depression and anxiety (Riskind et al., 1991; Somoza, Steer, Beck, & Clark, 1994; Woody, Taylor, McLean, & Koch, 1998). In summary, the CCL-D discriminated depression from anxiety in a number of studies, whereas the CCL-A did not consistently discriminate anxiety from depression or one anxiety disorder from another (R. Beck & Perkins, 2001; Somoza et al., 1994).

Limitations of Questionnaire Methods

Cognition questionnaires require individuals to endorse thoughts from a list and often specify a timeframe. Idiosyncratic thoughts may not be captured by questionnaires and/or the timeframe of assessment may not be optimal. Further, endorsing an item on a cognition questionnaire may not accurately reflect the frequency of the cognition.

According to Dunkley et al. (2010), individuals may answer a question by converting their experience of an emotion into a verbal statement. The individual may also rate items based on how the thought matches their view of themselves or how important they think the thought is rather than how often it occurs (Dunkley et al., 2010). Additionally, cognitions may consist of images or parts of a sentence and not full sentences as they appear in questionnaires (Arnkoff & Glass, 1982; Dunkley et al., 2010). Issues that relate generally to questionnaire methods are covered in detail in Arnkoff and Glass (1982), D. A. Clark (1988), and Glass and Arnkoff (1997) and have been further discussed recently by Dunkley et al. (2010).

A dysfunctional thought record can be used to identify relevant cognitions; however, this method also has limitations. Individuals may report cognitions based on what they consider to be a plausible response to a given situation (Nisbett & Wilson, 1977). Also, catastrophic cognitions such as "I am about to have a heart attack" may occur with other cognitions such as thoughts relating to loss (i.e., "I lost my friend to a heart attack"). Therefore, identifying the cognitions relevant to the emotional response under consideration may be difficult. Further, both questionnaires and thought records sample cognitions at a point in time, whereas thinking occurs across time as a process with one thought triggering another. Finally, it is unclear whether there is a frequency threshold for an automatic thought to elicit an emotional response. For example, an aggregation of thoughts may be required before an emotional response is elicited. In summary, self-report cognition questionnaires have a number of limitations that make precise assessment of cognitions difficult.

Measurement of Cognitions by Methods Other Than Questionnaires

R. Beck and Perkins (2001) highlighted that shared method variance may have been responsible for inconsistent findings in correlational studies that assess the CCSH. They suggested that future research could address this by assessing cognitions by methods other than questionnaire. Alternative methods include think-aloud, thought-listing, and thought-sampling approaches (Davison, Best, & Zanov, 2009). Most of these methods have been employed in research generally, but not necessarily to test the CCSH, and have not been fully integrated into clinical practice. (We briefly discuss some of these approaches, as a detailed discussion is presented in Chapter 3 by Haaga and Solomon.)

In a think-aloud procedure, the individual says whatever comes to mind while speech is recorded (Zanov & Davison, 2010). This approach has recently been used to assess progress in exposure therapy for panic disorder (Meuret, Wolitzky-Taylor, Twohig, & Craske, 2012). The CCSH could be assessed using a predetermined coding protocol within the think-aloud procedure. Although this procedure has high face validity, it may lead to changes in attentional resources; in turn, this affects the ecological validity of the assessment (Rozendaal, Buijzen, & Valkenburg, 2012). Thought-listing approaches avoid problems associated with vocalization; however, these approaches introduce recall bias (Cacioppo & Petty, 1981).

The articulated thoughts in simulated situations (ATSS) paradigm incorporates the strengths of think-aloud and thought-listing methods (Davison, Robins, & Johnson, 1983; Zanov & Davison, 2010) and can be adapted to assess cognitive content-specificity. The approach is laboratory-based and involves an audio simulation that is stopped for 30-second periods to allow thought recording (see Zanov & Davison,

2010, for a detailed history of the use of the ATSS paradigm). The ATSS has been used in more than 60 studies (Zanov & Davison, 2010) and has already been used in studies examining relationships between cognitive content and emotional states. For example, the ATSS was used to assess changes in irrational thinking in response to rational-emotive therapy for depression (Szentagotai, David, Lupu, & Cosman, 2008) and was used in a fear-of-flying study that produced results supportive of Beck et al.'s (1985) cognitive theory of anxiety (Moller, Nortje, & Helders, 1998).

Thought-sampling methods may improve the assessment of cognitions when used in conjunction with questionnaires. Nevertheless, assessing cognitive content using multiple methods has resulted in divergent results in some studies (e.g., Eckhardt, Barbour, & Davison, 1998). Eckhardt et al. assessed three groups using ATSS and cognitive questionnaires: maritally violent men, maritally unsatisfied and nonviolent men, and men who were satisfied in their marriage and nonviolent. Cognitive distortions elicited through the ATSS paradigm were not correlated with cognitive distortions on questionnaires. The cognitive distortions that were elicited through the ATSS provided better discrimination of groups than cognitive distortions identified in questionnaires. The development of specific protocols for production methods may facilitate further testing of the CCSH. We see potential in standardizing protocols to be used with the ATSS, so cognitions can be reliably elicited under controlled conditions and then systematically coded.

Assessment of Emotional Response

The Beck Depression Inventory–II (BDI-II; Beck, Steer, & Brown, 1996) and the Beck Anxiety Inventory (BAI; Beck, Steer, & Brown, 1993) have been used in numerous studies testing the CCSH (e.g., see R. Beck & Perkins, 2001; Lamberton & Oei, 2008); they assess symptoms on a continuous scale, which increases the measurement sensitivity when compared to employing a categorical diagnosis. Nevertheless, the BAI and BDI-II contain cognitive items that may inflate the relationship between cognitions and emotional response. Additionally, when questionnaires such as the BDI-II and BAI are used to differentiate anxiety and depression, the association may be affected by common variance associated with negative affectivity and the overlap of anxiety and depression (T. R. Norman, Judd, & Burrows, 1992). Finally, symptom measures may differ in sensitivity and specificity across normal and psychiatric populations. For example, the BDI-II was designed to measure symptom severity and shows good specificity at severe levels of depression, but not at lower levels (Rudd & Rajab, 1995). These issues place limitations on the extent to which the uniqueness component of the CCSH can be detected in cognitive-affective relationships.

Assessment of Emotional Disorders

The use of categorical diagnoses in the assessment of emotional disorders may reduce the ability to detect relationships between cognitive content and affective states, because the aspect of dimensionality is removed and diagnostic categories can be narrow; this may be more of an issue in relation to testing the CCSH with anxiety disorders than depressive disorders. By contrast to the range of diagnostic categories for anxiety outlined in the DSM, a diagnosis of major depressive disorder may include different subtypes of the disorder under the same label. The reliability of categorical diagnoses may also be affected by interrater reliability (D. A. Clark et al., 1999).

Other Methodological Issues in Assessing the CCSH

A further methodological issue in CCSH research has been referred to as state–trait or occasion–stability confounding (Smith & Mumma, 2008). Specifically, cross-sectional studies are unable to distinguish between trait and state mood disturbance. Therefore, the sensitivity to detect cognitive-affective relationships will be reduced in cross-sectional studies compared to studies with multiple data points and a specified recall timeframe (see Figure 8.2). According to Smith and Mumma (2008), the issue of trait–state confounding is particularly important to consider in nonclinical samples, due to the mood variation that occurs in response to daily events in this population (Smith & Mumma, 2008; Stader & Hokanson, 1998). Smith and Mumma (2008) highlight that 6 out of the 13 studies in a meta-analysis by R. Beck and Perkins (2001) were nonclinical and hence may have been affected by state–trait confounding. Variation in symptom reporting over the recall period is depicted in Figure 8.2. Differences in the timeframes assessed by symptom and cognitive measures also make a precise test of the CCSH difficult (see Figure 8.2; Smith & Mumma, 2008).

The statistical techniques used to analyze the CCSH have implications for conclusions that can be drawn. Group comparison studies typically use null hypothesis significance testing to compare groups. This type of analysis does not indicate the strength of a relationship and thus cannot test the CCSH adequately. Correlational studies allow the strength of the relationship between cognitions and affective states to be assessed. Meta-analysis can then be performed (e.g., R. Beck & Perkins, 2001) to determine the strength and consistency of these associations

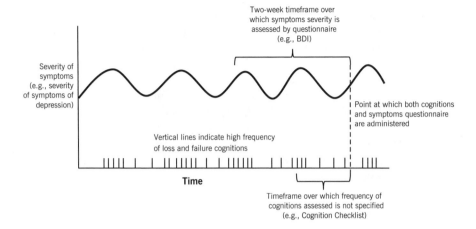

FIGURE 8.2. Timeframe mismatch and state–trait confounding. Fluctuations in symptom severity in a nonclinical sample across a 2-week timeframe may lead to confounding state and trait-symptom severity when a self-report measure such as the Beck Depression Inventory (BDI) is administered. Difference in timeframes assessed by symptom questionnaire and cognition questionnaire reduces measurement precision.

over multiple studies. Hierarchical linear regression and partial correlation can be used to determine whether cognitive content has a unique relationship with the corresponding affective state, after the effect of cognitions common across disorders are accounted for (Smith & Mumma, 2008). Nevertheless, linear regression allows only one dependent measure in the model and therefore requires that the CCSH is assessed in relation to one affective state at a time. More recently, structural equation modeling (SEM) has been used to assess the CCSH (see Cho & Telch, 2005; Smith & Mumma, 2008). SEM allows estimation of error and the ability to simultaneously test multiple independent and dependent variables within the same model. Although SEM is a promising statistical technique for testing the CCSH across affective states, only a small number of studies have employed the technique.

Evidence Supporting the CCH and CCSH for Anxiety and Depression

Early investigation of the CCSH in relation to anxiety and depression confirmed a cognitive-affective relationship in normal populations; in these studies loss and failure cognitions were associated with depressive symptoms, and danger and threat cognitions were associated with anxiety symptoms (D. M. Clark, 1983; Wickless & Kirsch, 1988). Arguably, the utility of the CCSH is in the application to clinical assessment and the differentiation of affective disorders. Different methodologies have been employed to test the CCSH in clinical populations (Lamberton & Oei, 2008). Some researchers have used group comparative approaches with groups defined by diagnosis or cutoff scores on psychometric measures (Beck et al., 1987; Ingram, Kendall, Smith, Donnell, & Ronan, 1987), whereas others have employed correlational designs in populations with mixed disorders and utilized statistical techniques such as multiple regression (D. A. Clark et al., 1989; Jolly & Dykman, 1994; Lamberton & Oei, 2008).

Group Comparison Studies

Studies using a group comparative approach have shown support for the relationship between loss/failure cognitions and depression at the level of the CCH and the CCSH (e.g., Beck, Riskind, Brown, & Steer, 1988). By contrast, support for discrimination between threat/danger cognitions and anxiety has been consistently demonstrated for the CCH in group comparison studies (e.g., Somoza et al., 1994), but only partial support for the CCSH has been found (e.g., Woody et al., 1998). Researchers who adopted a comparative approach began by comparing diagnostic groups on cognition questionnaires. For example, hopelessness was shown to be significantly higher in a group diagnosed with major depressive disorder than a group diagnosed with generalized anxiety disorder (Beck et al., 1988). D. A. Clark, Beck, and Stewart (1990) used the CCL in a study comprising three groups based on DSM-III diagnosis: depression, anxiety, and mixed anxiety–depression. The mixed group displayed both anxious and depressed cognitions, and the CCL successfully discriminated between the anxiety and depression groups (D. A. Clark et al., 1990). Nevertheless, the CCL-A has not consistently discriminated between anxiety and depression in group comparison research. A large outpatient study ($N = 518$; Riskind et al., 1991) found that while the CCL-D differentiated generalized anxiety disorder and dysthymic disorder, the CCL-A did not differentiate between groups (Riskind et al., 1991). D. A. Clark, Beck, and J. S. Beck (1994) also found that threat and danger did not adequately distinguish generalized anxiety disorder from depression, whereas loss and failure could differentiate between the groups. Similarly, Somoza et al. (1994) found that the CCL-D discriminated between panic disorder and major depressive disorder; however, the CCL-A did not. Subsequently, Woody et al. (1998) found that to differentiate anxiety from depression using anxious cognitions, cognitive content specific to the anxiety disorder was required. They found that the CCL-A did not differentiate between adults diagnosed with panic disorder and adults with major depressive disorder but found panic cognitions did successfully discriminate between the two disorders.

Group comparison studies have also been conducted with children and adolescents. Laurent and Stark (1993) obtained partial support for the CCSH in a sample of children ages 9–14, using a modified version of the CCL. There were no statistically significant differences between groups consisting of mixed anxiety–depression, depression, and anxiety. On a measure of depressive cognitions (Cognitive Triad Inventory for Children [CTI-C]; Kaslow, Stark, Printz, Livingston, & Ling Tsai, 1992), children with depression endorsed more items on the measure, but the difference was largely due to a lower frequency of positive thoughts in the depression group rather than to differences in the frequency of negative cognitions. Developmental factors may affect the presentation of depression and anxiety. Consequently, when testing the CCSH in adolescent and preadolescent samples using a group comparison approach, it may be appropriate to define groups based on categories that are applicable to psychopathology in this age group. For example, Epkins (2000) showed that in a preadolescent group aged 8–12 years, young people who were categorized as showing internalizing behaviors or both internalizing and externalizing behaviors on the basis of scores on the Child Behavior Checklist (Achenbach, 1991) reported more cognitive disturbance (as measured by the Cognitive Triad Inventory for Children and CCL) than both a group who displayed externalizing behaviors only and a control group.

In summary, threat- and danger-related content did not consistently discriminate anxiety and depressive disorders in early comparative studies. A possible explanation for this finding is that anxiety disorders are more heterogeneous than depressive disorders, and therefore disorder-specific anxious cognitions may be required to consistently differentiate between depressive and anxiety disorders (R. Beck, Benedict, & Winkler, 2003). In child and adolescent samples, the CCSH has been supported.

Correlational Studies

R. Beck and Perkins (2001) conducted a meta-analysis of 13 studies that reported correlations between anxious and depressed cognitions and anxious and depressed symptoms. Nine out of the 13 studies in the analysis used the CCL. Seven studies used clinical samples, and all except two assessed adults. The results showed significant relationships between depressive cognitions and depressive symptoms; depressive cognitions and anxiety symptoms; anxiety cognitions and anxiety symptoms; and anxiety cognitions and depressive symptoms (R. Beck & Perkins, 2001). Overall, the correlation between depressive symptoms and depressive cognitions was significantly larger than the correlation between depressive cognitions and anxiety symptoms; R. Beck and Perkins (2001) concluded support for the CCSH in the case of depression. By contrast, anxiety cognitions and anxiety symptoms also showed a statistically significant correlation, but this was not significantly different from the correlation between anxious cognitions and depressive symptoms. Therefore, the CCH was supported for anxiety, but the CCSH was not. A comparison of effect sizes for clinical and nonclinical studies showed that the relationship between depressive cognitions and anxiety symptoms was stronger in nonclinical samples than clinical samples. This finding is in keeping with Ambrose and Rholes (1993), who found a curvilinear relationship between cognitions and affective symptoms, such that the specificity of depressive cognitions improved as the frequency of the cognitions increased. By contrast, anxious cognitions showed greatest specificity at low frequency (Ambrose & Rholes, 1993). Although D. A. Clark, Steer, Beck, and Snow (1996) found cognitive specificity in clinical samples, they did not find a curvilinear relationship between cognitions and affective symptoms in their study. Overall, correlational studies have provided clearer support for the CCSH in the case of depression (i.e., for a unique relationship between loss and failure cognitions and depression) than for anxiety (i.e., for a unique relationship between threat/danger-related cognitions and anxiety; R. Beck & Perkins, 2001; Salkovskis, 1996).

A number of studies have shown support for the CCSH in relation to anxiety. R. Beck et al. (2003) assessed 411 individuals on a measure of anxious and depressive cognitions as well as symptoms of anxiety, depression, and a measure of general distress common to both anxiety and depression. In accordance with the CCH, depression was associated with self-critical and hopeless automatic thoughts and anxiety with physiological hyperarousal and catastrophic thoughts. Importantly for the CCSH, incremental validity was demonstrated in the cognitive domain such that anxious thoughts were a unique predictor of anxiety, and depressive thoughts were a unique predictor of depression after controlling for common variance such as worry and negative affectivity. Cho and Telch (2005) further tested the CCSH in a student analogue sample and employed SEM. A sample of 507 Korean students completed the ATQ, the BDI, a social avoidance measure, and a measure of self-statements relating to social interaction. Cognitive content about social interaction was unique to symptoms of social anxiety. The depressive cognitions measured by the ATQ were unique to depressive symptoms.

Positive cognitions measured by the ATQ-P were associated with both depression and social anxiety. In a subsequent study, Lamberton and Oei (2008) found that both anxious and depressive cognitions showed specificity when using a correlational design and continuous measures of anxiety and depression. Lamberton and Oei (2008) used a sample selected on depression but with anxiety permitted to freely vary. Depressive cognitive content was a significant unique predictor of depressive symptoms, and anxious cognitive content was a significant unique predictor of anxiety symptoms.

One correlational study has also found that the CCSH can be extended to children and adolescents (Jolly, 1993); in a study using an adolescent sample ($N = 80$), the CCSH was supported for anxiety but only partially for depression. In another study of children and adolescents, Schniering and Rapee (2004) demonstrated that negative automatic thoughts as measured by the Children's Automatic Thoughts Scale (CATS) showed that cognitive content related to loss was the strongest predictor of depressive symptoms; social threat was the strongest predictor of anxiety symptoms; and revenge/hostility-related cognitions were the strongest predictor of aggression.

Few studies that test the CCSH have employed longitudinal designs. One attempt at a longitudinal design by Smith and Mumma (2008) recorded university students' responses on five occasions on a weekly basis. They also assessed whether the CCSH generalized to anger-related cognitions. The longitudinal design allowed an analysis of the relationship between cognitions and emotions for specific occasions after accounting for stability of the constructs across time. Results showed that occasion-specific cognitions relating to anger and depressive content were uniquely associated with their respective affective states. Consistent with previous research, cognitions relating to vulnerability to harm were not uniquely related to anxiety symptoms.

Further Research Related to the CCSH

Another area of evidence that relates to cognitive-affective relationships is the cognitive therapy mechanisms of change literature. Oei, Bullbeck, and Campbell (2006) found that a model showing a reduction in depressed mood driving a reduction in depressive cognitions was a better fit to depression treatment data than a model showing changes in cognitions leading to a reduction in depressed mood. Longmore and Worrell (2007) have discussed in detail whether cognitive change is necessary for symptom change. As a component of a broader discussion, Longmore and Worrell (2007) identified evidence (e.g., Jacobson et al., 1996) suggesting that the cognitive component does not add to the effectiveness of

CBT for depression and anxiety; they recommended further studies with stronger methodology to examine this issue.

There is also emerging evidence that particular types of CBT for depression may work via mechanisms other than cognitive change. For example, acceptance-based treatments, such as acceptance and commitment therapy (Hayes, Strosahl, & Wilson, 2012), may influence treatment outcomes by changing the believability of depressive thoughts rather than their frequency. This process has been described as changing the function of thoughts (Zettle, Rains, & Hayes, 2011). Zettle and Rains (1989) reported the results of a study that led to significant change in depression without a corresponding change in depressogenic automatic thoughts (as measured by the ATQ). These results highlight complexities in the cognitive-affective relationship that go beyond the concept of cognitive content causing and maintaining emotional disorders.

Implications of the CCH and CCSH for Clinical Practice

The CCSH can be used to guide clinicians to focus on thoughts relevant to the emotional response. First, a number of structured techniques can be used to elicit clinically relevant thoughts (e.g., J. S. Beck, 1995; Burns, 1999; Greenberger & Padesky, 1995; Wells, 1997). For example, individuals can be asked to recall a time when they last experienced a particular emotional response, and the thoughts can then be sampled. The same approach can be used to elicit imagery and is particularly important to assess in the case of anxiety (Riskind, Rector, & Taylor, 2012). Reliability of memory is a consideration when asking for recall of thoughts to a concrete example. Second, as thoughts with differing cognitive content may be present simultaneously, individuals should be encouraged to recall a number of thoughts in the situation rather than what they consider to be the one "causal" thought. Third, specific education about cognitive-affective relationships could then be provided to persons receiving treatment.

The recall of clinically relevant cognitions can be improved by watching for changes in mood within a session and then probing thoughts associated with affective changes (a concept referred to as catching the "hot cognition"; Greenberger & Padesky, 1995). Findings from the CCSH literature can then be used to identify cognitions relevant to the mood disturbance. It may also be helpful to evoke the clinically relevant mood state in individuals prior to filling in cognitive measures. Individuals could be asked to remember a situation when they last had a panic attack just prior to filling in the CCQ-M or before listing panic-related thoughts (see D. M. Clark, 1996, and Segal & Ingram, 1994).

Daily Records of Dysfunctional Thought (DRDTs) have long been used to identify cognitive-affective relationships. When using DRDTs, an emphasis should be placed on capturing a range of thoughts that occur in a given context as opposed to what the client thinks is the most plausible explanation for the mood disturbance. Once the thoughts are obtained, CCH and CCSH concepts can be used to determine thoughts that are more or less relevant to the mood disturbance. Other strategies to assess cognitive content include exposure-based tasks in which thoughts and emotions are elicited, as well as role-plays and audio–video feedback. In addition to clinic-based thought identification, voice recordings of context-specific thoughts and emotions *in vivo* could be obtained via technology, such as smartphones. Cognitions have previously been sampled (i.e., Kenardy, Evans, & Oei, 1989). Nevertheless, the widespread use of mobile technology creates new possibilities.

Mumma (2004, 2011) and Haynes, Mumma, and Pinson (2009) described a validation process that consists of eliciting cognitions, integrating a person's idiosyncratic thoughts into a case conceptualization, and then examining the convergent and divergent validity of the formulation with data collected across the course of treatment. The initial selection of relevant cognitive content could be guided by findings from CCSH research. The clinician may attempt to elicit the person's idiosyncratic catastrophic thoughts that precede a panic attack. Hypotheses about cognitive-affective relationships could then be compared with treatment data. Although the previous suggestions may benefit clinical practice, a major disadvantage is that some of these methods can be time-consuming and may not be practical for routine clinical use.

The CCSH and Diagnosis

In clinical practice, the differentiation of emotional disorders can be difficult. Eliciting cognitive content may help rule out differential diagnoses, especially in the case of anxiety disorders, where cognitive content is incorporated into the diagnostic criteria. Sadock and Sadock (2007) note that anxiety experienced between panic attacks in panic disorder can be similar to anxiety experienced in generalized anxiety disorder. Conversely, panic attacks may occur within generalized anxiety disorder. Cognitively, generalized anxiety disorder is characterized by a perception of threat about a number of events or activities (Riskind, 2004), whereas panic disorder is characterized by the fear of having another panic attack. Therefore, cognitive content may be used to identify the diagnostic boundaries of generalized anxiety disorder and panic disorder.

The CCSH may have greater direct benefit in differentiating between anxiety disorders (as defined in DSM) than in differentiating between depressive disorders. In the case of major depressive disorder, DSM places emphasis on motivational and behavioral levels of depression. Nevertheless, the CCL-D and ATQ have shown a strong positive association with measures of depressive symptoms and depressive disorders, as well as successfully discriminating between depressive and anxious emotional states. Therefore, the presence of loss cognitions and negative self-worth measured by questionnaires could support a diagnosis of depression. However, in the absence of physiological and behavioral symptoms, a diagnosis of a major depressive episode cannot be made on the basis of cognitive content alone. Consequently, psychometric profiles can give us confidence that we have the diagnosis correct when there are noncognitive symptoms of depression present. If there are discrepancies between the provisional diagnosis and the cognitive content is elicited, then examination of the cognitive content may assist in suggesting a differential diagnosis.

There has been debate in the literature about the reliability and validity of categorical systems of mental disorders (Pilgrim & Bentall, 1999). D. A. Clark et al. (1999) have summarized the arguments about whether depression is best represented as continuous or discontinuous. These debates are beyond the scope of this chapter. We mention these issues because uncertainty about the validity and reliability of diagnostic categories presents a further challenge to the statement and assessment of the CCSH. The precision to which the CCSH can be stated in relation to diagnosis is limited not only by the validity of measures of cognition, but also by the validity of the diagnostic system itself.

Future Research

The CCL was developed to distinguish anxiety from depression on the basis of cognitive content and has received the most attention in CCSH research. An alternative research strategy may be to refine the search for cognitions that are strongly associated with depression rather than those that discriminate depression from anxiety (Smith & Mumma, 2008). For example, a specific item that relates to failure, such as "I have failed at many things in my life," may have a stronger association with depression than another item, such as "Things do not work out for me" (D. A. Clark, personal communication, January 2013). This is an area where differentiation of the CCH and CCSH may assist conceptualization of research questions.

A challenge for research in this area is to establish whether there are instances when depression is present without depressive cognitions. A significant problem for both the CCH and CCSH would be presented if a diagnosis of depression was not consistently correlated with depressive thinking. Some authors have suggested that cognitive disturbance is not an essential feature of depression (Hamilton & Abramson, 1983; Norman, Miller, & Klee, 1983). However, previous findings in support of this concept may be a result of the measures of cognition lacking sufficient sensitivity (D. A. Clark et al., 1999); a cognitive measure with high sensitivity may assist in this area of research.

Future research could further examine the CCSH in relation to anxiety and other disorders. In the case of anxiety disorders, measures that are more specific to each disorder may improve the discriminant validity. Finally, if the CCSH is to be considered in relative terms rather than in an all-or-nothing way (R. Beck & Perkins, 2001), then null hypothesis significance testing may not be the best way to assess and present findings, as these methods promote dichotomous thinking (Cumming, 2012, 2013). The relationship between cognitive content and an affective state could be visually represented with confidence intervals placed around point estimates.

SUMMARY

Over the past 40 years, the CCSH has been a key component of the cognitive model of emotional disorders. The CCSH has generated a large volume of research and has helped clinicians formulate and conceptualize presenting problems. We have distinguished between the CCSH and what we have termed the CCH. The CCH can be conceptualized as the sensitivity component of the CCSH, whereas the defining feature of the CCSH is specificity: the uniqueness of the relationship between cognitive content and a specific emotional response. The CCSH has been assessed in several ways, with group and correlational designs being the two major approaches. The uniqueness component can be conceptualized in either strict or relative terms. Testing different thresholds for the uniqueness component using different statistical techniques will aid understanding of the limits of sensitivity and specificity of cognitive measures in the assessment of mood disturbance. Visual presentation methods such as presenting group means with confidence intervals may assist practitioners to move away from dichotomous thinking about cognitive-affective relationships when comparing groups.

At present, the CCH and CCSH are useful heuristics for clinicians, provided that their limitations are considered. In particular, regard for the particular type of emotions under consideration and whether the affective state under consideration is an emotional response or an emotional disorder is important to avoid overgeneralizing or oversimplifying empirical findings. Loss and failure cognitions have been shown to be both strongly associated with and relatively unique to depressive states, whereas threat cognitions have been shown to be strongly associated with anxiety but have not consistently shown a unique relationship with anxiety. Therefore, threat cognitions may be common to depression and anxiety; however, specificity may be improved if cognitions specific to the type of disorder are sampled. With an awareness of the complexities of the relationship between cognitions and emotional response, clinicians can help individuals identify cognitions and explore their likely association with affective states. Insights from CCSH research can assist in the diagnostic process by providing support for the diagnosis or suggesting an alternative.

Despite the practical applications we have described, evidence for the CCSH is inconclusive. In particular, there is more evidence for the CCH than the CCSH. Further, evidence for the CCSH is likely to remain inconclusive because of the problems with conceptualization of the model and the inadequacy of current research methodology. The use of questionnaire methods will likely continue to result in a lack of certainty. Statistical techniques that help to move away from dichotomous thinking may assist clinicians in conceptualizing cognitive-affective relationships. New methodology may lead to further insights in a research context. Nevertheless, new clinical applications of this research may be limited.

KEY POINTS

FOR PRACTITIONERS

- From a practical standpoint, the CCSH has heuristic value. Nevertheless, given the limitations of the model, assessment should occur across behavioral, affective, and cognitive domains.
- When identifying clinically relevant cognitions, a number of thoughts should be sampled, not just the one the individual perceives to be the primary trigger thought.
- Loss and failure content (negative self-view) has utility in discriminating depression from anxiety.
- Danger and threat cognitions may be observed in a range of anxiety disorders as well as in depression. Therefore, when diagnosing, close attention should also be paid to the specific types of actual and perceived threat, as well as the behavioral and affective symptoms.

FOR RESEARCHERS

- Despite 40 years of research, evidence supporting the CCSH is mixed.
- Current methodology that predominantly involves the use of question-naires is insufficient and/or incapable of fully testing the CCSH.
- Research investigating the CCSH for emotional states other than anxiety and depression is limited.

FOR STUDENTS AND EDUCATORS

- The evidence to support the CCH is stronger than the evidence to support the CCSH.
- Loss and failure cognitions may show greatest specificity for depression at high frequencies.
- Threat and danger cognitions (catastrophic cognitions) may show greatest specificity for anxiety at low frequencies.

REFERENCES

Achenbach, T. M. (1991). *Child Behavior Checklist/4–18*. Burlington: University of Vermont.

Ambrose, B., & Rholes, W. S. (1993). Automatic cognitions and the symptoms of depression and anxiety in children and adolescents: An examination of the content-specificity hypothesis. *Cognitive Therapy and Research, 17*(3), 289–308.

American Psychiatric Association. (2013). *Diagnostic and statistical manual of mental disorders* (5th ed.). Arlington, VA: Author.

Arnkoff, D. B., & Glass, C. R. (1982). Clinical cognitive constructs: Examination, evaluation, and elaboration. In P. C. Kendall (Ed.), *Advances in cognitive-behavioral research* (pp. 1–34). New York: Academic Press.

Beck, A. T. (1967). *Depression: Clinical, experimental, and theoretical aspects*. New York: Harper & Row.

Beck, A. T. (1976). *Cognitive therapy and the emotional disorders*. New York: International Universities Press.

Beck, A. T. (1987). Cognitive models of depression. *Journal of Cognitive Psychotherapy, 1*, 5–37.

Beck, A. T. (2008). The evolution of the cognitive model of depression and its neurobiological correlates. *American Journal of Psychiatry, 165*, 969–977.

Beck, A. T., Brown, G., Steer, R. A., Eidelson, J. I., & Riskind, J. H. (1987). Differentiating anxiety and depression: A test of the cognitive content-specificity hypothesis. *Journal of Abnormal Psychology, 96*, 179–183.

Beck, A. T., Colis, M. J., Steer, R. A., Madrak, L., & Goldberg, J. F. (2006). Cognition Checklist for Mania—Revised. *Psychiatry Research, 145*(2), 233–240.

Beck, A. T., Emery, G., & Greenberg, R. (1985). *Anxiety disorders and phobias: A cognitive perspective.* New York: Basic Books.

Beck, A. T., Epstein, N., Brown, G., & Steer, R. A. (1988). An inventory for measuring clinical anxiety: Psychometric properties. *Journal of Consulting and Clinical Psychology, 56*(6), 893–897.

Beck, A. T., Freeman, A. M., & Davis, D. D. (2004). *Cognitive therapy of personality disorders* (2nd ed.). New York: Guilford Press.

Beck, A. T., Riskind, J. H., Brown, G., & Steer, R. A. (1988). Levels of hopelessness in DSM-III disorders: A partial test of content specificity in depression. *Cognitive Therapy and Research, 12,* 459–469.

Beck, A. T., Steer, R. A., & Brown, G. (1993). Dysfunctional attitudes and suicidal ideation in psychiatric outpatients. *Suicide and Life-Threatening Behavior, 23*(1) 11–20.

Beck, A. T., Steer, R. A., & Brown, G. K. (1996). *Beck Depression Inventory–II manual.* San Antonio, TX: Psychological Corporation.

Beck, J. S. (1995). *Cognitive therapy: Basics and beyond.* New York: Guilford Press.

Beck, R., Benedict, B., & Winkler, A. (2003). Depression and anxiety: Integrating the tripartite and cognitive content-specificity assessment models. *Journal of Psychopathology and Behavioral Assessment, 25*(4), 251–256.

Beck, R., & Perkins, T. S. (2001). Cognitive content-specificity for anxiety and depression: A meta-analysis. *Cognitive Therapy and Research, 25,* 651–663.

Burns, D. D. (1999). *The feeling good handbook.* New York: Penguin Group.

Butler, A. C., Chapman, J. E., Forman, E. M., & Beck, A. T. (2006). The empirical status of cognitive-behavioral therapy: A review of meta-analyses. *Clinical Psychology Review, 26*(1), 17–31.

Cacioppo, J. T., & Petty, R. (1981). Social psychological procedures for cognitive response assessment: The thought-listing technique. In T. V. Merluzzi, C. R. Glass, & M. Genest (Eds.), *Cognitive assessment* (pp. 309–342). New York: Guilford Press.

Cho, Y., & Telch, M. J. (2005). Testing the cognitive content-specificity hypothesis of social anxiety and depression: An application of structural equation modeling. *Cognitive Therapy and Research, 29*(4), 399–416.

Clark, D. A. (1988). The validity of measures of cognition: A review of the literature. *Cognitive Therapy and Research, 12*(1), 1–20.

Clark, D. A., & Beck, A. T., with Alford, B. A. (1999). *Scientific foundations of cognitive theory and therapy of depression.* New York: Wiley.

Clark, D. A., Beck, A. T., & Beck, J. S. (1994). Symptom differences in major depression, dysthymia, panic disorder, and generalized anxiety disorder. *American Journal of Psychiatry, 151*(2), 205–209.

Clark, D. A., Beck, A. T., & Brown, G. (1989). Cognitive mediation in general psychiatric outpatients: A test of the content-specificity hypothesis. *Journal of Personality and Social Psychology, 56*(6), 958–964.

Clark, D. A., Beck, A. T., & Stewart, B. (1990). Cognitive specificity and positive–negative affectivity: Complementary or contradictory views on anxiety and depression? *Journal of Abnormal Psychology, 99,* 148–155.

Clark, D. A., Steer, R. A., Beck, A. T., & Snow, D. (1996). Is the relationship between anxious and depressive cognitions and symptoms linear or curvilinear? *Cognitive Therapy and Research, 20,* 135–154.

Clark, D. M. (1983). On the induction of depressed mood in the laboratory: Evaluation and comparison of the Velten and musical procedures. *Advances in Behaviour Research and Therapy, 5,* 27–49.

Clark, D. M. (1996). Panic disorder: From theory to therapy. In P. M. Salkovskis (Ed.), *Frontiers of Cognitive Therapy,* (pp. 318–344). New York: Guilford Press.

Cumming, G. (2012). *Understanding the new statistics: Effect sizes, confidence intervals, and meta-analysis.* New York: Routledge.

Cumming, G. (2013). The new statistics: A how-to guide. *Australian Psychologist, 48,* 161–170.

Davison, G. C., Best, J. L., & Zanov, M. (2009). Think-aloud techniques. In W. T. O'Donohue & J. E. Fisher (Eds.), *General principles and empirically supported techniques of cognitive-behavior therapy* (pp. 648–654). Hoboken, NJ: Wiley.

Davison, G. C., Robins, C., & Johnson, M. K. (1983). Articulated thoughts during simulated situations: A paradigm for studying cognition in emotion and behavior. *Cognitive Therapy and Research, 7,* 17–40.

Dunkley, D. M., Blankstein, K. R., & Segal, Z. V. (2010). Cognitive assessment: Issues and methods. In K. S. Dobson (Ed.), *Handbook of cognitive-behavioral therapies* (3rd ed., pp. 133–171). New York: Guilford Press.

Eckhardt, C. I., Barbour, K. A., & Davison, G. C. (1998). Articulated thoughts of maritally violent and nonviolent men during anger arousal. *Journal of Consulting and Clinical Psychology, 66,* 259–269.

Epkins, C. (2000). Cognitive specificity in internalizing and externalizing problems in community and clinic-referred children. *Journal of Clinical Child Psychology, 29*(2), 199–208.

Epp, A. M., Dobson, K. S., & Cottraux, J. (2009). Applications of individual cognitive-behavioral therapy to specific disorders: Efficacy and indications. In G. O. Gabbard (Ed.), *Textbook of psychotherapeutic treatments* (pp. 239–262). Arlington, VA: American Psychiatric Publishing.

Glass, C. R., & Arnkoff, D. B. (1997). Questionnaire methods of cognitive self-statement assessment. *Journal of Consulting and Clinical Psychology, 65*(6), 911–927.

Greenberger, D., & Padesky, C. A. (1995). *Mind over mood: Change how you feel by changing the way you think.* New York: Guilford Press.

Hamilton, E. W., & Abramson, L. Y. (1983). Cognitive patterns and major depressive disorder: A longitudinal study in a hospital setting. *Journal of Abnormal Psychology, 92*(2), 173.

Hayes, S. C., Strosahl, K. D., & Wilson, K. G. (2012). *Acceptance and commitment therapy: The process and practice of mindful change* (2nd ed.). New York: Guilford Press.

Haynes, S. N., Mumma, G. H., & Pinson, C. (2009). Idiographic assessment: Conceptual and psychometric foundations of individualized behavioral assessment. *Clinical Psychology Review, 29,* 179–191.

Hollon, S. D., & Kendall, P. C. (1980). Cognitive self-statements in depression: Development of an Automatic Thoughts Questionnaire. *Cognitive Therapy and Research, 4*, 383–395.

Ingram, R. E., Kendall, P. C., Smith, T. W., Donnell, C., & Ronan, K. (1987). Cognitive specificity in emotional distress. *Journal of Personality and Social Psychology, 53*, 734–742.

Ingram, R. E., & Wisnicki, K. S. (1988). Assessment of positive automatic cognition. *Journal of Consulting and Clinical Psychology, 56*(6), 898–902.

Jacobson, N. S., Dobson, K. S., Truax, P. A., Addis, M. E., Koerner, K., Gollan, J. K., et al. (1996). A component analysis of cognitive-behavioral treatment for depression. *Journal of Consulting and Clinical Psychology, 64*(2), 295–304.

Jolly, J. B. (1993). A multimethod test of the cognitive content-specificity hypothesis in young adolescents. *Journal of Anxiety Disorders, 7*, 223–233.

Jolly, J. B., & Dykman, R. A. (1994). Using self-report data to differentiate anxious and depressive symptoms in adolescents: Cognitive content specificity and global distress? *Cognitive Therapy and Research, 18*, 25–37.

Kaslow, N. J., Stark, K. D., Printz, B., Livingston, R., & Ling Tsai, S. (1992). Cognitive Triad Inventory for Children: Development and relation to depression and anxiety. *Journal of Clinical Child Psychology, 21*(4), 339–347.

Kenardy, J., Evans, L., & Oei, T. P. S. (1989). Cognition and heart rate in panic disorders during everyday activity. *Journal of Anxiety Disorders, 3*, 33–43.

Kendall, P. C., Howard, B. L., & Hays, R. C. (1989). Self-referent speech and psychopathology: The balance of positive and negative thinking. *Cognitive Therapy and Research, 13*(6), 583–598.

Kendall, P. C., & Ingram, R. (1987). The future for cognitive assessment of anxiety: Let's get specific. In L. Michelson & L. M. Ascher (Eds.), *Anxiety and stress disorders: Cognitive-behavioral assessment and treatment* (pp. 89–104). New York: Guilford Press.

Khawaja, N. G., & Oei, T. P. S. (1992). Development of a Catastrophic Cognition Questionnaire. *Journal of Anxiety Disorders, 6*, 305–318.

Khawaja, N. G., Oei, T. P. S., & Baglioni, A. J. (1994). Modification of the Catastrophic Cognitions Questionnaire (CCQ-M) for normals and patients: Exploratory and LISREL analyses. *Journal of Psychopathological and Behavioral Assessment, 16*(4), 325–342.

Lamberton, A., & Oei, T. P. S. (2008). A test of the cognitive content specificity hypothesis in depression and anxiety. *Journal of Behavior Therapy and Experimental Psychiatry, 39*(1), 23–31.

Laurent, J., & Stark, K. D. (1993). Testing the cognitive content-specificity hypothesis with anxious and depressed youngsters. *Journal of Abnormal Psychology, 102*, 226–237.

Longmore, R. J., & Worrell, M. (2007). Do we need to challenge thoughts in cognitive-behavioral therapy? *Clinical Psychology Review, 27*, 173–187.

Meichenbaum, D. (1977). *Cognitive-behavior modification: An integrative approach.* New York: Plenum.

Meuret, A. E., Wolitzky-Taylor, K. B., Twohig, M. P., & Craske, M. G. (2012).

Coping skills and exposure therapy in panic disorder and agoraphobia: Latest advances and future directions. *Behavior Therapy, 43*(2), 271–284.

Moller, A. T., Nortje, C., & Helders, S. B. (1998). Irrational cognitions and the fear of flying. *Journal of Rational-Emotive and Cognitive-Behavior Therapy, 16*(2), 135–148.

Mumma, G. H. (2004). Validation of idiosyncratic cognitive schema in cognitive case formulations: An intraindividual idiographic approach. *Psychological Assessment 16*(3), 211–230.

Mumma, G. H. (2011). Validity issues in cognitive-behavioral case formulation. *European Journal of Psychological Assessment, 27*(1), 29–49.

Netemeyer, R. G., Williamson, D. A., Burton, S., Biswas, D., Jindal, S., Landreth, S., et al. (2002). Psychometric properties of shortened versions of the Automatic Thoughts Questionnaire. *Educational and Psychological Measurement, 62*, 111–129.

Nisbett, R. E., & Wilson, T. D. (1977). Telling more than we can know: Verbal reports on mental processes. *Psychological Review, 84*(3), 231–259.

Norman, T. R., Judd, F. K., & Burrows, G. D. (1992). New pharmacological approaches to the management of depression: From theory to clinical practice. *Australian and New Zealand Journal of Psychiatry, 26*(1), 73–81.

Norman, W. H., Miller, I. W., III, & Klee, S. H. (1983). Assessment of cognitive distortion in a clinically depressed population. *Cognitive Therapy and Research, 7*(2), 133–140.

Oei, T. P. S., Bullbeck, K., & Campbell, J. M. (2006). Cognitive change process during group cognitive behaviour therapy for depression. *Journal of Affective Disorders, 92*(2–3), 231–241.

Pilgrim, D., & Bentall, R. (1999). The medicalization of misery: A critical realist analysis of the concept of depression. *Journal of Mental Health, 8*(3), 261–274.

Riskind, J. H. (2004) Cognitive theory and research on generalized anxiety disorder. In R. L. Leahy (Ed.), *Contemporary cognitive therapy: Theory, research, and practice.* New York: Guilford Press.

Riskind, J. H., Moore, R. B., Jr., Harman, B., Hohnman, A. A., Stewart, B., & Beck, A. T. (1991). The relation of generalized anxiety disorder to depression in general and dysthymic disorder in particular. In R. M. Rapee & D. H. Barlow (Eds.), *Chronic anxiety: Generalized anxiety disorder and mixed anxiety–depression* (pp. 29–51). New York: Guilford Press.

Riskind, J. H., Rector, N. A., & Taylor, S. (2012). Looming cognitive vulnerability to anxiety and its reduction in psychotherapy. *Journal of Psychotherapy Integration, 22*(2), 137–162.

Rozendaal, E., Buijzen, M., & Valkenburg, P. (2012). Think-aloud process superior to thought-listing in increasing children's critical processing of advertising. *Human Communication Research, 38*(2), 199–221.

Rudd, M. D., & Rajab, M. H. (1995). Specificity of the Beck Depression Inventory and the confounding role of comorbid disorders in a clinical sample. *Cognitive Therapy and Research, 19*, 51–68.

Sadock, B. A., & Sadock, V. A. (2007). *Kaplan and Sadock's synopsis of psychiatry: Behavioral sciences/clinical psychiatry.* Philadelphia: Lippincott Williams & Wilkins.

Salkovskis, P. M. (1996). *Trends in cognitive and behavioural therapies.* Chichester, UK: Wiley.

Schniering, C. A., & Rapee, R. M. (2004). The relationship between automatic thoughts and negative emotions in children and adolescents: A test of the cognitive content-specificity hypothesis. *Journal of Abnormal Psychology, 113*(3), 464.

Segal, Z. V., & Ingram, R. E. (1994). Mood priming and construct activation in tests of cognitive vulnerability to unipolar depression. *Clinical Psychology Review, 14,* 663–695.

Smith, P. N., & Mumma, G. H. (2008). A multi-wave web-based evaluation of cognitive content-specificity for depression, anxiety, and anger. *Cognition Therapy Research, 32,* 50–65.

Somoza, E., Steer, R. A., Beck, A. T., & Clark, D. A. (1994). Differentiating major depression and panic disorders by self-report and clinical rating scales: ROC analysis and information theory. *Behaviour Research and Therapy, 32*(7), 771–782.

Stader, S. R., & Hokanson, J. E. (1998). Psychosocial antecedents of depressive symptoms: An evaluation using daily experiences methodology. *Journal of Abnormal Psychology, 107,* 17–26.

Szentagotai, A., David, D., Lupu, V., & Cosman, D. (2008). Rational emotive behavior therapy versus cognitive therapy versus pharmacotherapy in the treatment of major depressive disorder: Mechanisms of change analysis. *Psychotherapy: Theory, Research, Practice, Training, 45*(4), 523–538.

Wells, A. (1997). *Cognitive therapy of anxiety disorders: A practice manual and conceptual guide.* Chichester, UK: Wiley.

Wickless, C., & Kirsch, I. (1988). Cognitive correlates of anger, anxiety, and sadness. *Cognitive Therapy and Research, 12*(4), 367–377.

Woody, S. R., Taylor, S., McLean, P. D., & Koch, W. J. (1998). Cognitive specificity in panic and depression: Implications for comorbidity. *Cognitive Therapy and Research, 22,* 427–443.

Zanov, M. V., & Davison, G. C. (2010). A conceptual and empirical review of 25 years of cognitive assessment using the articulated thoughts in simulated situations (ATSS) think-aloud paradigm. *Cognition Therapy Research, 34,* 282–291.

Zettle, R. D. (2010). *Psychometric properties of the Automatic Thoughts Questionnaire—Believability Scale.* Manuscript in preparation.

Zettle, R. D., & Hayes, S. C. (1986). Dysfunctional control by client verbal behavior: The context of reason-giving. *Analysis of Verbal Behavior, 4,* 30–38.

Zettle, R. D., & Rains, J. C. (1989). Group cognitive and contextual therapies in the treatment of depression. *Journal of Clinical Psychology, 45,* 436–445.

Zettle, R. D., Rains, J. C., & Hayes, S. C. (2011). processes of change in acceptance and commitment therapy and cognitive therapy for depression: A mediation reanalysis of Zettle and Rains. *Behavior Modification, 35*(3), 265–283.

9

Transdiagnostic Cognitive Assessment and Case Formulation for Anxiety

A New Approach

Angela H. Smith, Chelsea G. Ratcliff,
and Peter J. Norton

CASE EXAMPLE OF COMPLEX ANXIETY

Marie[1] is a 24-year-old single European American woman enrolled as a student at a large state university in the midwestern United States. Marie relocated to the Midwest 1 year prior to her initial appointment, after living for many years in a large metropolitan city on the West Coast. She indicated that she had moved to "get away from some bad history," although she initially declined to elaborate further. Marie also indicated that she had recently become engaged to be married to a 25-year-old man whom she had begun dating after her move to the Midwest.

---

[1]The case example is an editorially modified and highly disguised representation of a client seen by one of us at a specialty clinic treating anxiety disorders. Modifications of specific case details to protect client confidentiality were made in accordance with the recommendations put forth by Clifft (1986).

Presenting Problems

Upon intake, Marie underwent a traditional diagnostic assessment using the Anxiety Disorders Interview Schedule for DSM-IV (ADIS-IV; Brown, Di Nardo, & Barlow, 1994). Marie met diagnostic criteria for several anxiety disorders and other Axis I disorders, including panic disorder with agoraphobia, generalized anxiety disorder, obsessive–compulsive disorder (OCD), specific phobia, posttraumatic stress disorder, and possible anorexia nervosa. Confirming the diagnostic assessment, the results from Marie's self-reported questionnaire assessments indicated significant elevations on symptoms indicative of all of these disorders.

Panic Disorder with Agoraphobia

Marie reported experiencing recurrent, nearly daily, panic attacks characterized by racing/pounding heart, shortness of breath, feelings of shakiness, nausea and stomach distress, and fears of losing control. Her primary interoceptive trigger was unusual stomach sensations that she feared might be a sign that she will vomit. She expressed a strong fear that the panic attacks could also cause her to vomit. As a result, Marie engaged in situational avoidance due to both (1) fears of being away from a toilet or a "safe place" if she felt nauseous or about to vomit, and (2) fears of being in crowded places where others may have an infectious, potentially vomit-inducing illness such as influenza.

Generalized Anxiety Disorder

Marie reported that she spent over 80% of her waking day engaged in excessive and uncontrollable worry. Most of her worry revolved around themes of vomit, including worry about possibly vomiting, seeing others vomit, the health of herself and others (e.g., influenza), and public or world health issues (e.g., viral pandemics), although she also worried about possible consequences of her vomit-related concerns such as the financial consequences of her inability to maintain employment due to her vomit-related fears and whether her fiancé would continue to love her despite these fears.

Obsessive–Compulsive Disorder

Marie reported frequent recurrent intrusive thoughts related to illness and vomiting and engaged in excessive rituals to negate these intrusive thoughts. Specifically, Marie indicated that she showered four times per day, washed her hands with soap over 20 times per day for over 5 minutes per episode, and very frequently used antibacterial gels. She indicated that her washing compulsions were highly ritualized, and that she would sometimes have to repeat her washing routine if she felt she did not complete it correctly. She also reported rituals regarding food storage and preparation, and the cleaning of food preparation and serving instruments. She also engaged in other germ avoidance behaviors such as opening doors with her elbow.

Anorexia Nervosa

Although Marie's body mass index was not medically verified, her self-reported height and weight indicated that she was below 80% of her expected body weight. While she did not report any body image disturbance, she indicated significant voluntary calorie restriction. She indicated that her food restriction was to (a) reduce the possibility of eating spoiled or infected foods that might make her vomit and (b) reduce feelings of "fullness" or bloating that she associates with needing to vomit. She also indicated that she only ate specific bland foods (i.e., plain tofu) because she felt that she had a sensitive stomach and that spicy or "harsh" foods might upset her stomach.

Posttraumatic Stress Disorder

Marie disclosed a repeated history of sexual assault during her young adult years while she worked as an exotic dancer. During the initial assessment, she declined to divulge details, but reported repeated unwanted recollections, hypervigilance to reminders of the assault, and emotional numbing resulting from the sexual assault.

Specific Phobia

As can be assumed from the above information, Marie also met criteria for a specific phobia of vomiting.

The Clinical Case for Transdiagnostic Assessment

Based on administration of the ADIS-IV (Brown et al., 1994), a widely employed diagnostic assessment tool, Marie met diagnostic criteria for several Axis I disorders. When approaching a client with an array of diagnoses, the clinician is left with several questions, including the validity of the diagnoses and how to approach symptoms over the course of treatment. The clinician is left wondering about the extent to which symptoms across diagnoses are related to each other and how these relationships will impact the course of treatment and treatment response. Specifically, the clinician may question whether it would be better to implement separate treatment hierarchies or a single hierarchy that includes triggers related to each concern. Questions such as these will be addressed throughout the chapter as we discuss a transdiagnostic perspective to the assessment and conceptualization of anxiety disorders.

A TRANSDIAGNOSTIC PERSPECTIVE
TO ASSESSMENT AND TREATMENT

The scientific approach to mental health is relatively young, and as such, the parameters of assessment and classification continue to evolve. In the early years (e.g., DSM-I [American Psychiatric Association, 1952], DSM-II [American Psychiatric Association, 1968]), clinicians and researchers treated symptoms, which were more descriptive than scientifically classified. The introduction of the third edition of the DSM (DSM-III; 1980) led to a clearly defined classification of diagnoses, and the treatment of distinct diagnoses became the zeitgeist. However, in recent years the utility of the classification system for treating many forms of psychopathology, including anxiety, has come into question (McManus, Shafran, & Cooper, 2010). Regarding anxiety symptomology, changes to the DSM over the past several decades have led to the expansion of anxiety disorder diagnoses from 3 (American Psychiatric Association, 1952, 1968) to 12 (American Psychiatric Association, 1994). Accounting for specifiers and subtypes, the current manual (DSM-5; American Psychiatric Association, 2013) encompasses over 18 distinct anxiety diagnoses, in addition to those disorders now classified under "obsessive–compulsive and related disorders" and "trauma- and stressor-related disorders." In recent years, these numerous distinctions have come under scrutiny as empirical findings have elucidated etiological similarities (Barlow, 2000; Brown & Barlow, 2009; Clark & Watson, 1991) as well as similar treatment responses across diagnoses (Norton & Price, 2007). These findings, in addition to other criticisms of the current diagnostic system (Watson, 2005), have motivated several research teams to take a transdiagnostic perspective as they consider the classification of anxiety and mood disorders.

Transdiagnostic approaches to psychopathology have been described as "those that transcend the diagnostic boundaries set out by classification schemes such as DSM-IV-TR" (McManus et al., 2010, p. 495). These are often applied to broad diagnostic categories that share clinical features and that are maintained by similar processes. Transdiagnostic conceptualizations of anxiety (Norton, 2006; Norton & Hope, 2005), anxiety and mood disorders (Barlow, Allen, & Choate, 2004), and psychopathology in general (Harvey et al., 2004) emphasize a core pathology underlying diagnostic distinctions. Although there is a growing body of literature related to transdiagnostic treatments of anxiety and mood disorders (Norton & Philipp, 2008), literature that assesses anxiety from a transdiagnostic perspective is sparse.

The case example of Marie illustrates how a diagnosis-specific assessment may hinder the development of a parsimonious case conceptualization and efficient treatment plan. However, researchers have also relied on disorder-specific assessments before conducting transdiagnostic treatments, seemingly without complication. Thus in this chapter we discuss the implications of the current assessment framework and provide suggestions for the development of transdiagnostic assessments. First, we briefly review the theoretical and empirical support for adopting a transdiagnostic conceptualization of anxiety.

CONCEPTUAL FRAMEWORK FOR ADOPTING A TRANSDIAGNOSTIC PERSPECTIVE TO ANXIETY

An examination of anxiety disorder risk factors and latent factor structure as well as comorbidity, clinical presentation, and response to treatment provides a case for a transdiagnostic conceptualization of anxiety disorders over discrete disorder-specific conceptualizations.

Shared Risk Factors

There is strong evidence suggesting shared risk factors for the development of anxiety disorders. Several genetic studies demonstrating increased heritability for affective disorders in general, but not for specific anxiety disorders (Andrews, Stewart, Morris-Yates, & Holt, 1990; Barlow, 2000; Hettema, Prescott, Myers, Neale, & Kendler, 2005) support the argument for a common underlying risk for anxiety. Additionally, early learning experiences, which inform temperament, also serve as risk factors for the development of anxiety disorders (Davidson, 2000; Rapee, 2002). Specifically, there is evidence that early environmental factors including parental overprotection, intrusive involvement, and low parental warmth lead to increased threat perception and an inhibited temperament as well as low self-efficacy in one's ability to cope with stressful or threatening events (Chorpita, Brown, & Barlow, 1998; Rapee, 2002). Together these studies indicate that a common genetic and environmental diathesis may underlie the anxiety disorders.

Comorbidity and Latent Factor Structure

Over half of all individuals with a primary diagnosis of an anxiety disorder have a secondary anxiety or mood disorder diagnosis as well

(Kessler, Chiu, Demler, & Walters, 2005). This overlap occurs at a rate that is far greater than chance, challenging the categorical notion that each disorder has a discrete biologically based etiology (Kessler et al., 2005). The most parsimonious explanation for extremely high comorbidity rates across anxiety disorders and between anxiety and mood disorders is that the "discrete" disorders spring from a common higher-order pathology (Barlow, 2000; Clark & Watson, 1991). This underlying pathology has been characterized as "neuroticism" (Eysenck, 1957) or "behavioral inhibition" (McNaughton & Gray, 2000), but is most commonly referred to as "negative affectivity" (NA; Clark & Watson, 1991). NA is described as chronic generalized stress accompanied by low self-efficacy in terms of one's ability to cope with future threats (Brown & Barlow, 2009). Factor analyses performed by Chorpita et al. (1998) supported the role of NA as a common factor to all the affective disorders tested, including depression, generalized anxiety disorder, panic disorder, obsessive–compulsive disorder, and social phobia.

Common Clinical Presentation

Unified conceptualizations of anxiety and affective disorders highlight the common clinical features present across diagnostic categories, such as overestimation of threat (regardless of the content) and underestimation of one's ability to cope with the threat (Barlow, 2000). Additionally, theorists have delineated common maintaining processes for anxiety and affective disorders, such as cognitive distortions (Harvey et al., 2004), avoidance patterns (Bar-Hiam, Lamy, Pergamin, Bakermans-Kranenburg, & van IJzendoorn, 2007), hypervigilance to threat, and poor emotion regulation (Barlow et al., 2004). Similarly, while these broad, underlying factors of anxiety and NA exist across cultures, there is no evidence to suggest that the "idioms of distress," such as are outlined in the DSM, exist cross-culturally (Good & Kleinman, 1985).

Common Response to Treatment across Diagnoses

McManus and colleagues (2010) note that systematic desensitization, exposure therapy, and cognitive theory and therapy were originally developed for the emotional disorders more generally, including all the current subtypes of anxiety. The specific disorder at hand was inconsequential to the treatment process. These authors acknowledge the benefits of disorder-specific treatment, and also recognize the relatively limited utility they have provided comorbid disorders and complex clinical cases. Perhaps not surprisingly, diagnostically diverse anxiety disorders respond to very similar treatments (Bandelow, Zohar, Hollander,

Kasper, & Moller, 2002; Norton & Price, 2007). Although a majority of the current cognitive-behavioral therapy (CBT) protocols are designed for specific diagnoses, their treatment components are remarkably similar, all involving psychoeducation, cognitive restructuring, and exposure. Norton and Philipp (2008) note that the differences across diagnosis-specific CBT protocols are superficial, relating to the content of the targeted fears rather than the function of the treatment components. Additionally, the efficacy of CBT is relatively similar across different anxiety disorders (Norton & Price, 2007). Likewise, the most effective pharmacological treatments are the same for diverse anxiety diagnoses, with selective serotonergic reuptake inhibitors at similar recommended doses being the front-line treatment across diagnoses (Bandelow et al., 2002).

In summary, evidence from multiple sources indicates that a transdiagnostic conceptualization of anxiety disorders, rooted in the assumption that anxiety disorders are driven by a common pathology, is appropriate and empirically grounded. Assessment born of this conceptualization then must focus on identifying the functional relationships between the individual's thoughts, behaviors, and emotions, rather than on identifying the particular category to which symptoms belong.

EMPIRICAL EVIDENCE FOR TRANSDIAGNOSTIC CBT: ADVANTAGES OVER DISORDER-SPECIFIC CBT

Several transdiagnostic, or unified, treatment protocols have been developed and tested over the past decade. In general, these protocols aim for flexible application of cognitive-behavioral skills on diverse manifestations of the core pathology underlying anxiety disorders. Norton and Philipp (2008) describe seven independently developed CBT transdiagnostic protocols (Allen, Ehrenreich, & Barlow, 2005; Barlow et al., 2003; Erickson, Janeck, & Tallman, 2007; Garcia, 2004; Larkin, Waller, & Combs-Lane, 2003; McEvoy & Nathan, 2007; Norton & Hope, 2005; Schmidt, 2003), and note that psychoeducation, cognitive restructuring, exposure to feared stimuli, and relapse prevention are common among the treatments, with other elements (e.g., relaxation training, behavioral activation) varying across protocols. The research evidence in support of the effectiveness of transdiagnostic CBT is unequivocal. Meta-analytic (Norton & Price, 2007) and benchmarking studies (McEvoy & Nathan, 2007) as well as direct comparison trials (Norton & Barrera, 2012) indicate that transdiagnostic CBT for anxiety results in large pre- to posttreatment change with improvements maintained at follow-up, results that are statistically equivalent to diagnosis-specific treatments.

Treating Core Pathology versus Specific Diagnoses: Effect on Comorbid Diagnoses

Beyond theoretical soundness, a transdiagnostic approach may provide practical benefits to both patients and providers. Due to the frequency with which patients seeking treatment for anxiety disorders meet diagnostic criteria for multiple disorders, the ability of a treatment protocol to address comorbid anxiety disorders is of critical importance. There is evidence suggesting that diagnosis-specific treatments benefit the nontargeted disorder (Blanchard et al., 2003; Borkovec, Abel, & Newman, 1995; Brown, Antony, & Barlow, 1995; Tsao, Mystkowski, Zucker, & Craske, 2002), and these results are not surprising, in light of the theoretical conceptualization that anxiety disorders share a common underlying factor (i.e., negative affect). However, there is also evidence to suggest that the ancillary benefits resulting from diagnostic-specific protocols are not as lasting as the benefits to the targeted disorder (Borkovec et al., 1995; Brown et al., 1995). Emerging evidence suggests that transdiagnostic protocols for treating anxiety can exert benefits on nontargeted affective disorders (Ellard, Fairholme, Boisseau, Farchione, & Barlow, 2010; Farchione et al., 2012; Norton, Hayes, & Hope, 2004; Titov, Andrews, Johnston, Robinson, & Spence, 2010), and indeed may be more effective than diagnosis-specific CBT at treating comorbid disorders (Norton et al., 2013).

MODELS FOR TRANSDIAGNOSTIC CONCEPTUALIZATION AND ASSESSMENT

The late Hans Eysenck once remarked that "a bad theory in science is never killed by criticism, but only by a better theory" (1957, p. 2). In light of the evidence supporting a transdiagnostic model of anxiety disorders, several leaders in the field have proposed new models of and methods for assessing the anxiety disorders. We consider several models here (see Figure 9.1).

Tripartite Model

Over 20 years ago, Clark and Watson (1991) proposed an empirically based and parsimonious structure of anxiety disorders in their tripartite model. This hierarchical model suggests that high NA underlies the pathology common to affective (anxiety and depressive) disorders, low positive affectivity (PA) is a second-order factor that results in symptoms such as anhedonia (or mania, if high), and physiological hyperarousal (PH) is a second-order factor underlying the expression of physiological

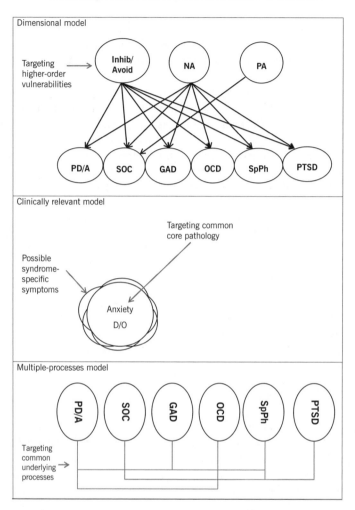

FIGURE 9.1. Schematic of approaches to the transdiagnostic conceptualization of anxiety disorders. Inhib/Avoid, inhibited/avoidant; NA, negative affectivity; PA, positive affectivity; PD/A, panic disorder with agoraphobia; SOC, social phobia; GAD, generalized anxiety disorder; OCD, obsessive–compulsive disorder; SpPh, specific phobia; PTSD, posttraumatic stress disorder.

anxiety, such as evident in panic disorder. This structure has been empirically supported by several research teams (e.g., Chorpita et al., 1998; Philipp, Washington, Raouf, & Norton, 2008). There have also been some criticisms of the model, specifically that PH is typical in panic disorder, but not in all anxiety disorders (Watson, 2005). Other researchers have suggested that the third factor involved in the expression of affective disorders is not PH, but rather a regulatory system that determines the extent to which an individual is inhibited or impulsive (Harkness & Lilienfeld, 1997).

In recent years, theorists have utilized these tripartite factors of high NA, low PA, high PH, and/or high inhibition to formulate a diagnostic scheme. Watson (2005) proposed a new categorical system based on the tripartite model in which all affective disorders are considered "emotional disorders." Within the emotional disorders, Watson outlines three subtypes based on factor analytic results, with "distress disorders" consisting of generalized anxiety disorder, major depressive disorder, and dysthymia; "fear disorders" consisting of panic disorder, agoraphobia, social phobia, and specific phobia; and "bipolar disorders" consisting of bipolar I, bipolar II, and cyclothymia. Although a conceptualization of anxiety disorders based on statistical analysis is appealing, it is not without problems. Watson notes the difficulty in categorizing posttraumatic stress disorder and obsessive–compulsive disorder, as they did not clearly "fall out" of the factor analysis in one of the three subgroups. Subsequently, researchers have proposed new diagnostic categories for obsessive–compulsive spectrum disorders (Stein et al., 2010) and traumatic stress disorders (Spitzer, First, & Wakefield, 2007).

Dimensional Model

Brown and Barlow (2009) proposed an interesting, more radically dimensional, alternative to Watson's categorical scheme. They emphasize that though NA underlies all affective disorders, it is expressed differently in individuals. For example, NA can be expressed as somatic complaints, as in a person with panic disorder-like symptoms, or intrusive cognitions, as in a person with OCD-like symptoms. In accordance with the tripartite model, they also discuss the implications of low PA (e.g., the dysphoric symptoms seen in individuals with depression and social phobia), and high inhibition or avoidance. They suggest that clinicians assess the three factors of NA, PA, and inhibition and then plot a profile, similar to the profiles generated by the Minnesota Multiphasic Personality Inventory. The resulting diagnostic profiles would communicate information about temperament (as indicated by NA and PA levels), the focus of anxiety (as indicated by the way in which NA is expressed), and the type of avoidance exhibited (e.g., behavioral, interoceptive, cognitive, or emotional avoidance). Brown and Barlow acknowledge that the primary hurdle with this conceptualization of diagnosis and treatment is the lack of an adequate assessment tool for determining such a diagnostic profile. Additionally, from a practical standpoint "cutpoints" and labels would need to be established, which would reintroduce many of the concerns of a categorical model.

Clinically Relevant Model

Norton (2006) proposed a transdiagnostic model for anxiety disorders, emphasizing the need for a clinically relevant model. While recognizing the utility of the current disorder-specific classification model for research purposes, Norton argues that this conceptualization of anxiety disorders has no clear clinical advantage over a transdiagnostic model on the basis of diagnostic reliability, case conceptualization, and treatment decisions. Recognizing the importance of clinical utility, Norton's model 1 is a dimensional diagnostic system that is optimized for use in a clinical setting. Norton (2006) suggests seven diagnostic criteria for a diagnosis of "anxiety disorder," including five primary criteria: (1) persistent and unreasonable fear of specific stimuli; (2) excessive and unreasonable anticipatory anxiety about potential encounters with feared stimuli; (3) use of cognitive or behavioral strategies to manage anxiety, such as avoidance, safety signals, worry, or preparation; (4) insight that the fear is excessive or unreasonable; and (5) anxiety, fear, or distress management strategies cause interference or distress. These criteria highlight the important distinctions between anxiety and fear (e.g., Barlow, 2002; Blanchard & Blanchard, 1990; Craske, 1999) and the importance of maladaptive coping strategies, such as avoidance and rituals, but deemphasize the specific stimulus or stimuli triggering the emotional states. Additionally, although evidence suggests that a dimensional model is warranted, cut-points for clinical decision making may still be necessary. Thus this model proposes that use of Clinical Severity Ratings (CSR; Brown et al., 1994) on a 9-point (0–8) scale of diagnostic severity with scores of 4 or greater considered clinically significant. This method provides a balance between the more appropriate dimensional structure and the practical need for clinical cutoffs. Furthermore, the CSR has been evaluated psychometrically and shows good reliability when used by trained diagnosticians (Brown, Di Nardo, Lehman, & Campbell, 2001).

This one-dimensional model is parsimonious and evidence-based, but does not provide individualized information that is essential for treatment planning. Norton (2006) acknowledges that, in any clinical setting, clinicians are capable of, and expected to, collect information about their clients beyond a diagnosis. Indeed, this model ensures that diagnosis is not a proxy for functional analyses of behavior and individualized case formulations, enabling clinicians to develop a person-centered, empirically based treatment plan.

Multiple-Process Model

Harvey and colleagues (Harvey, Watkins, Mansell, & Shafran, 2004; Mansell, Harvey, Watkins, & Shafran, 2009) proposed a process-driven model of psychopathology that focuses on the broad domains of attention, memory, reasoning, thoughts, and behaviors. This research group notes that the effective implementation of CBT with a transdiagnostic approach does not require a diagnostic assessment, unlike disorder-specific approaches (Mansell et al., 2009). This viewpoint leads to assessment focused on the processes related to the development and maintenance of psychological disorders and treatment that immediately begins to target these processes rather than on the specific symptom content. However, while some processes seem to be transdiagnostic (e.g., self-absorption and poor emotion regulation), others may be diagnosis-specific (e.g., overgeneral memory), suggesting that any clinical presentation may reflect a combination of transdiagnostic and disorder-specific processes (Mansell et al., 2009). Thus, this offers some justification for conducting traditional disorder-specific assessments such as the ADIS-IV or SCID-IV in addition to transdiagnostic assessments.

In summary, a large body of empirical evidence supports the adoption of a transdiagnostic conceptualization of anxiety and mood disorders. Yet the field is lacking in empirically derived transdiagnostic assessment tools, and transdiagnostic case conceptualizations are limited by near universal adoption of a categorical diagnostic classification system (i.e., ICD-10, DSM-5).

TRANSDIAGNOSTIC COGNITIVE ASSESSMENT

Transdiagnostic Assessment: New Methods for New Models

Over 50 years ago, the Hamilton Anxiety Rating Scale (HARS; Hamilton, 1959) was developed to assess anxiety irrespective of diagnosis. The HARS has demonstrated insufficient internal consistency, suggesting that the scale items may not be referring to the same construct (Maier, Buller, Philipp, & Heuser, 1988; Norton & Robinson, 2010), and—less problematic for a transdiagnostic assessment—it has shown poor discriminative ability between generalized anxiety disorder and major depression (Moras, Di Nardo, & Barlow, 1992). Since this initial attempt, there has been a relative void in the development of comprehensive transdiagnostic assessment for anxiety and mood disorders. Currently, a clinician-administered interview assessing for the common underlying pathology of anxiety disorders is not available, making transdiagnostic assessment an area ripe for development.

Despite compelling evidence for a transdiagnostic model of anxiety, the current "gold standard" diagnostic tools are rooted in the categorical DSM-based model of anxiety disorders (e.g., the ADIS-IV [Brown et al., 1994]; the Structured Clinical Interview for DSM-IV [SCID-IV; First, Spitzer, Gibbon, & Williams, 1997]). However, advances in transdiagnostic research and potential benefits to clients are dependent upon new methods of diagnosis and treatment evaluation that are consistent with a common pathology framework. While formal principles of transdiagnostic assessment have yet to be developed, here, we propose points for consideration. First, Mansell et al. (2009) suggest that transdiagnostic assessment focus on maintenance processes rather than diagnostic symptoms. If maintaining processes such as NA, PH, attentional biases, avoidance behavior, and others are to be the focus of treatment, these processes should also be the focus of assessment. Because there are a wide range of processes and factors that have been implicated in anxiety and emotional disorders, it is critical to determine which of the maintaining factors are central for each individual. Second, transdiagnostic assessment should determine the overall severity of and interference from anxiety. Current assessments such as the ADIS-IV and SCID-IV result in discrete diagnoses but are ill-equipped to determine the additive impact of having multiple disorders. Use of traditional assessment methods renders it difficult to determine the overall severity and functional impact of having several disorders. This also hinders comparison of severity and functionality across individuals. For example, how does a person with mild panic disorder, moderate social phobia, and mild-to-moderate generalized anxiety compare to someone with severe social phobia? Are multiple diagnoses necessarily indicative of greater overall severity or simply symptoms that manifest themselves in a variety of settings? High rates of anxiety symptom comorbidity contribute to the need for transdiagnostic assessments that capture overall severity and interference globally.

Transdiagnostic Cognitive Case Formulation for Anxiety

Persons (2008) describes case formulation as "a hypothesis about the psychological mechanisms and other factors *that are causing and maintaining* all of a particular patient's disorders and problems" (p. 5; emphasis added). The cognitive-behavioral case formulation is a guide for therapists, rooted in evidence-based practices, which informs treatment decisions that meet the unique, individualized needs of clients. An effective case formulation begins with effective assessment and leads to planning, treatment, continued progress monitoring, and eventually termination (Persons, 2008).

Consistent with transdiagnostic theory and treatment, the cognitive-behavioral case formulation is more concerned with the mechanisms underlying the disorder and the functional relationship between events and behaviors than it is with the particular symptoms of a disorder. Further, a transdiagnostic case formulation accounts for the fact that several common processes take place across diagnostic categories, resulting in disparate symptoms that are intertwined by a core pathology. Such a consideration leads to treatment based on psychological analysis rather than psychiatric diagnosis (Whitefield-Alexander & Edwards, 2009). The following section further describes the transdiagnostic cognitive-behavioral case formulation and illustrates this process with a transdiagnostic case conceptualization of the client, Marie, described at the beginning of the chapter.

Assessment and Treatment Planning

An individualized case formulation includes qualitative data derived from interviews as well as quantitative data gathered from psychometrically sound assessments (Persons, 2008). Both types of data provide valuable information that lend utility of the case formulation. Qualitative information obtained through structured and semistructured interviews highlights the client's symptoms as well as the cognitive and behavioral patterns that bind symptoms across diagnoses. Quantitative data that capture the frequency and intensity of symptoms provide an indication of symptom severity and overall life impact. Several self-report measures we describe later may be utilized to assess the severity of broad symptoms of emotional distress as well as the intensity of avoidance patterns and overall impact on quality of life. However, as previously noted, transdiagnostic assessments in the form of structured and semistructured interviews are almost nonexistent.

A thorough assessment results in a case formulation that leads to a treatment plan that targets the root of the anxiety and depressive experience. Rather than targeting specific behaviors, the treatment plan will broadly delineate avoidant and safety behaviors and maladaptive thought processes (e.g., overestimation of threat, catastrophizing, low self-efficacy) as the treatment targets. Taking a transdiagnostic perspective has clear benefits for the treatment process. First, the transdiagnostic fear hierarchy includes a variety of situations that span many diagnoses. For example, social, health, and interoceptive fears are listed and ranked on the same hierarchy and are addressed in a fluid and flexible manner throughout the treatment process. Flexibility in the approach to feared stimuli is thought to contribute to the client's understanding of discrete symptoms as being related to similar processes. Second, overarching cognitive and behavioral patterns rather than syndrome-specific concerns become the focus of treatment. For example, clients with co-occurring panic and somatic complaints may relay that they chose to not drive alone because they feared having a panic attack. Here, the therapist would suggest that the avoidant behavior was a function of anxiety about the physiological symptoms of anxiety, which is a process parallel to the clients' behaviors of researching somatic symptoms on the Internet—both are rooted in anxiety about physiological experiences. Encouraging clients to adopt a more global perspective on their anxiety aids the process of generalizing treatment gains from one symptom cluster to another. Similarly, for clients who experience symptoms related to a single disorder, discussing the underlying mechanisms helps to reduce the likelihood that the problem will manifest itself through a different symptom presentation in the future.

Transdiagnostic Self-Report Measures of Anxiety and Depression

Additionally, there are several widely used self-report measures designed to assess global anxiety. A brief discussion of some of the current options available for transdiagnostic assessment of disordered anxiety follows.

The Mood and Anxiety Symptom Questionnaire (MASQ; Clark & Watson, 1991) is an instrument designed to measure components of Clark and Watson's (1991) tripartite model (e.g., negative affect [NA], positive affect [PA], and physiological hyperarousal [PH]). It consists of four subscales: the General Distress: Anxious Symptoms (NA), General Distress: Depressive Symptoms (NA), Anxious Arousal (PH), and Anhedonic Depression (PA) subscales. Factor-analytic examinations of the MASQ with student, community, and patient samples have consistently yielded three-factor solutions (General Distress, Anhedonic Depression, and Somatic Anxiety) that broadly correspond to the instrument's conceptually derived subscales of NA, PA, and PH (Watson et al., 1995).

The Anxiety Disorder Diagnostic Questionnaire (ADDQ; Norton & Robinson, 2010) was developed as a screening tool for the presence of clinical fear and anxiety irrespective of diagnoses and is based on the transdiagnostic anxiety criteria outlined by Norton (2006). It is a brief four-section measure developed to assess fear, anxiety/worry, escape/avoidance behaviors, physiological symptoms, and associated distress and interference. Factor-analytic examination of the ADDQ in student and outpatient populations indicate a one- or two-factor solution, with a two-factor solution differentiating between the experience of fear/anxiety from the experience of physiological and cognitive symptoms of fear/anxiety (Norton & Robinson, 2010). Additionally, data from outpatients who completed a transdiagnostic CBT program indicated a very strong concordance between change on the ADDQ and change in clinician severity ratings from a structured diagnostic interview.

Other common measures used to assess for the general presence of anxiety include the Depression, Anxiety, and Stress Scales (DASS; Lovibond & Lovibond, 1995), the Beck Anxiety Inventory (BAI; Beck, Epstein, Brown, & Steer, 1988), and the Spielberger State–Trait Anxiety Inventory (STAI; Spielberger, Gorsuch, Lushene, Vagg, & Jacobs, 1983). These self-report measures have the advantages of being adequately reliable, brief, and commonly used, enabling comparisons of diagnostic-specific treatments to transdiagnostic treatments. However, some research suggests each of these scales may be more valid for some diagnoses than others. For example, although the BAI was developed to assess for global anxiety, the measure has extensive loading of anxiety presentations with a greater emphasis on panic or fear responses than those with a greater tendency toward anxious apprehension (Cox, Cohen, Direnfeld, & Swinson, 1996; Erickson et al., 2007). Additionally, some have raised concerns that the STAI is more strongly correlated with depression than with anxiety, calling into question its accuracy for measuring anxiety (Bieling, Antony, & Swinson, 1998; Creamer, Foran, & Bell, 1995).

Other construct-based approaches that may assess common anxiety disorder pathology include measures of emotion regulation (e.g., Difficulties in Emotion Regulation Scale, Gratz & Roemer, 2004; Emotion Regulation Questionnaire, Gross & John, 1998); locus of control (e.g., Locus of Control of Behavior, Craig, Franklin, & Andrews, 1984); self-esteem (e.g., Rosenberg Self-Esteem Scale, Rosenberg, 1979); quality of life (e.g., Quality of Life Inventory, Frisch, 1994), and overall measures of distress and disability (e.g., Fear and General Symptom Questionnaire, Hafner, 1981; Hallam & Hafner, 1978; Wing et al., 1998). Assessing these varied constructs may provide further information about treatment outcomes beyond symptom change.

Although continued work on developing and disseminating standard transdiagnostic clinical interviews is needed, many self-report tools are currently available for assessing the common constructs underlying anxiety disorders. Use of these transdiagnostic measures will assist in the transdiagnostic case conceptualization, treatment planning, and treatment evaluation by capturing baseline levels of and changes in underlying processes throughout treatment.

A Transdiagnostic Case Formulation of Marie

The complexity of Marie's presentation led to a diagnostic and treatment paradox. If conceptualized as six disparate conditions, treatment of this case would be daunting for the therapist and frustrating for the client, and difficulty would have arisen about which diagnoses to target and in which order to target them. In contrast, the diagnoses could be reduced to a single more parsimonious diagnosis: specific phobia, with an admittedly complex presentation. However, this option was limited by the fact that established evidence-based CBT protocols for specific phobias may not include strategies such as interoceptive exposure for her fear of stomach sensations, imaginal exposure for her intrusive thoughts or pathological worries, response prevention strategies for reducing her compulsive behaviors, or any established strategies for addressing her body weight and feared foods. From a transdiagnostic perspective, however, this case was seen as a complex interaction of triggers and behavioral responses, all centering around her beliefs that she was at risk for easily vomiting, that vomiting would be intolerable, and that she could not cope if she vomited. She also evidenced a very pervasive attentional bias toward interpreting most events and stimuli through a lens of how they might relate to the probability of vomiting.

Assessing the common factors and processes underlying Marie's many diagnoses would aid the development of a transdiagnostic case formulation. As there were no evidence-based instruments that adequately assessed all facets of her specific anxiety disorder manifestation, a collection of brief measures—including measures of bodily sensation fears, agoraphobic avoidance, compulsive hand washing, worry, and so forth—was developed and periodically completed by Marie throughout treatment to monitor changes in these processes. Additionally, in a collaboration between Marie and her therapist, a hierarchy of feared triggers and consequent safety behaviors was drafted, and specific evidence-based interoceptive, *in vivo*, and imaginal exposure strategies were identified to specifically elicit those triggers in a mutually agreed upon gradual schedule. When, for example, it became time to begin addressing her fear of gastrointestinal sensations, interceptive exposure strategies were incorporated. Similarly, later in treatment, when Marie became more comfortable with the therapist and explained that her sexual assault history involved the male manager of the exotic dancing establishment forcibly making her perform oral sex—resulting in her gagging and vomiting—treatment was able to incorporate prolonged imaginal exposure and cognitive processing of her rape-related memories, rather than needing to discontinue the current treatment and begin a treatment protocol for posttraumatic stress disorder. With the shift in treatment focus, it became necessary to incorporate a self-report measure of intrusive recollections into the assessment protocol.

In the real clinical case of Marie, transdiagnostic processes revealed themselves through the course of treatment. Had a transdiagnostic interview assessment been available at the time of intake, the clinician would have been able to target the underlying problems from the beginning. As it was, several weeks were spent trying to identify the common ties across the various diagnoses and attempting to adapt the most efficient treatment plan for addressing the myriad symptoms.

CONCLUSIONS AND FUTURE DIRECTIONS

With the publication of DSM-5, an examination of the implications of a transdiagnostic perspective as they relate to the new diagnostic system is warranted. Watson (2005) describes three assumptions of a psychiatric classification which may be untenable for anxiety disorder diagnoses. Namely, DSM-5 assumes that diagnoses in different classes are empirically unrelated, disorders in the same diagnostic class are significantly related, and diagnostic subtypes are more closely related than indicators of different disorders. The various benefits of conceptualizing anxiety and depressive disorders from a transdiagnostic perspective have become more evident in recent years. However, the practical implications of adopting a transdiagnostic perspective to assessment and case formulation can only be realized fully if the diagnostic classification system changes accordingly.

As noted throughout the chapter, there is a strong theoretical and empirical argument for the transdiagnostic conceptualization of anxiety. A transdiagnostic perspective appears to be the most parsimonious explanation of comorbidity among anxiety and depressive disorders as well as nonspecific heritability of mood disorders. Transdiagnostic approaches to the treatment of anxiety appear promising and may be a more efficient way of training clinicians to treat an array of anxiety and mood symptoms. However, issues of assessment cannot be ignored without endangering the further development of transdiagnostic CBT.

Currently, transdiagnostic treatment is often preceded by diagnosis-specific assessment. While the research groups conducting transdiagnostic treatment have realized treatment success, it is unclear to what extent the lack of transdiagnostic assessments has impacted potential treatment improvements. Using a global index of anxiety severity provides a way of assessing overall severity, but a single rating relies on the subjectivity of the clinician. The development of a more thorough transdiagnostic interview, possibly based on the ADDQ, may prove to be a more useful transdiagnostic assessment.

This chapter has provided an overview of the extant assessments that aim to elucidate the higher order factors that underlie anxiety disorders. However, much work remains to develop a comprehensive structured assessment tool. The changes proposed by several impactful researchers in the field of anxiety suggest that the new diagnostic system emphasize the underlying pathologies that drive pathological anxiety more generally, benefiting evidence-based assessment, case conceptualization, and treatment.

--- **KEY POINTS** ---

FOR PRACTITIONERS

- Strong empirical evidence supports a transdiagnostic conceptualization of anxiety.
- Targeting the core pathology for anxiety may be more efficient and comprehensive than targeting specific anxiety disorder symptoms.
- Transdiagnostic measures should be used during the assessment process to assist the formulation of a transdiagnostic case conceptualization and treatment plan.

FOR RESEARCHERS

- Transdiagnostic assessment of anxiety is not as advanced as transdiagnostic treatment.
- Current transdiagnostic measures capture the pathology reflected in certain specific disorders better than others.
- Clinical trials for anxiety disorders will benefit from the development of a structured interview capturing underlying anxiety constructs.

FOR STUDENTS AND EDUCATORS

- Transdiagnostic measures should be used during the assessment process to help develop an individualized transdiagnostic case conceptualization and treatment plan.
- Transdiagnostic assessment and treatment plans may be more efficient in training clinicians by defining a unified approach rather than proposing assessment and treatment plans for each diagnosis.
- Transdiagnostic assessment tools are still limited in number and will benefit from further development and empirical evaluation.

REFERENCES

Allen, L. B., Ehrenreich, J. T., & Barlow, D. H. (2005). A unified treatment for emotional disorders: Applications with adults and adolescents. *Japanese Journal of Behavior Therapy*, *31*, 3–31.

American Psychiatric Association. (1952). *Diagnostic and statistical manual of mental disorders*. Washington, DC: Author.

American Psychiatric Association. (1968). *Diagnostic and statistical manual of mental disorders* (2nd ed.). Washington, DC: Author.

American Psychiatric Association. (1980). *Diagnostic and statistical manual of mental disorders* (3rd ed.). Washington, DC: Author.

American Psychiatric Association. (1994). *Diagnostic and statistical manual of mental disorders* (4th ed.). Washington, DC: Author.

American Psychiatric Association. (2013). *Diagnostic and statistical manual of mental disorders* (5th ed.). Arlington, VA: Author.

Andrews, G., Stewart, G., Morris-Yates, A., & Holt, P. (1990). Evidence for a general neurotic syndrome. *British Journal of Psychiatry, 157,* 6–12.

Bandelow, B., Zohar, J., Hollander, E., Kasper, S., & Moller, H. J. (2002). World Federation of Societies of Biological Psychiatry guidelines for the pharmacological treatment of anxiety, obsessive–compulsive and posttraumatic stress disorders. *World Journal of Biological Psychiatry, 3,* 171–199.

Bar-Hiam, Y., Lamy, D., Pergamin, L., Bakermans-Kranenburg, M. J., & van IJzendoorn, M. H. (2007). Threat-related attentional bias in anxious and non-anxious individuals: A meta-analytic study. *Psychological Bulletin, 133,* 1–24.

Barlow, D. H. (2000). Unraveling the mysteries of anxiety and its disorders from the perspective of emotion theory. *American Psychologist, 55,* 1247–1263.

Barlow, D. H. (2002). *Anxiety and its disorders* (2nd ed.). New York: Guilford Press.

Barlow, D. H., Allen, L. B., & Choate, M. L. (2003, November). A unified treatment protocol for the emotional disorders. In P. J. Norton (Chair), *Integrative treatment approaches across anxiety and related disorders.* Symposium conducted at the annual meeting of the Anxiety Disorders Association of America, Toronto, Ontario, Canada.

Barlow, D. H., Allen, L. B., & Choate, M. L. (2004). Toward a unified treatment for emotional disorders. *Behavior Therapy, 35,* 205–230.

Beck, A. T., Epstein, N., Brown, G., & Steer, R. A. (1988). An inventory for measuring clinical anxiety: Psychometric properties. *Journal of Consulting and Clinical Psychology, 56,* 893–897.

Bieling, P. J., Antony, M. M., & Swinson, R. P. (1998). The State–Trait Anxiety Inventory, Trait version: Structure and content re-examined. *Behaviour Research and Therapy, 36,* 777–788.

Blanchard, E. B., Hickling, E. J., Devineni, T., Veazey, C. H., Galovski, T. E., Mundy, E., et al. (2003). A controlled evaluation of cognitive behavioural therapy for posttraumatic stress in motor vehicle accident survivors. *Behaviour Research and Therapy, 41,* 79–96.

Blanchard, R. J., & Blanchard, D. C. (1990). An ethnoexperimental analysis of defense, fear, and anxiety. In N. McNaughton & G. Andrews (Eds.), *Anxiety* (pp. 124–133). Dunedin, New Zealand: University of Otago Press.

Borkovec, T. D., Abel, J. L., & Newman, H. (1995). Effects of psychotherapy on comorbid conditions in generalized anxiety disorder. *Journal of Consulting and Clinical Psychology, 63,* 479–483.

Brown, T. A., Antony, M. M., & Barlow, D. H. (1995). Diagnostic comorbidity in panic disorder: Effect on treatment outcome and course of comorbid diagnoses following treatment. *Journal of Consulting and Clinical Psychology*, *63*, 408–418.

Brown, T. A., & Barlow, D. H. (2009). A proposal for a dimensional classification system based on the shared features of the DSM-IV anxiety and mood disorders: Implications for assessment and treatment. *Psychological Assessment*, *21*, 256–271.

Brown, T. A., Di Nardo, P. A., & Barlow, D. H. (1994). *Anxiety Disorders Interview Schedule for DSM-IV (Adult Version)*. Albany, NY: Graywind.

Brown, T. A., Di Nardo, P. A., Lehman, C. L., & Campbell, L. A. (2001). Reliability of DSM-IV anxiety and mood disorders: Implications for the classification of emotional disorders. *Journal of Abnormal Psychology*, *110*, 49–58.

Chorpita, B. F., Brown, T. A., & Barlow, D. H. (1998). Perceived control as a mediator of family environment in etiological models of childhood anxiety. *Behavior Therapy*, *29*, 457–476.

Clark, L. A., & Watson, D. (1991). Tripartite model of anxiety and depression: Psychometric evidence and taxonomic implications. *Journal of Abnormal Psychology*, *100*, 316–336.

Clifft, M. A. (1986). Writing about psychiatric patients: Guidelines for disguising case material. *Bulletin of the Menninger Clinic*, *50*, 511–524.

Cox, B. J., Cohen, E., Direnfeld, D. M., & Swinson, R. P. (1996). Does the Beck Anxiety Inventory measure anything beyond panic attack symptoms? *Behavior Research and Therapy*, *34*, 949–954.

Craig, A., Franklin, J., & Andrews, G. (1984). A scale to measure locus of control of behaviour. *British Journal of Medical Psychology*, *57*, 173–180.

Craske, M. G. (1999). *Anxiety disorders: Psychological approaches to theory and treatment*. Boulder, CO: Westview Press.

Creamer, M., Foran, J., & Bell, R. (1995). The Beck Anxiety Inventory in a nonclinical sample. *Behaviour Research and Therapy*, *33*, 477–485.

Davidson, R. J. (2000). Affective style, psychopathology, and resilience: Brain mechanisms and plasticity. *American Psychologist*, *55*, 1196–1214.

Ellard, K. K., Fairholme, C. P., Boisseau, C. L., Farchione, T. J., & Barlow, D. H. (2010). Unified protocol for the transdiagnostic treatment of emotional disorders: Protocol development and initial outcome data. *Cognitive and Behavioral Practice*, *17*, 88–101.

Erickson, D. H., Janeck, A., & Tallman, K. (2007). Group cognitive-behavioral group for patients with various anxiety disorders. *Psychiatric Services*, *58*, 1205–1211.

Eysenck, H. J. (1957). *The dynamics of anxiety and hysteria: An experimental application of modern learning theory to psychiatry*. London: Routledge & Kegan Paul.

Farchione, T. J., Fairholme, C. P., Ellard, K. K., Boisseau, C. L., Thompson-Hollands, J., Carl, J. R., et al. (2012). Unified protocol for transdiagnostic treatment of emotional disorders: A randomized controlled trial. *Behavior Therapy*, *43*, 666–678.

First, M. B., Spitzer, R. L., Gibbon, M., & Williams, J. B. W. (1997). *Structured*

Clinical Interview for DSM-IV Axis I Disorders, Clinician Version (SCID-CV). Washington, DC: American Psychiatric Press.

Frisch, M. B. (1994). *Manual and treatment guide for the Quality of Life Inventory.* Minneapolis, MN: NCS Pearson.

Garcia, M. S. (2004). Effectiveness of cognitive-behavioral group therapy in patients with anxiety disorders. *Psychology in Spain, 8,* 89–97.

Good, B. J., & Kleinman, A. M. (1985). Culture and anxiety: Cross-cultural evidence for the patterning of anxiety disorders. In A. Tuma & J. D. Maser (Eds.), *Anxiety and the anxiety disorders* (pp. 297–323). Hillsdale, NJ: Erlbaum.

Gratz, K. L., & Roemer, L. (2004). Multidimensional assessment of emotion regulation and dysregulation: Development, factor structure, and initial validation of the Difficulties in Emotion Regulation Scale. *Journal of Psychopathology and Behavioral Assessment, 26,* 41–54.

Gross, J. J., & John, O. P. (1998). Mapping the domain of emotional expressivity: Multi-method evidence for a hierarchical model. *Journal of Personality and Social Psychology, 74,* 170–191.

Hafner, R. (1981). Agoraphobia in men. *Australian and New Zealand Journal of Psychiatry, 15,* 243–249.

Hallam, R., & Hafner, R. (1978). Fears of phobic patients: Factor analyses of self-report data. *Behaviour Research and Therapy, 16,* 1–6.

Hamilton, M. (1959). The assessment of anxiety states by rating. *British Journal of Medical Psychology, 32,* 50–55.

Harkness, A. R., & Lilienfeld, S. O. (1997). Individual differences science for treatment planning: Personality traits. *Psychological Assessment, 9,* 349–360.

Harvey, A., Watkins, E., Mansell, W., & Shafran, R. (2004). *Cognitive-behavioral processes across psychological disorders: A transdiagnostic approach to research and treatment.* Oxford, UK: Oxford University Press.

Hettema, J. M., Prescott, C. A., Myers, J. M., Neale, M. C., & Kendler, K. S. (2005). The structure of genetic and environmental risk factors for anxiety disorders in men and women. *Archives of General Psychiatry, 62,* 182–189.

Kessler, R. C., Chiu, W., Demler, O., & Walters, E. E. (2005). Prevalence, severity, and comorbidity of 12-month DSM-IV disorders in the National Comorbidity Survey Replication. *Archives of General Psychiatry, 62,* 617–627.

Larkin, K. T., Waller, S., & Combs-Lane, A. (2003, March). Anxiety management group therapy for multiple anxiety disorder diagnoses. In P. J. Norton (Chair), *Integrative treatment approaches across anxiety and related disorders.* Symposium conducted at the annual meeting of the Anxiety Disorders Association of America, Toronto, Ontario, Canada.

Lovibond, P. F., & Lovibond, S. H. (1995). The structure of negative emotional states: Comparison of the Depression Anxiety Stress Scales (DASS) with the Beck Depression and Anxiety Inventories. *Behaviour Research and Therapy, 33,* 335–343.

Maier, W., Buller, R., Philipp, M., & Heuser, I. (1988). The Hamilton Anxiety

Scale: Reliability, validity and sensitivity to change in anxiety and depressive disorders. *Journal of Affective Disorders, 14,* 61–68.

Mansell, W., Harvey, A., Watkins, E., & Shafran, R. (2009). Conceptual foundations of the transdiagnostic approach to CBT. *Journal of Cognitive Psychotherapy, 23,* 6–19.

McEvoy, P. M., & Nathan, P. (2007). Effectiveness of cognitive behaviour therapy for diagnostically heterogeneous groups: A benchmarking study. *Journal of Consulting and Clinical Psychology, 75,* 344–350.

McManus, F., Shafran, R., & Cooper, Z. (2010). What does a "transdiagnostic" approach have to offer the treatment of anxiety disorders? *British Journal of Clinical Psychology, 49,* 491–505.

McNaughton, N., & Gray, J. A. (2000). Anxiolytic action on the behavioral inhibition system implies multiple types of arousal contribute to anxiety. *Journal of Affective Disorders, 61,* 161–176.

Moras, K., Di Nardo, P. A., & Barlow, D. H. (1992). Distinguishing anxiety and depression: Reexamination of the reconstructed Hamilton scales. *Psychological Assessment, 4,* 224–227.

Norton, P. J. (2006). Toward a clinically-oriented model of anxiety disorders. *Cognitive Behaviour Therapy, 35,* 88–105.

Norton, P. J., & Barrera, T. L. (2012). Transdiagnostic versus diagnosis-specific CBT for anxiety disorders: A preliminary randomized controlled trial. *Depression and Anxiety, 29*(10), 874–882.

Norton, P. J., Barrera, T. L., Mathew, A. R., Chamberlain, L. D., Szafranski, D. D., Reddy, R., et al. (2013). Effect of transdiagnostic CBT for anxiety disorders on comorbid diagnoses. *Depression and Anxiety, 30*(2), 168–173.

Norton, P. J., Hayes, S. A., & Hope, D. A. (2004). Effects of a transdiagnostic group treatment for anxiety on secondary depressive disorders. *Depression and Anxiety, 20,* 198–202.

Norton, P. J., & Hope, D. A. (2005). Preliminary evaluation of a broad-spectrum cognitive-behavioral group therapy for anxiety. *Journal of Behavior Therapy and Experimental Psychiatry, 36,* 79–97.

Norton, P. J., & Philipp, L. M. (2008). Transdiagnostic approaches to the treatment of anxiety disorders: A meta-analytic review. *Psychotherapy: Theory, Research, Practice, and Training, 45,* 214–226.

Norton, P. J., & Price, E. C. (2007). A meta-analytic review of adult cognitive-behavioral treatment outcome across the anxiety disorders. *Journal of Nervous and Mental Disease, 195,* 521–531.

Norton, P. J., & Robinson, C. M. (2010). Development and evaluation of the Anxiety Disorder Diagnostic Questionnaire. *Cognitive Behaviour Therapy, 39,* 137–149.

Persons, J. B. (2008). *The case formulation approach to cognitive-behavior therapy.* New York: Guilford Press.

Philipp, L. M., Washington, C., Raouf, M., & Norton, P. J. (2008). Cross-cultural examination of the tripartite model in adults. *Cognitive Behaviour Therapy, 37,* 221–232.

Rapee, R. M. (2002). The development and modification of temperamental risk for anxiety disorders: Prevention of a lifetime of anxiety? *Biological Psychiatry, 52,* 947–957.

Rosenberg, M. (1979). *Conceiving of the self.* New York: Basic Books.

Schmidt, N. B. (2003, November). Unified CBT for anxiety: Preliminary findings from false safety behavior elimination therapy (F–SET). In D. F. Tolin (Chair), *Increasing the cost-effectiveness and user-friendliness of cognitive behavior therapy for anxiety disorders.* Symposium conducted at the 37th annual convention of the Association for Advancement of Behavior Therapy, Boston.

Spielberger, C. D., Gorsuch, R. L., Lushene, R., Vagg, P. R., & Jacobs, G. A. (1983). *Manual for the State–Trait Anxiety Inventory.* Palo Alto, CA: Consulting Psychologists Press.

Spitzer, R. L., First, M. B., & Wakefield, J. C. (2007). Saving PTSD from itself in DSM-V. *Journal of Anxiety Disorders, 21,* 233–241.

Stein, D. J., Fineberg, N. A., Bienvenu, O., Denys, D., Lochner, C., Nestadt, G., et al. (2010). Should OCD be classified as an anxiety disorder in DSM-V? *Depression and Anxiety, 27,* 495–506.

Titov, N., Andrews, G., Johnston, L., Robinson, E., & Spence, J. (2010). Transdiagnostic Internet treatment for anxiety disorders: A randomized controlled trial. *Behaviour Research and Therapy, 48,* 890–899.

Tsao, J. I., Mystkowski, J. L., Zucker, B. G., & Craske, M. G. (2002). Effects of cognitive-behavioral therapy for panic disorder on comorbid conditions: Replication and extension. *Behavior Therapy, 33,* 493–509.

Watson, D. (2005). Rethinking the mood and anxiety disorders: A quantitative hierarchical model for DSM-V. *Journal of Abnormal Psychology, 114,* 522–536.

Watson, D., Clark, L. A., Weber, K., Assenheimer, J., Strauss, M. E., & McCormick, R. A. (1995). Testing a tripartite model: II. Exploring the symptom structure of anxiety and depression in student, adult, and patient samples. *Journal of Abnormal Psychology, 104,* 15–25.

Whitefield-Alexander, V., & Edwards, D. (2009). A case of effective single-session treatment for attention deficit and learning problems in a routine clinical practice: The value of a transdiagnostic approach to case formulation. *Journal of Child and Adolescent Mental Health, 21,* 61–72.

Wing, J. K., Beevor, A. S., Curtis, R. H., Park, S. B., Hadden, S., & Burns, A. (1998). Health of the Nation Outcome Scales (HONOS): Research and development. *British Journal of Psychiatry, 172,* 11–18.

10

Beyond DSM Diagnosis

The Pros and Cons
of Cognitive Case Formulation

Brenda Key and Peter J. Bieling

In this chapter we set out to review the definition and purpose of cognitive case formulation, as well as to review key areas of assessment in the development of a case formulation. We also discuss the current state of empirical evidence for cognitive case formulation and we hypothesize about the future role of case formulation in the next wave of cognitive therapy treatment. A comprehensive description of how to develop and use a cognitive case formulation is beyond the scope of this chapter; there are a number of excellent resources available that describe the details of how to create and use a case formulation (e.g., Eells, 2007; Persons, 2008). We focus here on larger questions of function and utility, beginning with definitions.

WHAT IS CASE FORMULATION?

At the broadest level, "case formulation" is a tool that therapists use to assist in the treatment of clients. More specifically, "case formulation is a hypothesis about the causes, precipitants and maintaining influences of a person's psychological, interpersonal, and behavioral problems"

(Eells, 2007, p. 4). A closer look at this definition reveals that case formulation involves both describing a client's current problems and also making inferences about how these problems developed and are maintained. These inferences are based on a theoretical foundation and inform intervention choices.

Regardless of the theoretical orientation, case formulations share several unifying elements: a description of the presenting problems; relevant developmental history; causal factors (distal and proximal); maintaining factors; coping strengths and weaknesses; and implications for intervention (Bieling & Kuyken, 2003). The formulation should describe these factors, but even more important should focus the practitioner on hypotheses about the mechanisms that link these factors together in a coherent way. In cognitive case formulation, cognitive theory is used to derive these inferences and develop an explanation of how learning principles have led to the client's systems of beliefs, behaviors, and thoughts. Where specific models of cognitive case formulation differ is in their emphasis on the various components of the case formulation (i.e., behaviors, thoughts, underlying beliefs) and the methods and structure used to develop the formulation. Three commonly cited cognitive-behavioral case formulation models are those developed by Nezu, Nezu, and Lombardo (2004), Persons (2008), and J. S. Beck (1995). In their case formulation model, Nezu et al. (2004) emphasize the role of the clinician in solving problems and identifying the client's unique style of orienting to difficulties. This model applies a multistep problem-solving strategy to reach defined goals. Persons's (2008) model emphasizes adapting empirical evidence regarding mechanisms, underlying symptoms, and disorders to the specific client. Persons's approach focuses on two levels in creating a formulation: overt problems and underlying cognitive mechanisms. The hypothesized underlying mechanisms are used to explain how the cognitions, beliefs, and behaviors cause and maintain problems. Additionally, Persons's model stresses the importance of identifying core beliefs and triggers to make the client less vulnerable to relapse. J. S. Beck's (1995) model similarly emphasizes the identification of problematic core beliefs. This model furthermore incorporates a focus on dysfunctional assumptions and maladaptive compensatory strategies, as well as elements of the client's history that may have led to the development of maladaptive core beliefs.

All of these cognitive case conceptualization approaches are quite structured and directive, and tend toward the diagrammatic, especially when compared to formulation approaches from other schools of psychotherapy. Cognitive therapists in practice often use an eclectic approach to formulation that is based on concepts consistent with these models, and perhaps other types of formulation as well, but in a less formalized manner. The "prevalence" of formulation use by cognitive therapists is relatively difficult to ascertain, in part because formulation methods are so diverse. The diversity in approaches derives from the fact that there are several different cognitive formulation models, with no particular data-driven "best practice" identified to date. Without the empirical evidence to support the benefits of a comprehensive, structured case formulation approach, the costs in terms of client and clinician time may be seen as unjustified. The feasibility of structured case formulation relies on this cost–benefit analysis, and both the costs and benefits have not been systematically evaluated and remain unclear. Thus the approaches clinicians choose to use in their everyday practice likely contain a certain amount of creativity and clinical wisdom and may also reflect a desire for efficiency rather than comprehensiveness.

Finally, we have observed that formulation methods are rarely taught at an introductory level and are more likely to be included as an "advanced" aspect of cognitive therapy training for more seasoned clinicians. Moreover, training in formulation tends to emphasize more difficult and challenging cases. It may be that formulation methods have a particular resonance with cases that go beyond standard protocols, at which point the potential benefits of better organizing clinical information outweigh the costs of spending extra time in creating the formulation. This has been expressed in a maxim whose origin is unknown: "Three most important things for a difficult case? Formulate, formulate, formulate!" In the next sections, we attempt to test this maxim by focusing in a more detailed way on the context, content, and validity of cognitive formulation.

WHAT ARE THE ROLE AND FUNCTIONS OF CASE FORMULATION?

The central role of cognitive case formulation is to translate nomothetic cognitive theory and research into idiographic treatment. Formulation therefore requires building and sustaining an up-to-date understanding of factors contributing to the development and maintenance of psychopathology. While previous knowledge of cognitive theory remains a useful base to build on, theories have been refined over time in important ways that may alter formulation, and therefore it is a clinician's responsibility to stay abreast of the current literature. A solid understanding of current cognitive theory lays the foundation for quality inputs into the formulation and a clear, coherent understanding of the case.

A good case formulation should also result in high-quality outputs by providing clear implications for treatment planning and suggesting variables to be assessed for monitoring treatment progress and outcome.

The utility of formulation is more clearly seen through the treatment implications produced by the formulation, but these outputs rely heavily on a coherent understanding of psychopathology theory. Therefore the quality of a case formulation relies on both high-quality inputs and outputs.

The proposed benefits of case formulation are numerous, at least in theory. A case formulation aspires to provide a systematic framework for hypothesizing about a client's presenting problems, and can help to improve the description and understanding of the presenting problem for both the client and the therapist. This enhanced understanding of the client's problems facilitates greater therapist empathy for the client and improves the therapeutic alliance. Moreover, a comprehensive formulation also helps to focus therapeutic interventions on key factors underlying or maintaining the client's problems. When impasses or plateaus in treatment occur, a case formulation explains the reasons for these difficulties and suggests courses of action. Finally, a case formulation approach to treatment leads to enhanced outcomes for clients. While these potential benefits are comprehensive and far-reaching, unfortunately there is currently little empirical evidence regarding the impact of formulation on treatment.

And while the evidence for the benefits of formulation is relatively embryonic, the evidence for the efficacy and effectiveness of manualized cognitive-behavioral therapy (CBT) is strong (Beck & Dozois, 2011; Chambless & Ollendick, 2001; Leichsenring, Hiller, Weissberg, & Leibing, 2006). This observation could lead to the following critical question: If manualized CBT works so well, why would anyone formulate an individual case at all? There are several important points to be made here. First, it is important to note that manualized treatment and case formulation need not be mutually exclusive. While a manual can be applied without a case formulation, the insights gained through the development of a formulation can be used within the framework of a standardized treatment. Treatment protocols typically specify mainly what the therapist does in treatment; a formulation can shed light on what the client is likely to do, say, and feel during treatment. Second, empirically supported treatments do not provide guidance in several difficult situations that clinicians commonly face, and a case formulation can provide a framework for making such decisions. Among the most common of these situations are comorbid problems. When there are multiple presenting problems, clinicians must decide whether to target problems sequentially or simultaneously and what to focus on first. A cognitive case formulation can help to guide these decisions. Third, a formulation can provide guidance when there are multiple treatment providers by clarifying the goals and roles of various treatment components. Fourth, when there is no empirically supported treatment available for the client's disorder or the problem is not a diagnosable disorder (e.g., perfectionism), then a formulation can provide a framework for selecting suitable treatment components. Even when a suitable evidence-based treatment is available for a client's presenting problem, a clinician has to make many decisions beyond the scope of information provided in a treatment protocol. For example, treatment protocols typically outline classes of problematic behaviors and cognitions, but the clinician must identify which specific behaviors and cognitions are problematic for a specific client, as the same behavior may be adaptive for one client but problematic for another. Case formulation may also help predict, prevent, and understand nonadherence to treatment. Persons (2008) explains that the "case formulation approach can prevent or reduce nonadherence because the therapist works to adapt to the patient rather than the other way around" (p. 8). Finally, a case formulation can provide guidance in choosing an alternative treatment if an empirically supported treatment protocol is not resulting in improvements of the client's symptoms. In summary, whereas a treatment manual provides the skeleton of the treatment plan, the case formulation can guide the decisions involved in filling in this framework with an individualized treatment suitable to a specific client.

The degree to which an individualized case formulation is utilized can best be conceptualized as lying on a continuum with an entirely nomothetic approach at one end and a tailored idiographic approach at the other end. As already described, even within a manualized treatment there is a role for case formulation in guiding decisions, though we would suggest that for straightforward cases, a manual is likely to be completely sufficient for good-quality cognitive therapy to occur. Highly structured interventions for simple problems and "curriculum" group-based interventions likely rely less on a formal individualized case conceptualization. But even in highly manualized CBT protocols, therapists are likely to anticipate the kinds of thoughts, behaviors, and beliefs that clients present with in sessions, and to tailor the delivery of interventions based on these predictions. Although it is not formalized, the ability to make such predictions accurately implies that a therapist has actually created an implicit formulation. To some extent, formalizing one's skills in formulation is simply extending this ad hoc, implicit work into something more thoughtful, formal, and planned, and it seems reasonable to suggest that this could have benefits for treatment efficiency, alliance, and adherence.

That case formulation becomes particularly useful as complexity increases is a claim that could be subjected to empirical scrutiny. Unfortunately, we do not have the empirical evidence to support this claim. Evidence from effectiveness CBT trials that emphasize the dissemination of CBT to community therapists, who hypothetically have less thorough knowledge of CBT and less ability to create a CBT case formulation, suggests that manualized CBT can be effective without a detailed formulation (explicit or implicit). However, this line of reasoning relies on several assumptions and direct evidence regarding the value of CBT formulation, particularly in complex cases, is needed.

OPTIMIZING CASE FORMULATION THROUGH ASSESSMENT

As previously noted, a case formulation has several components, and the approaches used in developing each of these components vary. These components can be translated into five tasks for the therapist:

1. Developing the problem list.
2. Creating hypotheses regarding causal mechanisms.
3. Creating inferences regarding the distal origins and the proximal precipitants of the mechanisms.
4. Tying the hypotheses and inferences together into a coherent explanation of the client's problems.
5. Deducing the implications for treatment and continuing to refine the formulation during treatment.

Each of these components is discussed in more detail below.

Developing a Problem List

The central challenge in developing a problem list is ensuring that the list is comprehensive—going beyond symptoms, and considering multiple domains such as interpersonal functioning, physical health problems and access to treatment. The problem list will, of course, overlap with symptoms associated with DSM diagnoses, but it should be more individualized and client-driven. Tools for obtaining information to develop the problem list include clinical interview (e.g., Structured Clinical Interview for DSM-IV-TR [First, Spitzer, Gibbon, & Williams, 2002]), broad-based self-report measures (e.g., Short-Form-36 Health Survey [Ware, Snow, Kosinski, & Gandek, 1996]; Symptom Checklist 90—Revised [Derogatis, 2000]), symptom-focused self-report measures appropriate to the client's problem areas (e.g., Beck Depression Inventory-II [Beck, Steer, & Brown, 1996]; Penn State Worry Questionnaire [Meyer, Miller, Metzger, & Borkovec, 1990]), available reports from other health care providers, and information from other informants such as family members (with the client's permission). Several comprehensive sources can be consulted to guide the selection of measures appropriate to specific areas of clinical practice (e.g., Antony & Barlow, 2010; Antony, Orsillo,

& Roemer, 2001; Fischer & Corcoran, 2007; Hunsley & Mash, 2008; Nezu, Ronan, Meadows, & McClure, 2000). The selection of assessment tools used will vary, based on the client's presenting problems to ensure a comprehensive evaluation of the key areas. Objective assessment follows the scientific spirit of CBT. It encourages the development of case formulation hypotheses based on objective information and also facilitates openness to disconfirming evidence. This process of seeking information in objective ways is therefore essential to the CBT formulation process.

As important as such objective measures are, they need always to be paired with client-centered questions about what the clients are struggling with the most; which changes would mean that therapy has been successful for them; and what they would like to be able to change about themselves, their situations or their lives. Where there is a synergy between a client's own choices and objective measurement, a therapist is likely to find the most important and central issues to be worked on (see Haynes, Mumma, & Pinson, 2009, for a step-by-step guide to the development and evaluation of idiographic assessment tools).

Developing Mechanism Hypotheses

The psychological mechanisms that are hypothesized to cause and maintain the client's problem list are central to the cognitive case formulation. The formulation may additionally comment on biological or sociological aspects that contribute to the problem. Persons (2008) describes two main strategies for developing the mechanism hypotheses: using a disorder-specific theory associated with an empirically supported treatment, or using a more general psychological theory such as cognitive or learning theory. Regardless of the method chosen, the clinician identifies the nomothetic theory appropriate to the client and his or her problems, and with this in mind attempts to elicit information that will inform how this theory applies to the client. Within the context of cognitive case formulation, this assessment will involve a focus on the client's automatic thoughts, assumptions, and beliefs.

The tools to assist in this assessment process will vary, depending on the nomothetic theory chosen; however, a few broad measures may be applicable. The two most commonly used self-report scales that are applicable to the development of cognitive mechanism hypotheses are the Dysfunctional Attitude Scale (Weissman & Beck, 1978) and the Young Schema Questionnaire: Short Form (Young, 1998). Self-report tools related to a theory of a specific disorder may also be used. For example, the Thought–Action Fusion Scale measures beliefs that are thought to be key mechanisms in the development and maintenance of obsessive–compulsive disorder (Shafran, Thordarson, & Rachman, 1996). Interview questions that probe for thoughts in problematic situations or beliefs about the self, the world, and others may also be used. Client self-monitoring of thoughts and behaviors can also provide information about possible cognitive mechanisms contributing to current problems. In choosing the assessment measures, the clinician should be guided by CBT theory regarding automatic thoughts, beliefs, and assumptions potentially related to the development and maintenance of the client's primary symptoms. Ideally, the clinician should utilize both standardized measures and more subjective assessment methods (such as open-ended interview questions) to determine which problematic cognitions are in operation for the client.

Identifying Distal Origins and Proximal Precipitants of Mechanisms

The focus for assessment of the next component of formulation is on identifying how the client learned or acquired the mechanisms that are causing the symptoms and identifying any activating stressors that may have led to the presentation of the client's problems at this time. Information related to distal origins is typically gathered through clinical interview, particularly the client's reports of his or her early upbringing, relationships with parents and other caregivers, significant childhood events (especially traumas, neglect, abuse), and information about psychiatric illness in relatives. One of the challenges for the clinician in eliciting this history is to ensure that it does not become overwhelming; another is to relate the current problems the client has identified to early life experiences. The task is less to obtain a complete biographical overview than it is to identify the particular people, times, and places from which the client learned to understand his or her experiences in a way that is related to the current symptoms and impairments.

Proximal precipitants are typically assessed through clinical interview, as most clinicians ask clients about recent stressors and changes at initial assessment. A simple life events survey (listing common stressful life events) may also be used as a tool to evaluate possible precipitants. In many cases, the precipitants are specifically related to cognitive vulnerabilities (e.g., a relationship breakup in a person with unlovability beliefs).

Tying Case Formulation Together, Deducing Treatment Implications, and Continuing to Refine the Formulation

The process of tying the case formulation together and deducing treatment implications does not involve additional assessment, but rather an integration of the information already collected with reference to etiological theory. The continued refinement of the formulation does involve ongoing assessment. This ongoing assessment may initially take the form of discussing the formulation with the client and getting his or her feedback. As treatment proceeds, self-report measures of symptoms may be used for ongoing measurement of problems. For example, the Penn State Worry Questionnaire (Meyer et al., 1990) may be used to measure the severity of worry symptoms for a client with generalized anxiety disorder (GAD). Cognitive factors contributing to the maintenance of the problem may be assessed through client self-monitoring, self-report measures, and direct questioning in session. For example, for a client with excessive worry, in-session discussion of the client's beliefs about worry as well as the Meta-Cognitions Questionnaire (Cartwright-Hatton & Wells, 1997) could be used to measure positive beliefs about worry, negative beliefs about the controllability of thoughts, and negative beliefs about cognitive confidence (cognitive factors thought to contribute to the maintenance of GAD). Client self-monitoring records of daily activities, exposure practice, hierarchies, and associated subjective ratings of distress can also be used to monitor treatment progress and to continue evaluating the mechanisms that may be contributing to the client's problems. As additional information is presented regarding the mechanisms of the client's problems, this information should be checked against the initial hypotheses, and the formulation should be refined as necessary. The utility of a high-quality case formulation becomes clear as treatment moves forward, because the formulation helps guide the assessment of progress and can also provide avenues for adjusting treatment when the client is not improving. For example, suppose a progress assessment for a client with GAD reveals that the client has developed increased confidence in his or her ability to control worry, but still holds strong positive beliefs about the benefits of worry; this finding helps to explain why the client's symptom improvement has stalled. This knowledge helps the clinician understand why the client is resistant to changing worry behavior and guides the clinician toward interventions to challenge positive beliefs about worry. In contrast, if a clinician is choosing intervention strategies based on diagnosis alone and these techniques are not benefiting the client, then the clinician cannot rely on the formulation for guidance regarding why the treatment is falling short or what adjustments should be made.

Initial attention to assessing possible cognitive factors contributing to the development and maintenance of the client's problems will provide greater quantities of data on which to base case formulation hypotheses. This assessment process may lead to a more accurate and comprehensive formulation, and potentially to enhanced inferences regarding treatment. In the next section, we review the evidence related to the impact of case formulation.

EMPIRICAL EVIDENCE FOR CASE FORMULATION

While the benefits of case formulation have been broadly stated across theoretical orientations (e.g., Binder, 2004; Hersen & Porzelius, 2002), there has been a relatively small amount of research investigating its importance (Eells et al., 2011). When looking at the evidence for cognitive case formulation, we can look at not only how case formulation influences treatment, but also whether case formulations are reliable and valid (Bieling & Kuyken, 2003).

Reliability and Validity of Case Formulation

The limited available evidence for case formulation reliability suggests that the descriptive and informational aspects of the formulation (such as the problem list) may be obtained reliably, but that it is more difficult for clinicians to agree on the elements that tie the factors of the formulation together, such as hypothesized underlying beliefs (Bieling & Kuyken, 2003). Some research suggests that reliability (Kuyken, Fothergill, Musa, & Chadwick, 2005) and the quality of case formulations (Kendjelic & Eells, 2007) can be improved with training. Evidence also indicates that expert therapists produce higher-quality formulations (Eells et al., 2011), supporting the notion that increased training may enhance formulation. Among the barriers to establishing the reliability and validity of case formulations are difficulties in systematically validating case formulations to ensure that the inferences within the formulation are well founded and accurate. A proposed method for validating case formulations has been developed (Mumma, 2004). Unfortunately, this method is time-consuming and requires the client to provide extensive data. Overall, the current state of the literature suggests that reliability and validity of case formulation may be improved through clinician training and experience; however, further research is needed to establish whether cognitive case formulation approaches meet an acceptable level of reliability and validity.

Impact of Case Formulation on Treatment Outcome

Although the benefits claimed for case formulation are many, there is a surprising lack of data regarding the impact of formulation on treatment outcome. For example, one randomized controlled trial (Ghaderi, 2006) compared formulation-guided versus manual-based CBT in the treatment of 50 clients with bulimia nervosa. The formulation guided treatment used logical functional analysis (Hayes & Follette, 1992) as a structured method for developing an individualized conceptualization and treatment. Logical functional analysis is an approach where the assessment and conceptual analysis components are specified in a decision tree with four branches: (1) inadequate antecedent stimulus control, (2) inadequate consequential control, (3) inadequate motivational conditions, and (4) restricted repertoire of behaviors. The manual-based treatment followed Fairburn and colleagues' manual on CBT for bulimia nervosa (Fairburn, Marcus, & Wilson, 1993). Treatments were matched in terms of duration and frequency of sessions. Results indicated that the formulation-guided intervention was associated with greater improvements; however, both groups achieved sustained improvements. Additionally, the majority of nonresponders (80%) were in the manualized treatment condition. This trial provides promising support for the role of case formulation, but further evidence with a variety of clinical populations is needed.

The answer to the question of whether using an individualized case formulation has substantial impact on treatment outcome is likely to be complicated. The impact of formulation on treatment outcome may be moderated by the characteristics of clients, with clients who have complex problems potentially receiving the most benefit. Initial evidence supports the proposal that clients who have multiple co-morbidities and require multiple therapies can benefit from empirically supported treatments guided by a case formulation (Persons, Roberts, Zalecki, & Brechwald, 2006). Unfortunately, the implications that can be drawn from this research are limited by the lack of inclusion of a comparison group that did not receive treatment guided by case formulation. Future research may support the benefits of idiographic cognitive case formulation with complex patients (as suggested by Persons et al., 2006), whereas an individualized intervention may be less important for patients with less complex problems.

CRITICAL RESEARCH ISSUES AND NEW DIRECTIONS IN CASE FORMULATION RESEARCH

Many questions regarding the reliability, validity, and treatment utility of cognitive case formulation are currently inadequately addressed by the literature. While it appears that increased training and experience lead to enhanced case formulations (Eells et al., 2011), there is not yet enough research to establish that specific training or a particular case formulation approach leads to reliable and valid cognitive case formulations. Research comparing multiple case formulation strategies with regard to their ease of use (e.g., how much training and time are required of the clinician), their reliability and validity (e.g., whether a formulation method leads multiple clinicians to arrive at similar formulations for the same client), and their impact on treatment outcome (e.g., whether symptom reduction is achieved) could help to refine and focus future investigations on the best formulation approaches. Valuable information regarding the relative benefits of case formulation would be gained by implementing randomized controlled trials comparing case-formulation-driven therapy with manual-driven therapy. Previous findings would suggest that it would be important to assess therapist expertise and skills in case formulation (Eells, Lombart, Kendejelic, Turner, & Lucas, 2005) whenever investigating the impact of case formulation on treatment outcomes. Furthermore, client characteristics may be an important moderator variable to assess, as preliminary evidence indicates that case formulation may be less important for routine cases (Persons et al., 2006). Assuming that this research suggests the benefits of case formulation, it would then be important to focus on what particular elements of the case formulation approach are most important or mediate the observed treatment benefits by using dismantling studies. For example, is a formulation that provides attention to all the components of formulation (i.e., the problem list, predisposing factors, stressors or triggering factors, and maintaining factors) superior to simply developing a comprehensive problem list? Ultimately, the goal of future research should be to establish that with specific training and/or experience clinicians can develop reliable and valid cognitive case formulations, and that this case formulation approach, or specific components of this approach,[1] are associated with enhanced treatment outcomes for all clients (or perhaps a subset of clients with complex problems).

CASE FORMULATION AND DSM-5

Diagnosis based on the *Diagnostic and Statistical Manual of Mental Disorders* (DSM) has long been the cornerstone of assessment, treatment planning, and empirical evaluation of treatment outcome for psychopathology. In many ways, case formulation stands in contrast to the DSM diagnostic system, although both approaches certainly focus on symptoms. A case formulation approach emphasizes a more detailed and comprehensive description of a client's problems, in comparison to a categorical diagnosis, which is focused on an overall syndrome that is either

---

[1] A "dismantling" approach to formulation may be particularly helpful to discern what components of the formulation exercise are related to improved outcomes—for example, construction of the problem list versus specifying distal beliefs. Such findings would have important implications for training practitioners.

present or absent. One approach will always be bottom-up (formulation) and the other top-down (DSM). Within case formulation, characteristics of clients that do not meet the level of diagnostic severity, or that are not typically considered in a diagnostic scheme (e.g., interpersonal patterns), may still be considered as playing an important role in the clients' problems. This stands in direct contrast with the circumscribed symptoms and thresholds of DSM, at least up until now. DSM-5 (American Psychiatric Association, 2013) has moved in the direction of a more continuous approach to conceptualizing psychopathology, though perhaps less than was originally intended when preliminary contents were first posted for feedback and comment. In the end, DSM-5 has largely maintained the categorical diagnostic system, though it has added a dimensional approach that allows clinicians to rate disorders along a continuum of severity. Also, the American Psychiatric Association originally proposed a hybrid dimensional–categorical model for personality within DSM-5; however, this was not included in the main text and was relegated to Section III of the manual as an area for future study (American Psychiatric Association, 2013). Nonetheless, any movement toward continuum-based measurement of psychopathology in DSM would begin to close some of the gaps between diagnosis and formulation. A final issue concerning DSM-5 with at least some implications for formulation is the loss of the multi-axial system, which (historically at least) has left some room for describing nonsymptom issues, including medical problems and stressors. Such issues have always had a place in most formulation approaches, so, with this reform, DSM-5 has actually created a larger gap between the diagnostic system and formulation schemes.

CASE FORMULATION AND THE NEW WAVE OF TREATMENTS

As new innovations and adaptations in CBT continue to emerge, the role of case formulation within these respective approaches may also change and evolve. Three recent areas of development for consideration are the increasing use of low-intensity CBT, transdiagnostic approaches, and mindfulness-based treatments.

Low-Intensity CBT

With increasing demands for evidence-based mental health treatment, low-intensity CBT can serve an important role in providing access to treatment. Low-intensity CBT is now being delivered in several formats, including guided use of self-help manuals, online CBT interventions, and large-group CBT. Across these interventions, a commonality is the assumption of less therapist time input for each individual client, and therefore also less emphasis on individualized case formulation. These low-intensity CBT approaches may therefore be generally said to take a nomothetic approach to conceptualization of client problems. With less therapist involvement, the onus is more on clients to decide how the CBT model and strategies apply to their difficulties. Some clients may create their own informal case formulations of their problems, while others may simply use the strategies suggested without understanding the rationale or mechanisms that they are targeting with the interventions. Most clients are likely to experience some increase in understanding of the factors that contributed to the development and maintenance of their problems. Consistent with a stepped-care approach, clients with less complex problems may be suitable for less intensive and less individualized treatment while the role of an individualized case formulation available in more intensive forms of CBT may be more important for clients with multiple and more severe difficulties. While this assertion is theoretically sound, the empirical basis for the benefits of case formulation in more complex cases has yet to be established.

Transdiagnostic Interventions

Transdiagnostic approaches to treatment, such as the unified protocol for the treatment of emotional disorders (Barlow et al., 2011), place less emphasis on diagnosis in determining treatment. At first impression, the assertion that variations in symptoms across disorders are "relatively trivial" (Barlow et al., 2011, p. 15) would suggest that the development of an idiographic formulation may not be highly valued in this treatment model. Conversely, the increased flexibility of the transdiagnostic approach—which uses treatment modules to allow for more emphasis on some areas and less on others, based on individual differences in patient presentations—suggests that there is a greater role for clinical decision making and therefore an associated role for individualized case conceptualization.

Mindfulness-Based Interventions

The number of interventions integrating mindfulness-based approaches, and the associated research on these interventions, have seen substantial growth in recent years. Interventions that incorporate mindfulness, such as mindfulness-based cognitive therapy (MBCT), dialectical behavior therapy (DBT), and acceptance and commitment therapy (ACT), each have their own theoretical foundations. For example, MBCT is based on the cognitive vulnerability model of depressive relapse (Lau, Segal, & Williams, 2004; Teasdale, 1988). Case formulation in mindfulness-based approaches share the elements of general case formulations; however, the hypotheses about the mechanisms that link these factors together are based on the relevant theoretical models. For example, in the case of a client with recurrent depression, a mindfulness-based formulation would emphasize the client's awareness of and relationship to negative thinking patterns as factors predisposing him or her to the development of current and future low-mood episodes. Following from this formulation, mindfulness-based treatment focuses on developing a new relationship to thoughts and feelings that is more open, accepting, and decentered from these experiences. In contrast, CBT would emphasize the content of thinking patterns that suggest underlying negative core beliefs, and therefore would focus on challenging the content of these negative thoughts in an effort to develop less distorted patterns of thinking and ultimately to shift core beliefs.

MBCT also helps clients construct a relapse prevention and wellness plan, which contains several aspects of formulation, including the kinds of thoughts and beliefs that might be triggered. In comparison to traditional CBT approaches, case formulation in the context of mindfulness-based intervention also places increased emphasis on identifying clients' vulnerabilities and coping strengths as opposed to current deficits. This is consistent with the wellness and preventative focus common to mindfulness-based interventions, and it is another component of a wellness plan in MBCT; however, it has not traditionally been a component of CBT, wherein the formulation usually focuses more on problems and relatively less on solutions and strengths. Additionally, when the mindfulness-based treatment is presented in a group format, the role of the therapist in creating an individualized formulation may be deemphasized, while clients' exploration and understanding of factors that may contribute to their difficulties is emphasized.

CONCLUSION

The role of case formulation within new forms of CBT will vary, depending on the emphasis placed on individualized conceptualization and treatment. The focus of the formulations will also vary, depending on the theoretical underpinning of the interventions. However, the potential role for case formulation in guiding clinical decisions with the goal of enhancing treatment process and outcome will remain constant. As more research emerges regarding the reliable and valid methods of developing cognitive case formulations and the impact of such formulations on treatment, it is hoped that cognitive case formulation will be established as an evidence-based technique that can be used to enhance already recognized, empirically supported forms of CBT, or to inform treatment when there is no evidence-based intervention available for a client's problems.

KEY POINTS

FOR PRACTITIONERS

- Valid and reliable assessment tools, paired with client-centered inquiries, should be used to assess current problems across multiple domains.
- Cognitive theory should guide the assessment of possible cognitive and behavioral factors contributing to the development and maintenance of problems.
- Case formulation hypotheses and inferences should be based on available client data.
- The general CBT model should be applied to this particular individual's current problems, precipitants, and early life events.
- A therapist should continue to refine the formulation and check hypotheses against the data that emerge over the course of therapy.
- Case formulation can help guide clinical decision making when empirical evidence or guidance from treatment manuals is lacking.
- A case-formulation-driven approach may be particularly helpful when clients have complex or multiple problems.

FOR RESEARCHERS

- Assessments of the current use of case formulation by clinicians in everyday practice, and of what forms this case formulation most commonly takes (e.g., methods used, models followed, time devoted to formulation), are needed.
- Studies should focus on the reliability and validity of case formulation. That is, how reliably and validly can clinicians produce the different components of case formulation (the problem list, predisposing factors, stressors or triggering factors, and maintaining factors), using a particular method of case formulation? Further research should compare methods and describe the clinician training and experience necessary to meet this standard.
- Dismantling studies focused on the efficacy of case formulation should evaluate the benefits of developing the various components of the case formulation. For example, is simply creating a comprehensive problem list beneficial over no case formulation at all? Does a comprehensive formulation that includes a problem list, predisposing factors, triggering factors, and maintaining factors result in superior symptom improvement compared to a problem list alone?
- Randomized controlled trials comparing manualized treatment (not

tailored to the client) with formulation-based treatment should assess therapist characteristics (expertise in case formulation) and client characteristics as possible moderator variables.

- Studies that provide cost–benefit analyses of case formulation are needed. Specifically, what time and resource investment is required to create a comprehensive case formulation versus standardized treatment (without a case formulation), and what is the magnitude of benefit to the client? Measures of benefit might include magnitude of symptom improvement, number of sessions required to reach symptom remission, or a measure of longer-term mental health morbidity (such as number of health care visits over 5 years).

FOR STUDENTS AND EDUCATORS

- Case formulation is a tool used in therapy that involves describing a client's current problems and also making hypotheses about how these problems developed and are maintained.
- Using a case formulation approach can help to improve the description and understanding of the presenting problems for both the client and the therapist.
- A good case formulation provides clear implications for treatment planning and suggests variables to be assessed for monitoring treatment progress and outcome.
- Case formulations can help to guide decisions during treatment and may be particularly helpful in working with clients with multiple complex problems.

REFERENCES

American Psychiatric Association. (2013). *Diagnostic and statistical manual of mental disorders* (5th ed.). Arlington, VA: Author.

Antony, M. M., & Barlow, D. H. (2010). *Handbook of assessment and treatment planning for psychological disorders* (2nd ed.). New York: Guilford Press.

Antony, M. M., Orsillo, S. M., & Roemer, L. (Eds.). (2001). *Practitioner's guide to empirically-based measures of anxiety*. New York: Kluwer Academic/Plenum.

Barlow, D. H., Farchione, T. J., Fairholme, C. P., Ellard, K. K., Boisseau, C. L. Allen, L. B., et al. (2011). *The unified protocol for transdiagnostic treatment of emotional disorders: Therapist guide*. New York: Oxford University Press.

Beck, A. T., & Dozois, D. J. A. (2011). Cognitive therapy: Current status and future directions. *Annual Review of Medicine, 62*, 397–409.

Beck, A. T., Steer, R. A., & Brown, G. K. (1996). *Beck Depression Inventory–II manual*. San Antonio, TX: Psychological Corporation.

Beck, J. S. (1995). *Cognitive therapy: Basics and beyond.* New York: Guilford Press.

Bieling, P. J., & Kuyken, W. (2003). Is cognitive case formulation science or science fiction? *Clinical Psychology: Science and Practice, 10,* 52–69.

Binder, J. L. (2004). *Key competencies in brief dynamic psychotherapy: Clinical practice beyond the manual.* New York: Guilford Press.

Cartwright-Hatton, S., & Wells, A. (1997). Beliefs about worry and intrusions: The Meta-Cognitions Questionnaire and its correlates. *Journal of Anxiety Disorders, 3,* 279–296.

Chambless, D. L., & Ollendick, T. H. (2001). Empirically supported psychological interventions: Controversies and evidence. *Annual Review of Psychology, 52,* 685–716.

Derogatis, L. R. (2000). *Symptom Checklist 90—Revised.* Washington, DC: American Psychological Association.

Eells, T. D. (2007). History and current status of psychotherapy case formulation. In T. D. Eells (Ed.), *Handbook of psychotherapy case formulation* (2nd ed., pp. 3–32). New York: Guilford Press.

Eells, T. D., Lombart, K. G., Kendjelic, E. M., Turner, L. C., & Lucas, C. (2005). The quality of psychotherapy case formulations: A comparison of expert, experienced, and novice cognitive-behavioral and psychodynamic therapists. *Journal of Consulting and Clinical Psychology, 73,* 579–589.

Eells, T. D., Lombart, K. G., Salsman, N., Kendejelic, E. M., Schneiderman, C. T., & Lucas, C. P. (2011). Expert reasoning in psychotherapy case formulation. *Psychotherapy Research, 21,* 385–399.

Fairburn, C. G., Marcus, M. D., & Wilson, G. T. (1993). Cognitive behavior therapy for binge eating and bulimia nervosa: A comprehensive treatment manual. In C. G. Fairburn & G. T. Wilson (Eds.), *Binge eating: Nature, assessment, and treatment* (pp. 361–404). New York: Guilford Press.

First, M. B., Spitzer, R. L., Gibbon M., & Williams, J. B. W. (1996). *Structured Clinical Interview for DSM-IV Axis I Disorders, Clinician Version (SCID-CV).* Washington, DC: American Psychiatric Press, Inc.

Fischer, J., & Corcoran, K. (2007). *Measures for clinical practice and research: A sourcebook* (Vol. 1). New York: Oxford University Press.

Ghaderi, A. (2006). Does individualisation matter?: A randomized trial of standardised (focused) versus individualized (broad) cognitive behaviour therapy for bulimia nervosa. *Behaviour Research and Therapy, 44,* 273–288.

Hayes, S. C., & Follette, W. C. (1992). Can functional analysis provide a substitute for syndromal classification? *Behavioral Assessment, 14,* 345–365.

Haynes, S. N., Mumma, G. H., & Pinson, C. (2009). Idiographic assessment: Conceptual and psychometric foundations of individualized behavioral assessment. *Clinical Psychology Review, 29,* 179–191.

Hersen, M., & Porzelius, L. K. (Eds.). (2002). *Diagnosis, conceptualization, and treatment planning for adults: A step-by-step guide.* Mahwah, NJ: Erlbaum.

Hunsley, J., & Mash, E. J. (Eds.). (2008). *A guide to assessments that work.* New York: Oxford University Press.

Kendjelic, E. M., & Eells, T. D. (2007). Psychotherapy case formulation training improves formulation quality. *Psychotherapy: Theory, Research, Practice, Training, 44*, 66–77.

Kuyken, W., Fothergill, C. D., Musa, M., & Chadwick, P. (2005). The reliability and quality of cognitive case formulation. *Behaviour Research and Therapy, 43*, 1187–1201.

Lau, M. A., Segal, Z. V., & Williams, M. G. (2004). Teasdale's differential activation hypothesis: Implications for mechanisms of depressive relapse and suicidal behaviour. *Behaviour Research and Therapy, 42*, 1001–1017.

Leichsenring, F., Hiller, W., Weissberg, M., & Leibing, E. (2006). Cognitive-behavioral therapy and psychodynamic psychotherapy: Techniques, efficacy, and indications. *American Journal of Psychotherapy, 60*(3), 233–259.

Meyer, T. J., Miller, M. L., Metzger, R. L., & Borkovec, T. D. (1990). Development and validation of the Penn State Worry Questionnaire. *Behavior Research and Therapy, 28*, 487–495.

Mumma, G. (2004). Validation of idiosyncratic cognitive schema in cognitive case formulations: An intraindividual idiographic approach. *Psychological Assessment, 16*, 211–230.

Nezu, A. M., Nezu, C. M., & Lombardo, E. (2004). *Cognitive-behavioral case formulation and treatment design: A problem solving approach.* New York: Springer.

Nezu, A. M., Ronan, G. F., Meadows, E. A., & McClure, K. S. (Eds.). (2000). *Practitioner's guide to empirically based measures of depression.* New York: Kluwer Academic/Plenum.

Persons, J. B. (2008). *The case formulation approach to cognitive-behavior therapy.* New York: Guilford Press.

Persons, J. B., Roberts, N. A., Zalecki, C. A., & Brechwald, W. A. G. (2006). Naturalistic outcome of case formulation-driven cognitive-behavior therapy for anxious depressed outpatients. *Behaviour Research and Therapy, 44*, 1041–1051.

Shafran, R., Thordarson, D. S., & Rachman, S. (1996). Thought–action fusion in obsessive compulsive disorder. *Journal of Anxiety Disorders, 10*, 379–391.

Teasdale, J. D. (1988). Cognitive vulnerability to persistent depression. *Cognition and Emotion, 2*, 247–274.

Ware, J. E., Snow, K. K., Kosinski, M., & Gandek, B. (1996). SF-36 Health Survey: Manual and interpretation guide. In I. McDowell & C. Newell (Eds.), *Measuring health: A guide to rating scales and questionnaires* (pp. 649–665). New York: Oxford University Press.

Weissman, A. N., & Beck, A. T. (1978). *Development and validation of the Dysfunctional Attitude Scale: A preliminary investigation.* Paper presented at the meeting of the Association for the Advancement of Behavior Therapy, Chicago.

Young, J. E. (1998). *The Young Schema Questionnaire: Short form.* Available at *www.schematherapy.com*.

PART III

CHALLENGES AND CONTINUING CONTROVERSIES

11

Toward a Validity Framework for Cognitive-Behavioral Therapy Self-Report Assessment

Nick Hawkes and Gary P. Brown

That self-report questionnaires are ubiquitous in cognitive-behavioral approaches has been noted by commentators both critical ("overreliance"; Coyne & Gotlib, 1983) and sympathetic ("almost exclusive reliance"; D. A. Clark, 1997). Therefore, it is undeniable that the validity of self-report measurement in cognitive-behavioral therapy (CBT) is a central concern in the development of theory and therapy in the field. Within CBT research, reviews of assessment have tended to be descriptive rather than prescriptive. Furthermore, while research on CBT assessment measures is informed by general assessment and measurement standards, there is scope for these standards to be examined more closely in relation to the specific aims of CBT research, in the hopes of making the goals of assessment and measurement more explicit and thereby helping accelerate advancement within the field. Brown and Clark (Chapter 2, this volume) provide a historically based account of endorsement methods within CBT research, focusing on the supportable inferences that can be drawn from existing self-report measures. The present chapter continues in the same vein by taking a forward-looking approach to self-report assessment anchored in considerations of validity—an approach that, it is hoped, can help guide research in the area out of its current relative stasis.

DEFINING THE DOMAIN OF INTEREST

According to a recent definition, "validity refers to the degree to which variation in scores on an instrument reflects variation in the psychological entity or process of interest" (Haynes, Smith, & Hunsley, 2011, p. 55). In cognitive therapy research and clinical assessment, the domain of interest is the role of cognition in psychopathology and the functional relationship of cognition to behavior, physiology, and affect. This general mapping is captured within available clinical assessment models widely used within CBT practice, such as the "five areas" approach (Williams & Garland, 2002; see Figure 11.1) and the "hot cross bun" didactic model (Padesky & Mooney, 1990). These applied frameworks have a theoretical counterpart in Lang's model of three response systems (Lang, 1979), which in turn has influenced several prominent theoretical formulations (e.g., Foa & Kozak, 1986).

Beyond characterizing and measuring cognition in order to investigate its relationship to other response systems and life circumstances, CBT assessment has also sought to differentiate types of cognitive variables to provide a means for determining which variables are etiological and causal, and which, in contrast, may be correlates or consequences of emotional disorders. The earliest approaches to classifying constructs of interest to CBT reflected the influence on CBT research of information-processing models and the computer metaphor, and associated research in experimental cognitive psychology and social cognition. A frequently applied taxonomy was presented by Hollon and Kriss (1984), who distinguished among cognitive "structures," "products," and "processes" (see also Ingram & Kendall, 1986). Structures are largely synonymous with the concept of "schemas"—a central etiological component of Beck's original cognitive formulations, particularly for depression, that function similarly to the schema concept in Piagetian theory. Schemas serve to store previously encoded knowledge, but, importantly, also play a role in processing new information, helping to determine which information will be attended to and which ignored, how much importance to attach to stimuli, and how to structure information (Hollon & Kriss, 1984, p. 37). Previously encoded enduring beliefs are considered to be reflections of schema structures in propositional form. In contrast, cognitive products are the conscious outputs of the information-processing system, and include momentary cognitions (e.g., automatic thoughts). Enduring beliefs when they have been retrieved and are in a person's awareness are also considered to be cognitive products (as such, Ingram & Kendall, 1986, distinguish between stored and accessed beliefs in their taxonomy; see also Brown & Clark, Chapter 2, this volume, for a related discussion). Finally, cognitive processes refer to the actual workings of

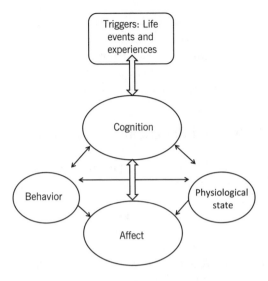

FIGURE 11.1. Basic CBT therapy assessment framework.

the system, whereby inputs are taken in and processed and outputs are produced. Biases to attention, interpretation, and memory are examples of processes of interest in CBT assessment and research.

In practice, cognitive products and structures have been the main targets of direct self-report assessment. Cognitive processes, on the other hand, have typically been studied experimentally in recognition of the fallibility of subjective reporting of thinking processes (e.g., Nisbett & Wilson, 1977). Kwon and Oei (1994) offered a more fundamental division of cognitive constructs into enduring and momentary types, with the initial target of treatment being to identify and correct momentary cognitions such as automatic thoughts: "As therapy progresses, the focus of therapy shifts to finding and changing depressogenic assumptions—the beliefs that predispose a person to depression. Changing the erroneous or dysfunctional assumptions has a direct effect on the patient's ability to avoid future depression" (p. 333).

In summary, at the broadest level, CBT assessment is concerned with the reciprocal relationships among the three response systems of cognition, behavior, and physiology and their joint roles in giving rise to aversive affect, against the background of relevant environmental triggers. Cognition is given precedence as an entry point into the interrelationships among the response systems, and a basic distinction is made between momentary discrete thoughts and appraisals occurring within a particular episode on the one hand, and more enduring ongoing attitudes and beliefs that persist across episodes on the other. A final central organizing principle is that each form of emotional disorder will have a distinctive cognitive content reflected in both momentary appraisals and enduring beliefs (see Baranoff & Oei, Chapter 8, this volume, for a focus on the cognitive content-specificity hypothesis).

CBT ASSESSMENT AND GENERAL VALIDATION STANDARDS

As Strauss and Smith (2009; see also Guller & Smith, Chapter 14, this volume) show in their historical review, advances in assessment in the field at large have been enabled by the articulation of testing standards, which themselves are then revised in reference to the subsequently accumulating knowledge base, in turn spurring further advances. The current set of standards was published in 1999 (American Educational Research Association, American Psychological Association, & National Council on Measurement in Education, 1999), with the most notable departure from the previously published standards being that they were no longer organized around different types of validity (content, criterion, discriminant, etc.), but rather subsumed these all within the definition of construct validity: "Validity is a unitary concept. It is the degree to which all the accumulated evidence supports the intended interpretation of test scores for the proposed purpose" (American Educational Research Association et al., 1999, p. 11). Instead, the standards identify different sources of validity evidence. Specifically, five categories are set out: evidence based on test content, evidence based on response processes, evidence based on internal structure, evidence based on relationship to other variables, and evidence based on the consequences of testing. In relation to CBT assessment, it is tempting to try to map the categories of validity evidence onto the matching categories of cognitive constructs (content/products, structure, and operations/processes) from Ingram and Kendall's (1986) classification of constructs. Although there might be some scope for considering these correspondences, this is not pursued as an expressed aim in the following discussion, which focuses instead on holding up CBT assessment as it is actually practiced against the established general standards.

Although not presented as such, the order in which the evidence categories are set out in the standards can readily be viewed as a pragmatic sequence of test development stages. We proceed through this sequence in the following discussion. We initially focus on one CBT measurement instrument, the Anxiety Sensitivity Index (ASI; Reiss, Peterson, Gursky, & McNally, 1986), as an exemplar and consider the issues related to the different sources of validity evidence. The ASI is one of the most widely used measures in the field (e.g., Naragon-Gainey, 2010). Moreover, it epitomizes the approach to assessment that is characteristic of many instruments in the field, and so the discussion naturally applies to the many other instruments that share common features. A summary of the central issues and extension of these to other key CBT measurement instruments follows consideration of the different validity evidence categories. This is followed by a section aimed at identifying potential methodological steps that can be taken to address the central issues previously identified.

Evidence Based on Content

The category of evidence based on content refers to "the themes, wording, and format of the items, tasks, or questions on a test, as well as the guidelines for procedures regarding administration and scoring" (American Educational Research Association et al., 1999, p. 11). Haynes, Richard, and Kubany (1995) define content validity as "the degree to which elements of an assessment instrument are relevant to and representative of the targeted construct for a particular assessment purpose" (p. 238). Although the latter definition is stated in terms of types of validity (rather than types of evidence), it has the advantage of providing an explicit basis for evaluating the sort of content evidence that is required. It is also consistent with Messick's (1989) identification of two main threats to content validity, "construct underrepresentation" and "construct-irrelevant variance." These threats are often illustrated within educational testing, where they have obvious practical consequences (e.g., omission of important subject matter from a topic or performing well on a test due to guessing rather than knowledge, respectively), but they are also central considerations in tests of more abstract psychological constructs.

In the context of prevailing validation practices, content considerations are usually underemphasized; however, it has been argued that evidence from content can be regarded as the essential foundation for establishing validity, and it figures more centrally in recent formulations of validity theory (e.g., Lissitz & Samuelsen, 2007). Along these lines, Haynes et al. (1995) argue that if an instrument omits measurement of important elements of a construct or produces systematic construct-irrelevant variance, all further applications of the instrument are compromised because variance in obtained scores cannot be ascribed with confidence to the putative underlying construct, and any inferences based on these scores will be suspect even if other indices of validity are satisfactory (p. 240). However, Haynes et al. (1995) also emphasize that validity evidence based on content needs to be evaluated with regard to a particular purpose. For example, whereas the Beck Depression

Inventory–II (BDI-II; Beck, Steer, & Brown, 1996) is considered a "gold standard" general measure of depression, its use for the specific purpose of testing predictions of the cognitive model, as represented by the assessment areas in Figure 11.1, entails additional considerations. In this regard, Hammen and Krantz (1985) pointed out that the BDI includes cognitive content, which limits it to an extent as a criterion measure for investigating the role of cognition in giving rise to depression. Moreover, the most obvious remedy for this issue of simply omitting potentially overlapping content would potentially compromise the validity of the BDI as a measure of the full syndrome of depression if the truncated scale no longer includes essential elements (see Nicholls, Licht, & Pearl, 1982, for a general discussion of predictor–criterion confounding in assessment).

Criterion–Predictor Overlap

The focus of the majority of research and assessment efforts within the CBT domain of interest is the functional relationship between cognition and emotion, and so establishing the boundary between cognition and affect is arguably the most basic challenge for CBT assessment. Whereas cognitive content in a measure of a diagnostic construct, such as the BDI, creates measurement overlap between predictor and criterion (as just discussed), the complementary problem, whereby a cognitive predictor measure captures variance in affect, can be a more insidious validity threat, and one that can spring from several sources. First, natural language use (e.g., "I feel," meaning "I think") does not always clearly distinguish semantically between affect and cognition, and so care must be taken in this regard with respect to item construction. More generally, as L. A. Clark and Watson (1995) argue, affect terms appear to be particularly salient and influential: "The inclusion of almost any negative mood term (e.g., 'I worry about . . . ,' or 'I am upset [or bothered or troubled] by . . . ') virtually guarantees that an item will have a substantial neuroticism component; the inclusion of several such affect-laden items, in turn, ensures that the resulting scale—regardless of its intended construct—will be primarily a marker of neuroticism" (p. 312). It follows that including affect terms within the scale content when affect is not the target of assessment would be susceptible to producing construct-irrelevant variance.

The ASI belongs to a class of cognitive vulnerability measures that would also include the Dysfunctional Attitude Scale (DAS) for depression (Weissman & Beck, 1978) and the Obsessive Beliefs Questionnaire (OBQ) for obsessive–compulsive disorder (Obsessive Compulsive Cognitions Working Group, 2003), all of which seek to quantify the trait-like tendency to interpret experience in a disorder-specific manner. The stated purpose of the ASI is to measure anxiety sensitivity, "an individual difference variable consisting of beliefs that the experience of anxiety/fear causes illness, embarrassment or additional anxiety" (Reiss et al., 1986, p. 1). The authors emphasize that the ASI "is not just another measure of anxiety but actually predicts an important outcome (fearfulness) that cannot be predicted as well by anxiety scales" (p. 2). Items in this category of scales typically reflect beliefs concerning experiences salient to the disorder and so often adopt an "if–then" ("if salient trigger, then consequence") format, as shown in the ASI item "When my chest feels tight, I get scared that I won't be able to breathe properly" (indicative items from the DAS and OBQ include "If I fail at my work, then I am a failure as a person," and "If I do not control my thoughts, I will be punished," respectively). In light of L. A. Clark and Watson's (1995) observation about affect terms, the use of the word "scared" in the ASI item is immediately notable. Furthermore, although ASI items on their face appear, indeed, to assess the fear of anxiety-related sensations, the operation of a corresponding belief is merely implied; that is, the belief is not manifest in the item content, but rather needs to be inferred. As one of the ASI's authors has acknowledged, those employing the scale "implicitly assumed that statements like 'It scares me when my heart beats rapidly' imply beliefs about the negative consequences of rapid heart rate. Whether this assumption is warranted remains an empirical question" (McNally, 1999, p. 10). Figure 11.2 depicts two potential alternative wordings to an ASI appraisal—the first one (a) containing the actual ASI item wording, and the second (b) showing how it could have been worded differently so as not to confound the criterion and predictor. The "and that scares me" in (b) is in parentheses to indicate that the content is not included in the item, as the affective reaction is the criterion to be predicted. In this regard, Lilienfeld, Turner, and Jacob (1993) remarked that "because the word 'scare' or 'scares' appears in eight of the ASI's 16 items, a more parsimonious explanation for the partial correlation between the ASI and the FSS-II [Fear Survey Schedule–II] is that one measure of fear is highly associated with another measure of fear" (p. 168).

It might be argued that affective content within a cognitive measure would merely produce construct-irrelevant variance; however, affect is decidedly not irrelevant within the CBT model, but is rather the very outcome that cognition is frequently intended to predict and explain. Everything else being equal, spurious, truly irrelevant variance will tend to diminish the validity coefficient; however, systematic affective variance in a putative cognitive measure will produce an in-built relationship to a corresponding criterion affect measure, resulting in artificially

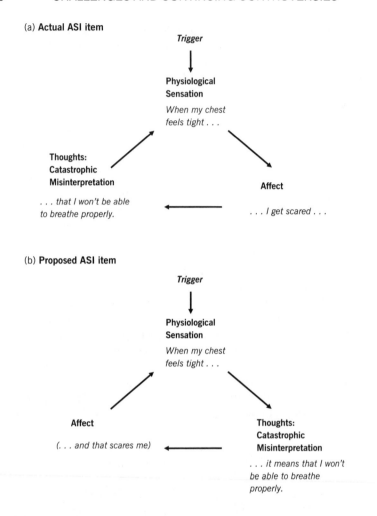

FIGURE 11.2. Anxiety Sensitivity Index (ASI) item mapped onto the panic cycle.

inflated validity estimates. In the complementary situation, where cognition items are included in a diagnostic measure such as the BDI-II, there is the justifiable view, already noted, that the overlap is substantive and therefore should not be removed arbitrarily. There is no such dilemma where cognitive measures are concerned; to the extent that there is overlapping variance with the criterion, this needs to be recognized as poor assessment design.

Cognitive Content Specificity and Applicability

A central principle of CBT theory is that emotional disorders have distinct cognitive content (Beck, 1976; see Baranoff & Oei, Chapter 8, this volume). As Brown and Clark (Chapter 2, this volume) note, it is important for a scale to relate meaningfully to respondents to whom the items do not apply as well as those to whom they apply, because inapplicability can lead to certain measurement anomalies that are not widely recognized. Measures intended to quantify the specific cognitive content of a particular disorder (e.g., the Automatic Thoughts Questionnaire [ATQ; Hollon & Kendall, 1980] for depression) will typically require respondents to rate the frequency or intensity of content typifying the disorder by means of endorsement methods. Someone to whom a thought such as the one in the ATQ item "My life is a mess" does not apply can usually choose a response such as "Never" or "Not at all." In contrast, scales like the ASI (along with the DAS and OBQ, as discussed above) are constructed around items that assess the joint or contingent occurrence of a disorder-relevant trigger and a resulting outcome. Items such as these that are compounds of two elements, in which one is conditioned on the other, are susceptible to the well-known test construction pitfall of being "double-barreled." L. A. Clark and Watson (1995) provide a general example: "I would never drink and drive for fear that I might be stopped by the police," which confounds the occurrence versus nonoccurrence of a behavior (drinking and driving) with a putative motive for that behavior (fear of legal complications) (p. 312). With regard to the ASI, Lilienfeld et al. (1993) point out that "items such as 'It scares me when I feel faint' or 'Other people notice when I feel shaky' may be largely or entirely irrelevant to subjects who rarely if ever feel faint or shaky. Such 'double-barreled' items are potentially problematic, because some subjects may respond 'No' to them because they never or virtually never have had the experience in question. This could produce a spurious correlation between the ASI and panic disorder (as well as similar criteria), because panic disorder patients are more likely than other subjects to experience anxiety-related symptoms, such as faintness and shakiness" (p. 167). In other words, the double-barreled structure makes it so that we cannot know which "barrel" a response reflects. A response of "Not at all" can mean either that the respondent is unconcerned about the body sensation in question (as the ASI intends), or that the respondent simply never experiences the sensation and so the item is inapplicable. The result is that the item may simply transmit selective applicability to those who have a panic disorder and so may be a marker of panic itself rather than a predictor. This is another form of criterion–predictor confounding, albeit an indirect one. Aside from this confounding, inclusion of respondents for whom items are inapplicable along with respondents for whom they are applicable can lead to measurement anomalies that are discussed further in the section on evidence based on structure.

Evidence Based on Response Processes

The category of evidence based on response processes relates to "the fit between the construct and the detailed nature of performance or response actually engaged in by examinees" (American Educational Research Association et al., 1999, p. 12). It follows naturally from the prior category, just discussed, which relates to the whether the content included is relevant to the construct of interest, sufficiently comprehensive, and structured in such a way that construct-relevant variance is likely to be transmitted by the ultimate response. The initial foundation represented by content evidence could either be preserved or compromised, depending on the processing subsequently engaged in by respondents in the course of developing a response. The full body of knowledge about cognitive processing can potentially be brought to bear to evaluate evidence in this category. Along these lines, for example, the analysis provided by Brown and Clark (Chapter 2, this volume) of endorsement methods broadly aims to weigh up the evidence for the validity of the endorsement approach based on a decomposition of the response processes entailed, as set out in Ericsson and Simon's (1980) verbal protocol approach.

No amount of processing can undo a flaw in the content of a scale; these are built in and intrinsic. However, processing can attenuate or amplify content flaws. Moreover, a scale that is seemingly valid in terms of content evidence might be compromised if the processes engaged in by respondents completing the scale generate responses that are at odds with the operation of the putative underlying construct. By the same token, evidence from response processes can potentially resolve ambiguities inherent in the content of a scale, such as the situation represented in Figure 11.2 with regard to the ASI. As previously discussed, the aim of measuring degree of belief is not self-evidently supported by the content of the ASI item; it is only implied by a rating of an affective reaction. It is possible that in practice, the rating of the affective reaction is invariably the result of processes rooted in the respondent's belief system, as presumed; but this would need to be settled as an empirical matter, provided appropriate procedures for decomposing the underlying processes are available. Brown, Hawkes, and Tata (2009) directly examined this question in a cognitive interviewing (Willis, 2004) study (see "Process-Based Methods," p. 261, for further discussion of this method) and found that in fact, respondents most often based their responses to ASI items not on the ongoing appraisal of their experience relative to their beliefs, but rather on recollections of their previous anxiety reactions. When the basis for forming judgments was examined through analysis of think-aloud protocols for the ASI, 56.9% of responses were formed by respondents on the basis of gauging the intensity or frequency of recollected anxiety reactions rather than the strength of the presumed prevailing belief. Beliefs about the harmful consequences of body sensations were found to be expressed explicitly in only 20.8% of ASI protocols. As such, the more parsimonious explanation regarding response processes was supported: Eliciting responses about anxiety reactions recruited cognitive processing concerned with anxiety reactions that was not reflective of the implied beliefs.

The category of process-based validity evidence would appear to be at least as fundamental as content-based evidence, but has similarly been relatively neglected in validation practices (see Bornstein, 2011, for a discussion). Embretson (1983) ascribed the neglect of the study of processes that give rise to test responses as a basis for understanding validity to the nature of the dominant validity paradigm originated by Cronbach and Meehl (1955), according to which the validity of a measure of a construct is inferred from the pattern of associations with theoretically related and unrelated constructs—the so-called "nomological network" of the construct. "When Cronbach and Meehl . . . initially elaborated the construct validation concept, the functionalist paradigm that guided psychological research was not compatible with construct representation as a separate research goal. In experimental psychology, the main emphasis was antecedent/consequent relationships, with little interest in the intervening mechanisms" (Embretson, 1983, p. 180). However, the sufficiency of this view of validity is increasingly being questioned. As Borsboom (2005) argues, patterns of findings are incapable of fixing the meaning of a construct: "One does not get anywhere by saying that 'intelligence is whatever is positively related to general knowledge and negatively to criminal behavior,' because there are too many theoretical terms that satisfy this description, and many of them will evidently not be the same as intelligence" (p. 157). On this basis, Embretson (1983) argued that validation also requires the decomposition of the processes leading to a response, and that this constitutes a distinct basis for validity, which she named "construct representation." Embretson cited intelligence as an example of a construct that has strong evidence of validity in terms of its nomothetic span (the relationships within its nomological network), whereas the theoretical basis for intelligence in terms of the processes that produce IQ scores is still largely unknown. What form construct representation validation might take for tests of constructs of interest to CBT will require considerable effort to work out. The section "Methods for Improving Validity of CBT Assessment," below, provides a preliminary idea of the sorts of procedures that might be entailed and what issues these will address.

Evidence Based on Internal Structure

The category of evidence based on internal structure is concerned with "the degree to which the relationships among test items and test components conform to the construct on which the proposed test score interpretations are based" (American Educational Research Association et al., 1999, p. 13). Where an item is relevant in its content, well constructed, and sound from the standpoint of construct representation in terms of the intervening mechanisms it involves, there remains the task of properly assigning it to the scale to which it best fits. Summing together items that are construct-irrelevant along with relevant ones, though not irreversible, has the same effective outcome as constructing confounded items. As Smith and colleagues (see Guller & Smith, Chapter 14, this volume) have extensively shown, in the absence of compelling reasons to the contrary, the aim should be to devise scales that reflect a unitary, homogeneous construct. Such scales are more likely to be theoretically meaningful and to provide a basis for clearer inferences for both applied and empirical purposes. One context in which heterogeneous scales are intentionally used is to measure symptom severity relative to a defined syndrome, such as major depression. Scales such as the BDI-II draw together items from the different response systems represented in Figure 11.1. As Smith and Zapolski (2009) point out, quoting McGrath (2005), these scales intentionally seek to capture covariance between the underlying component univariate constructs. However, the utility of such scales in capturing a heterogeneous syndrome in a single dimension needs to be offset against the measurement ambiguities this creates: "Assessments of anxiety, for example, may combine measures of subjective emotional states, physiological arousal, cognitive worry, and approach/avoidance behavior into an aggregate index of anxiety. . . . A drawback to this aggregation of data is that it forestalls questions about the possible functional relations among distinct psychological systems that underlie the distinct measures" (Cervone, 2004, p. 120).

Questionable validity evidence with regard to content or process can have ramifications for the structure of a scale. In considering the content validity evidence for the ASI, the issue of inapplicability was identified as an underrecognized validity threat. Waller (1989) studied the general case in which items are inapplicable because they share an unmet prerequisite (e.g., never experiencing shakiness) and found that as small an inapplicable rate as 5% can lead to substantially inflated correlations between items and the resulting extraction of spurious or distorted factors. Schwarz and colleagues (see Schwarz, 1999, for a review) have shown that individuals responding to items that are less applicable to them are much more likely to be affected by the context, sequencing, and wording of items than individuals for whom the subject matter is more continually accessible, resulting in greater instability of measurement in the former populations and lack of measurement invariance across populations. Consistent with this premise, Deacon, Abramowitz, Woods, and Tolin (2003) found in a factor analysis of the revised and expanded ASI cross-validated in two large undergraduate samples that items concerned with somatic sensations loaded on factors that appeared to differ on the basis of item wording (being scared of anxiety symptoms vs. being worried about the potentially catastrophic consequences of such symptoms), as compared to Taylor and Cox's (1998) original analysis in a clinical population, in which items loaded according to domain of somatic sensation (cardiovascular, gastrointestinal, etc.). Deacon et al. (2003) attribute this to the inapplicability of these items in a nonclinical sample: "it is possible that individuals without clinically significant anxiety symptoms may have difficulty identifying specific feared consequences of somatic sensations, even when these sensations are feared" (p. 1446). Indeed, it has proven difficult to identify a stable factor structure of the ASI within nonclinical populations, let alone one that is related to the structure found in clinical populations (e.g., Zvolensky et al., 2003). The potential for the factor scores of the ASI to be unstable and substantially based on spurious statistical artifacts is a serious concern, and particularly so for the ASI-R, as arguments for its validity are in large part based upon studies of its factor structure (Taylor et al., 2007; Zinbarg, Barlow, & Brown, 1997).

It should be noted that evidence based on structure is derived from patterns of correlations and so has the same inferential limitations as nomothetic span of being an insufficient basis for fixing meaning. As such, although it is tempting to view the derivation of underlying dimensions that are consistent with the theoretical constructs as support for the preferred theory (as is the case with intelligence), there may be any number of alternative accounts that are consistent with a particular set of latent variables. With regard to the ASI, because there is evidence that what is being transmitted through response processes has at least as much to do with affect as cognition, the apparent structure is likely to be highly informed by affect. In general, "the issue of when it is appropriate to aggregate is inherently a conceptual rather than statistical matter, since a statistically reliable scale can be generated by combining a sufficiently large sample of any collection of highly correlated indicators regardless of whether or not they share the same referent" (McGrath, 2009, p. 28).

Evidence Based on Relationships with Other Variables

The next category addresses "questions about the degree to which these relationships are consistent with the construct underlying the proposed test interpretation" (American Educational Research Association et al., 1999, p. 13). It is worth noting that all previous forms of evidence are internal to the test, and yet, according to the prevailing construct validity paradigm, external relationships with other variables (Cronbach & Meehl's [1955] nomological network, discussed earlier) the primary means for establishing the meaning of the construct measured by a test. To the majority of the field, this type of validity is synonymous with construct validity. However, it should be self-evident from the previous sections that validity evidence based on patterns of association needs to be predicated upon clear validity evidence for the categories of content, process, and structure. As Smith and Zapolski (2009) note,

> If my measure of A performs as expected by my theory, then I am likely to have increased confidence in both my theory and my measure of A. However, I cannot be certain that both my theory is correct and my measure is accurate. Suppose, instead, my new measure of A inadvertently overlaps with B (known not to correlate with C), and my supportive results are really due to the measures of A and B partly reflecting the same construct. Thus, positive results increase one's confidence in one's measure and in one's theory, but they do not constitute either proof of a theory or full validation of a measure. (p. 84)

Evidence Based on the Consequences of Testing

The last category of evidence directly reflects the influence of Messick's (1989) unified view of validity: "Validity is an integrated evaluative judgment of the degree to which empirical evidence and theoretical rationales support the adequacy and appropriateness of inferences and actions based on test scores" (p. 13). This view of validity unites the question of whether a test measures what it purports to with the question of its utility for the uses to which it is put. More recent writings among certain validity theorists argue that this approach conflates principles (e.g., values such as fairness and lack of bias) with empirical issues that are best kept separate at the risk of obscuring validity questions (see Markus &

Borsboom, 2013, for a summary of this debate). Clearly, consideration of the uses to which particular measures can be put (supporting formulation, making a demonstrable difference in treatment decisions, and adding meaningfully to knowledge about the etiology and development of disorders, etc.) is critical and arguably a more immediate consideration than strict scientific validity in applied settings. One approach to this might be to distinguish test validity, which is the focus of this chapter, from clinical validity or clinical utility, which has test validity as a prerequisite but then extends to issues that are the focus of evidence-based assessment (see Hunsley & Elliott, Chapter 6, this volume).

SUMMARY AND EXTENSION

The focus to this point has been on the ASI as an exemplar of a number of validity issues. Table 11.1 contains a selective sample of other, mostly anxiety-related questionnaires that reflect similar issues. These are mainly confined to content evidence and issues related to criterion–predictor overlap with regard to cognition and affect. Similar examples can be compiled for overlap among the other response systems represented in Figure 11.1. Content issues are fairly easy to detect from a relatively rapid examination of item content. Issues concerned with process evidence require more in-depth analysis but are also likely to be prevalent among these scales, given the nearly complete neglect of construct representation in validation studies.

To the extent that CBT research continues to rely on self-report assessment, further progress will depend on improving measurement and assessment so that they afford a basis for addressing the clinical and empirical issues of interest. On the basis of the foregoing survey of measurement and validity issues in the area, it is reasonable to suppose that the relative stasis within the field stems from a state of affairs whereby the prevailing approach to measurement has provided all that it can provide with regard to the sorts of questions seen as worth addressing within CBT research and assessment. This is not particular to CBT, but rather is a situation shared with the field at large as a consequence of the limitations of the current validation paradigm, which emphasizes post hoc inferences of meaning based on associations with external criteria, at the expense of efforts to verify that measurement procedures produce scores that accurately and faithfully represent the construct of interest. In other words, the field at large finds itself at the sort of juncture described in Strauss and Smith's (2009) review as having previously led to a fundamental redefinition of standards. McGrath (2005) concisely summarizes what is at stake:

TABLE 11.1. Validity Issues in CBT Self-Report Measures

Scale	Item	Content
		Cognitive content on diagnostic measures
DASS	17	I felt I wasn't worth much as a person.
BAI	5	Fear of the worst happening.
FSQ	3	If I saw a spider now, I would think it will harm me.
CBOCI	13	I am convinced that any obsessional intrusions that I might have are HARMLESS thoughts, images, or impulses.
		Automatic thoughts measures with affect terms
SSPSS	9	Instead of worrying I could concentrate on what I have to say.
STBS	20	People can easily see when I am nervous.
STBS	15	If I am around someone I am interested in, I am likely to get panicky or do something to embarrass myself.
ACQ	14	I am going to be paralyzed by fear.
		Affective content on belief measures
MCQ	19	If I do not stop my worrying thoughts, they could come true.
MCQ	7	If I did not control a worrying thought, and then it happened, it would be my fault.
COWS	19	Worry increases my anxiety.
COWS	9	Worry acts as a stimulant.
COWS	5	When I worry, it stops me taking decisive action.
		Beliefs inferred from affective consequences
IUS	6	Uncertainty makes me uneasy, anxious, or stressed.
IUS	17	Uncertainty makes me vulnerable, unhappy, or sad.
SATI	5	When others are not paying attention to my speech, I worry that the audience is thinking poorly of me.
COWS	14	Worrying gets me worked up.
RAS	5	I worry a great deal about the effects of things which I do or don't do.
		Double-barreled items: potential for inapplicability
AnxCQ	3	When I am put under stress, I am likely to lose control.
AnxCQ	5	When I am frightened by something, there's generally nothing I can do.

(continued)

TABLE 11.1. (*continued*)

AAQ	5	I rarely worry about getting my anxieties, worries, and feelings under control.
OBQ	13	If I have aggressive thoughts or impulses about my loved ones, this means I may secretly want to hurt them.
ACS	4	If I get depressed, I am quite sure that I'll bounce right back.

Note. ACS, Affective Control Scale; AAQ, Acceptance and Action Questionnaire; ACQ, Agoraphobic Cognitions Questionnaire; AnxCQ, Anxiety Control Questionnaire; BAI, Beck Anxiety Inventory; COWS, Consequences of Worry Scale; DASS, Depression Anxiety Stress Scale; IUS, Intolerance of Uncertainty Scale; MCQ, Metacognitions Questionnaire; OBQ, Obsessive Beliefs Questionnaire; OCI, Clark–Beck Obsessive Compulsive Inventory; RAS, Responsibility Attitudes Scale; SATI, Speech Anxiety Thoughts Inventory; SSPSS, Self Statements during Public Speaking Scale; STBS, Social Thoughts and Beliefs Scale. For references and copies of the scales, see Antony, Orsillo, and Roemer (2001).

> Any time a scale is used as a criterion or dependent variable, or for descriptive purposes, or for the estimation of parameters, the representational accuracy of the measurement is paramount because some rough equivalence between placement on the variable and placement on the construct is required. If the meaning of the scores on a scale is unclear, then the accuracy of any inferences about constructs made on the basis of that scale is in doubt. Scales that correspond poorly with the constructs they are intended to represent cannot provide the basis for clear answers to empirical questions. (p. 113)

Lack of clarity, as undesirable as it is, represents the relatively more benign end of the spectrum of potential difficulties stemming from the limitations of current assessment measures. As documented above, a number of the validity threats endemic in current assessment instruments raise the very real possibility that a good number of positive research findings are artifacts of flawed measures that produce inflated validity estimates. If this is true, it would potentially require wholesale reconsideration of the state of evidence in areas that rely on this type of measurement.

METHODS FOR IMPROVING VALIDITY OF CBT ASSESSMENT

If the shortcomings of current measurement instruments outlined in the present chapter are given credence, it is tempting to conclude that this approach should be completely abandoned as a serious scientific venture in favor of more experimental paradigms. There are several difficulties with this conclusion, as documented elsewhere in this volume. First, as Roefs, Huijding, Smulders, Jansen, and MacLeod (Chapter 13, this volume) demonstrate, experimental paradigms have their own limitations and can only hope to complement rather than replace self-report assessment. Second, as discussed by Brown and Clark (Chapter 2, this volume), particular central phenomena of interest are only ascertainable through self-report. Finally, self-report instruments are irreplaceable in applied contexts, such as clinical assessment and treatment, due to their unmatched utility. Fortunately, various researchers have begun to develop methods that can potentially serve as vehicles for the implementation of the developing and changing conceptualization of validity. An overview of these approaches is provided below in relation to the three forms of validity evidence previously discussed (content, process, and structure) that have been relatively neglected in light of the dominance of evidence based on relationships with other variables.

Content-Based Methods

The relative emphasis on establishing meaning and validating putative measures empirically on the basis of external patterns of associations has served to deemphasize considerations earlier in the process of test construction, particularly those surrounding content. A wide range of measure construction shortcomings reviewed above (double-barreled items, confounded items, problems of inapplicability) have been identified in the area of content evidence. A relevant methodology literature already exists with regard to survey methodology that can be readily applied to self-report assessment in clinical psychology—specifically, the research movement known as Cognitive Aspects of Survey Methodology (CASM; see Presser et al., 2004, for a review). The CASM movement was spurred by Ericsson and Simon's (1980) groundwork on the validity of verbal reports and parallel efforts in social psychology (e.g., Schwarz, 1999), and seeks to characterize the full sequence of cognitive processes involved in responding to test items. Much of the basis of CASM was developed at a conference in 1984 and was crystallized in a paper by Loftus (1984; Loftus, Fienberg, & Tanur, 1985) that made explicit the link between Ericsson and Simon's conceptual analysis and questionnaire response. Tourangeau (1984) summarized the overall framework for organizing the sequence of operations set into motion when one is making an item response, and this still forms the core of most CASM approaches. Specifically, he proposed that to answer a question, one has to (1) attend to and comprehend it, (2) recall whatever facts are relevant, (3) make any required judgments, and, (4) format and select a response. In one widely used pretesting system (questionnaire analysis [QA]; Lessler & Forsyth, 1996), an instrument is evaluated against a comprehensive checklist derived from Tourangeau's cognitive model. Content problems such as those discussed previously would potentially be identified in the course of considering the reference set type of the individual questions—that is, what class of phenomenon the instrument is intended to elicit from the respondent. With regard to CBT assessment, these would likely be drawn from the response systems and environmental factors summarized in Figure 11.1. Table 11.2 illustrates the use of QA in the development of a revised Anxiety Attitude and Belief Scale (Brown, Hawkes, Cooper, Jonsdottir, & Tata, 2013).

Process-Based Methods

The testing standards include a specific suggestion regarding process evidence: "Questioning test takers about their performance strategies or responses to particular items can yield evidence that enriches the definition of a construct" (American Educational Research Association et al., 1999, p. 12). One such approach, cognitive interviewing (CI; Willis, 2005), is another CASM technique and can be seen as the process-oriented counterpart to QA that is carried out when a questionnaire is administered. It likewise draws on Tourangeau's model of survey response, but uses think-aloud protocols from actual respondents. CI is an application of Ericsson and Simon's (1980) protocol analysis methodology, which was geared to the general task of collecting valid verbal protocols, applied to the specific aim of evaluating self report instruments. An example of the application of CI has already been summarized above with regard to the ASI (Brown et al., 2009). Like production methods (see Haaga & Solomon, Chapter 3, this volume), CI elicits verbal protocols in response to set stimuli, and so can be seen as a means of capitalizing on some of advantages of production methods to enhance the validity of endorsement methods. CI, along with QA, has a straightforward application in potentially providing a means for implementing validation procedures in which construct representation is a coequal consideration, along with the usual understanding of construct validity in terms of patterns of external associations (please see Table 11.2 for an illustration of the application of CI in a CBT context). Another set of more specialized methods that can potentially provide process evidence uses experimental procedures rather than verbal protocols to examine individual responses to test items (Bornstein, 2011; Cervone, 2004; Haynes, Mumma, & Pinson, 2009). These approaches can potentially provide a bridge between self-report methods and more experimental approaches.

Methods for Investigating Evidence Based on Structure

The category of structure-based evidence bears on the questions of whether and how test items are to be aggregated. Smith and colleagues (e.g., Guller & Smith, Chapter 14, this volume) have written extensively

TABLE 11.2. Illustration of Questionnaire Analysis and Cognitive Interviewing for Enhancing Content and Process Validity with Items from the Anxiety Attitude and Belief Scale

Initial content	QA or CI information	Final content
If I feel anxious it is always a sign that something is wrong.	CI: First-person "I" results in retrievals of anxiety episodes. Use of "always" results in underendorsement.	Anxiety is generally a sign that something is wrong.
If I ignore my worries, then I am irresponsible.	CI: Varies from worry to worry, person to person. Elicits affect rather than cognition.	Item deleted.
If I feel something unusual happening in my body, it might not be anything dangerous now, but could develop into something serious later.	QA: Item comprises multiple propositions.	It is necessary to continually be aware of signs that a health problem is developing.
If I feel an unusual physical sensation, there must be something serious causing it.	CI: Elicits judgments based on frequency of occurrence of thoughts; "if" understood as "when."	An unusual physical sensation in your body is likely to be a sign that something is seriously wrong with you.
Not every unusual physical sensation is a sign of something seriously wrong with my body.	QA: Double negative created when coupled with "disagree" rating. Syntax confusing.	Item deleted.
Just because I can imagine something happening doesn't mean that it will come true.	CI: Syntax causes confusion about what is being asked.	Picturing something happening might cause it to really happen.
I need to avoid thinking about the bad things that I hear of happening to others as it will cause the same thing to happen to me.	QA: Item comprises two propositions. CI: First-person "I" results in episodic retrievals.	Thinking about bad things that have happened to other people could cause the same thing to happen to you.
Other people should not see you losing control of yourself in any way.	CI: Misconstrued as referring to whether others watching is proper or polite.	You should not allow yourself to be seen losing control of yourself in any way.
I prefer to carry out my activities when nobody is watching me.	CI: Form of statement and use of "prefer" elicits retrievals of instances of social anxiety.	It is better to carry out your activities when nobody is watching you.

Note. QA, questionnaire analysis; CI, cognitive interviewing.

on the desirability of homogeneous, single-construct scales. At the same time, techniques are emerging for potentially modeling the inherent complexity of clinical psychology constructs. For example, Naragon-Gainey and T. A. Brown (Chapter 12, this volume) discuss the use of bifactor models for use in the frequently encountered situation within the area in which a single common factor underlies the latent subscales of an instrument. A more recent development forgoes the use of latent variable models entirely and instead models overlapping constructs by using a network approach (e.g., Cramer, Waldorp, van der Maas, & Borsboom, 2010).

CONCLUSION

The present chapter has evaluated the capacity for the predominant approach to measurement within CBT research and assessment to address unresolved issues in the field and to provide a clear basis for clinical decision making. Numerous shortcomings of commonly used instruments have been argued to seriously curtail the capacity of the field to address these issues. Indeed, these shortcomings could point to the need for a fundamental reevaluation of taken-for-granted findings in the field. In common with the rest of the field at large, CBT research and assessment stand to profit from an emerging paradigm shift with regard to the concept of validity and validation practices that may serve to accelerate progress in addressing unresolved questions that stem from etiology and causality, which have remained largely unaddressed in a satisfactory manner to date.

KEY POINTS

FOR PRACTITIONERS

- Knowledge of validity standards should underpin the informed use of assessment instruments.
- So-called "gold standard" measures should not be immune to ongoing assessment of evidence that they meet validity standards.

FOR RESEARCHERS

- A fundamental principle in CBT assessment is the need to distinguish response systems and not introduce confounds based on content, process, and structure.

- Theories of validity are evolving, with particular focus on how meaning of scale scores is established. It is likely that the classic Cronbach and Meehl approach will be superseded over the course of time.
- Validation practices are likely to change along with the evolving theories of validity, which may lead to greater emphasis on establishing validity during scale construction, rather than in a post hoc manner following administration.

FOR STUDENTS AND EDUCATORS

- Informed use of assessment instruments requires a solid grounding in validity theory.
- Validity claims based on patterns of correlations offer only very basic evidence of what interpretations of scale scores can be supported and are premised on adequate content, process, and structure validity evidence.

REFERENCES

American Educational Research Association, American Psychological Association, & National Council on Measurement in Education. (1999). *Standards for educational and psychological testing.* Washington, DC: American Educational Research Association.

Antony, M. M., Orsillo, S. M., & Roemer, L. (2001). *Practitioner's guide to empirically based measures of anxiety.* New York: Springer.

Beck, A. T. (1976). *Cognitive therapy and the emotional disorders.* New York: International Universities Press.

Beck, A. T., Steer, R. A., & Brown, G. K. (1996). *Manual for Beck Depression Inventory–II.* San Antonio, TX: Psychological Corporation.

Bornstein, R. F. (2011). Toward a process-focused model of test score validity: Improving psychological assessment in science and practice. *Psychological Assessment, 23*(2), 532–544.

Borsboom, D. (2005). *Measuring the mind: Conceptual issues in contemporary psychometrics.* Cambridge, UK: Cambridge University Press.

Brown, G. P., Hawkes, N. C., Cooper, A., Jonsdottir, S., & Tata, P. (2013). The Anxiety Attitude and Belief Scale–2: Development, measurement model, and initial validity. *Clinical Psychology and Psychotherapy.*

Brown, G. P., Hawkes, N. C., & Tata, P. (2009). Construct validity and vulnerability to anxiety: A cognitive interviewing study of the revised Anxiety Sensitivity Index. *Journal of Anxiety Disorders, 23*(7), 942–949.

Cervone, D. (2004). Personality assessment: Tapping the social-cognitive architecture of personality. *Behavior Therapy, 35*(1), 113–129.

Clark, D. A. (1997). Twenty years of cognitive assessment: Current status and future directions. *Journal of Consulting and Clinical Psychology, 65*(6), 996–1000.

Clark, L. A., & Watson, D. (1995). Constructing validity: Basic issues in objective scale development. *Psychological Assessment, 7*(3), 309–319.

Coyne, J. C., & Gotlib, I. H. (1983). The role of cognition in depression: A critical appraisal. *Psychological Bulletin, 94*(3), 472–505.

Cramer, A. O. J., Waldorp, L. J., van der Maas, H. L. J., & Borsboom, D. (2010). Comorbidity: A network perspective. *Behavioral and Brain Sciences, 33*(2–3), 137–150.

Cronbach, L. J., & Meehl, P. E. (1955). Construct validity in psychological tests. *Psychological Bulletin, 52*(4), 281.

Deacon, B. J., Abramowitz, J. S., Woods, C. M., & Tolin, D. F. (2003). The Anxiety Sensitivity Index—Revised: Psychometric properties and factor structure in two nonclinical samples. *Behaviour Research and Therapy, 41*(12), 1427–1449.

Embretson, S. E. (1983). Construct validity: Construct representation versus nomothetic span. *Psychological Bulletin, 93*(1), 179–197.

Ericsson, K. A., & Simon, H. A. (1980). Verbal reports as data. *Psychological Review, 87*(3), 215–251.

Foa, E. B., & Kozak, M. J. (1986). Emotional processing of fear: Exposure to corrective information. *Psychological Bulletin, 99*(1), 20–35.

Hammen, C., & Krantz, S. E. (1985). Measures of psychological processes in depression. (Eds.). *Handbook of depression: Treatment, assessment, and research* (pp. 408–444). Homewood, IL: Dorsey Press.

Haynes, S. N., Mumma, G. H., & Pinson, C. (2009). Idiographic assessment: Conceptual and psychometric foundations of individualized behavioral assessment. *Clinical Psychology Review, 29*(2), 179–191.

Haynes, S. N., Richard, D. C., & Kubany, E. S. (1995). Content validity in psychological assessment: A functional approach to concepts and methods. *Psychological Assessment, 7*(3), 238–247.

Haynes, S. N., Smith, G. T., & Hunsley, J. D. (2011). *Scientific foundations of clinical assessment.* New York: Routledge/Taylor & Francis.

Hollon, S. D., & Kendall, P. C. (1980). Cognitive self-statements in depression: Development of an automatic thoughts questionnaire. *Cognitive Therapy and Research, 4*(4), 383–395.

Hollon, S. D., & Kriss, M. R. (1984). Cognitive factors in clinical research and practice. *Clinical Psychology Review, 4*(1), 35–76.

Ingram, R. E., & Kendall, P. C. (1986). Cognitive clinical psychology: Implications of an information processing perspective. In R. E. Ingram (Ed.), *Information processing approaches to clinical psychology* (pp. 3–21). Orlando, FL: Academic Press.

Kwon, S. M., & Oei, T. P. S. (1994). The roles of two levels of cognitions in the development, maintenance, and treatment of depression. *Clinical Psychology Review, 14*(5), 331–358.

Lang, P. J. (1979). A bio-informational theory of emotional imagery. *Psychophysiology, 16*(6), 495–512.

Lessler, J. T., & Forsyth, B. H. (1996). A coding system for appraising questionnaires. In N. Schwarz & S. Sudman (Eds.), *Answering questions:*

Methodology for determining cognitive and communicative processes in survey research (pp. 259–291). San Francisco: Jossey-Bass.

Lilienfeld, S. O., Turner, S. M., & Jacob, R. G. (1993). Anxiety sensitivity: An examination of theoretical and methodological issues. *Advances in Behaviour Research and Therapy, 15*(2), 147–183.

Lissitz, R. W., & Samuelsen, K. (2007). A suggested change in terminology and emphasis regarding validity and education. *Educational Researcher, 36*(8), 437–448.

Loftus, E. F. (1984). Protocol analysis of responses to survey recall questions. In T. Jabine, M. Straf, J. Tanur, & R. Tourangeau (Eds.), *Cognitive aspects of survey methodology: Building a bridge between disciplines* (pp. 61–64). Washington, DC: National Academy Press.

Loftus, E. F., Fienberg, S. E., & Tanur, J. M. (1985). Cognitive psychology meets the national survey. *American Psychologist, 40*(2), 175–180.

Markus, K. A., & Borsboom, D. (2013). *Frontiers of test validity theory: Measurement, causation, and meaning.* New York: Routledge/Taylor & Francis.

McGrath, R. E. (2005). Conceptual complexity and construct validity. *Journal of Personality Assessment, 85*(2), 112–124.

McGrath, R. E. (2009). On prototypes and paradigm shifts. *Measurement, 7*(1), 27–29.

McNally, R. J. (1999). Theoretical approaches to the fear of anxiety. In S. Taylor (Ed.), *Anxiety sensitivity: Theory, research, and treatment of the fear of anxiety* (pp. 3–16). Mahwah, NJ: Erlbaum.

Messick, S. (1989). Meaning and values in test validation: The science and ethics of assessment. *Educational Researcher, 18*(2), 5–11.

Naragon-Gainey, K. (2010). Meta-analysis of the relations of anxiety sensitivity to the depressive and anxiety disorders. *Psychological Bulletin, 136*(1), 128–150.

Nicholls, J. G., Licht, B. G., & Pearl, R. A. (1982). Some dangers of using personality questionnaires to study personality. *Psychological Bulletin, 92*(3), 572–580.

Nisbett, R. E., & Wilson, T. D. (1977). Telling more than we can know: Verbal reports on mental processes. *Psychological Review, 84*(3), 231–259.

Obsessive Compulsive Cognitions Working Group. (2003). Psychometric validation of the Obsessive Beliefs Questionnaire and the Interpretation of Intrusions Inventory: Part I. *Behaviour Research and Therapy, 41*(8), 863–878.

Padesky, C., & Mooney, K. (1990). Clinical tip: Presenting the cognitive model to clients. *International Cognitive Therapy Newsletter, 6*(1), 13–14.

Presser, S., Couper, M. P., Lessler, J. T., Martin, E., Martin, J., Rothgeb, J. M., et al. (2004). Methods for testing and evaluating survey questions. *Public Opinion Quarterly, 68*(1), 109–130.

Reiss, S., Peterson, R. A., Gursky, D. M., & McNally, R. J. (1986). Anxiety sensitivity, anxiety frequency and the prediction of fearfulness. *Behaviour Research and Therapy, 24*(1), 1–8.

Schwarz, N. (1999). Self-reports: How the questions shape the answers. *American Psychologist, 54*(2), 93–105.

Smith, G. T., & Zapolski, T. C. (2009). Construct validation of personality measures. In J. N. Butcher (Ed.), *Oxford handbook of personality assessment* (pp. 81–98). New York: Oxford University Press.

Strauss, M. E., & Smith, G. T. (2009). Construct validity: Advances in theory and methodology. *Annual Review of Clinical Psychology, 5*, 1–25.

Taylor, S., & Cox, B. J. (1998). Anxiety sensitivity: Multiple dimensions and hierarchic structure. *Behaviour Research and Therapy, 36*(1), 37–51.

Taylor, S., Zvolensky, M. J., Cox, B. J., Deacon, B., Heimberg, R. G., Ledley, D. R., et al. (2007). Robust Dimensions of Anxiety Sensitivity: Development and initial validation of the Anxiety Sensitivity Index–3. *Psychological Assessment, 19*(2), 176.

Tourangeau, R. (1984). Cognitive science and survey methods. In T. Jabine, M. Straf, J. Tanur, & R. Tourangeau (Eds.), *Cognitive aspects of survey methodology: Building a bridge between disciplines* (pp. 73–100). Washington, DC: National Academy Press.

Waller, N. G. (1989). The effect of inapplicable item responses on the structure of behavioral checklist data: A cautionary note. *Multivariate Behavioral Research, 24*(1), 125–134.

Weissman, A. N., & Beck, A. T. (1978). Development and validation of the Dysfunctional Attitude Scale: A preliminary investigation. Retrieved from *www.eric.ed.gov/ERICWebPortal/detail?accno=ED167619.*

Williams, C., & Garland, A. (2002). A cognitive-behavioural therapy assessment model for use in everyday clinical practice. *Advances in Psychiatric Treatment, 8*(3), 172–179.

Willis, G. B. (2005). *Cognitive interviewing: A tool for improving questionnaire design.* Thousand Oaks, CA: Sage.

Zinbarg, R. E., Barlow, D. H., & Brown, T. A. (1997). Hierarchical structure and general factor saturation of the Anxiety Sensitivity Index: Evidence and implications. *Psychological Assessment, 9*(3), 277–284.

Zvolensky, M. J., Arrindell, W. A., Taylor, S., Bouvard, M., Cox, B. J., Stewart, S. H., et al. (2003). Anxiety sensitivity in six countries. *Behaviour Research and Therapy, 41*(7), 841–859.

12

Enhancing Measurement Validation in Cognitive Clinical Research with Structural Equation Modeling and Item Response Theory

Kristin Naragon-Gainey and Timothy A. Brown

As in many areas of psychology, most of the variables of interest in cognitive-behavioral therapy (CBT) research and practice are constructs that are not directly observable. For example, researchers and clinicians may be interested in assessing depression levels over the past week, cognitive distortions that arise in specific social situations, a patient's perception of the therapeutic alliance, or subjective distress during an exposure. Because these constructs are not observable by the researcher or clinician, the value of conclusions drawn about them is limited by the validity of the measures and analyses used. Strong measurement validation is therefore essential at various stages of CBT assessment and research, including the creation and initial validation of new measures; the evaluation of measures' properties in different populations; and the use of advanced measurement techniques to model, analyze, and interpret data most appropriately.

Several analytic techniques are frequently used in measurement validation in CBT research. For example, a data reduction technique called exploratory factor analysis (EFA) is often used to develop a new scale or to assess the underlying structure (i.e., dimensions or factors) of a measure or construct. Correlational analyses and multiple regression can determine the strength and direction of the association among variables, with the latter analysis allowing for the assessment of the unique contribution of variables in predicting the dependent variable. In addition, analysis of variance (ANOVA) and related techniques are frequently used to evaluate group differences on measures of interest.

These analyses continue to be appropriate and valuable in many contexts, but they do have some notable limitations. First, with the exception of EFA, the above-described techniques cannot model "latent variables," which are variables formed from the shared variance among multiple measures. Latent variables represent the underlying construct of interest (e.g., intolerance of uncertainty) that one cannot measure directly or perfectly, whereas observed variables (e.g., total score on the Intolerance of Uncertainty Scale) are variables that exist in the data set and are proxies for the underlying construct. Latent variables are in theory "error-free," because the measure-specific error found in observed variables is statistically isolated into an error term or residual. Because latent variables have less error variance than single measures, measuring constructs with latent variables typically increases assessment validity and reliability. Although EFA includes latent variables (also called "factors"), it is limited, in that examining the associations among factors and covariates with regression can be somewhat cumbersome and problematic within the EFA framework (see Grice, 2001, for a discussion of the problem of factor score indeterminacy).

Second, these standard analyses cannot account for "method effects," or shared variance across constructs due to similar assessment approaches (e.g., scales from the same measure, measures all collected via semistructured interview, or negatively worded items). A failure to account for method effects can bias parameter estimates and standard errors, leading to inaccurate structural conclusions (Brown, 2015). The Penn State Worry Questionnaire provides an illustration of this issue. Although the measure was designed to be unidimensional, early factor analyses reported a two-factor structure, consisting of a Worry factor and an Absence of Worry factor formed by the reverse-worded items (see Fresco, Heimberg, Mennin, & Turk, 2002). Brown (2003) found that a single-factor model that allowed error correlations among the reverse-worded items provided a better fit to the data than either a one-factor model that did not account for method effects or the two-factor model just described. Thus, in this case, failing to account for method variance led to inaccurate conclusions about the underlying structure of the measure and resulted in poorer model fit. Finally, traditional techniques cannot directly model and compare properties of responses across different groups. For example, it is important to determine whether a test is biased so that the meaning of items differs across groups (e.g., by gender, race, or age). Traditional approaches do not easily allow for the comparison of mean levels of latent variables and associations among latent variables across different samples.

OVERVIEW OF LATENT VARIABLE APPROACHES TO MEASUREMENT

We focus on three established latent variable analytic techniques—structural equation modeling (SEM), confirmatory factor analysis (CFA), and item response theory (IRT)—that address many of the limitations of the commonly used techniques described above. Because SEM and CFA have been more frequently applied to clinical assessment and research than IRT, we emphasize the former two techniques. SEM consists of two parts: (1) a measurement model that prespecifies the number of latent variables, "indicators" (e.g., scales or items) for each latent variable, and the relationships among indicator error terms (also called "residuals" or "error variances," which quantify the variance of the indicator not accounted for by the latent variable) and (2) a structural model that prespecifies the associations among the latent variables. CFA is a special case of SEM that includes the measurement model portion, but does not focus on structural relations among latent variables.

For the CFA measurement model, the researcher assigns observed measures (e.g., Beck Depression Inventory–II, Hamilton Rating Scale for Depression) or single items as indicators of a particular factor (e.g., Depression) in the model. Thus, unlike in EFA, factor loadings—defined as the regression path linking the latent variable to the indicator—are not freely estimated for all indicators on all factors. Each indicator has an associated error term that is freely estimated, and error terms can be allowed to covary to account for method effects such as similar wording or substantive shared variance beyond that attributable to the latent variable. In addition, the measurement model can include information about mean values by estimating latent variable means and the indicator intercepts (i.e., the predicted value of the indicator when the latent variable is zero). The structural model includes regression paths (directional) and correlations as specified by the researcher on the basis of theory, resulting in parameter estimates interpreted similarly to betas and correlations in a standardized solution, as well as standard errors. Multiple fit indices with complementary information are computed for each model, and these can be used to assess absolute goodness of fit and to compare the relative fit of competing models. Figure 12.1 shows two

1a. Measurement Model

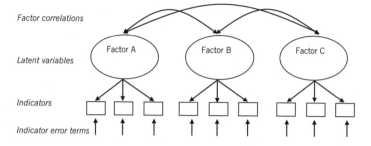

Factor correlations

Latent variables

Indicators

Indicator error terms

1b. Structural Model (built upon the measurement model above)

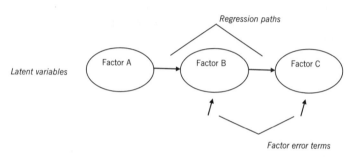

Regression paths

Latent variables

Factor error terms

FIGURE 12.1. Path diagram of a confirmatory factor analysis (CFA) measurement model and a structural model in structural equation modeling (SEM).

path diagrams that illustrate a sample measurement model and structural model. For a detailed presentation of SEM and CFA in the social sciences, see texts such as Brown (2015) or Kline (2010).

IRT is a latent variable technique with the basic premise that an individual's response to a questionnaire or test item is a function of his or her standing on the construct of interest (e.g., IQ, anxiety, or extraversion) and the characteristics of the item itself. As such, IRT can estimate an individual's score on the latent variable that the measure purportedly assesses. In addition, each item has up to three parameters that can be calculated: (1) discrimination parameter (referred to as a), which describes how well the item distinguishes different levels of the latent variable; (2) difficulty parameter (b), defined as the value on the latent variable at which an individual has a 50% chance of responding affirmatively or correctly; and (3) pseudoguessing parameter (c) or lower asymptote parameter, which is a correction that is most relevant when the "correct" answer can be guessed (c is often estimated in educational settings such as achievement testing, but rarely estimated in clinical applications). These parameters can be illustrated graphically in an item characteristic curve (ICC) that shows the probability of endorsement at different levels of the latent variable (see Figure 12.2 for an example of an ICC). For further details on IRT, see Embretson and Reise (2000) or de Ayala (2009); Thomas (2011) describes IRT in clinical assessment specifically. It is important to note that under certain conditions, IRT and CFA yield nearly identical results, wherein the discrimination parameters correspond to factor loadings and difficulty parameters correspond to indicator intercepts (e.g., Takane & de Leeuw, 1987). In fact, with current software implementations (e.g., Mplus; Muthén & Muthén, 1998–2012), IRT can be construed as a special case of CFA with categorical outcomes.

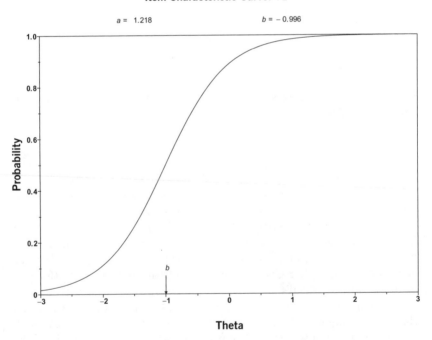

Item Characteristic Curve: Y1

a = 1.218   *b* = – 0.996

FIGURE 12.2. Sample item characteristic curve (ICC). *a*, discrimination parameter; *b*, difficulty parameter; probability, probability of endorsing the item; theta, latent variable the item assesses. Guessing parameter (*c*) is not shown here.

UTILIZING ADVANCED MEASUREMENT
TECHNIQUES IN CONSTRUCT VALIDATION

"Construct validation," as conceptualized by Cronbach and Meehl (1955), may be defined as the extent to which a measure assesses the construct it is intended to measure. Construct validity includes assessment of measure dimensionality, reliability, convergent and discriminant validity, criterion validity, and generalizability (see Strauss & Smith, 2009, for a review). Next, we highlight several ways in which advanced measurement techniques can be utilized to build evidence for construct validity.

Early Measurement Validation with Exploratory SEM

As described previously, EFA is typically used in the early stages of measure development, when the structure of the measure has not yet been established and the preliminary scale may require modifications. However, Marsh and colleagues (2009) point out that many psychopathology and personality measures have a robust, replicable structure when analyzed with EFA, but demonstrate poor fit when the same structure is assessed with CFA. Typically, extensive post hoc modifications are necessary for the CFA model to have acceptable fit to the data, including some modifications that seem arbitrary rather than aligned with theory. This discrepancy in structural analyses done with EFA versus CFA is likely due to the "congeneric" nature of CFA, meaning that (generally) indicators are assigned to load on one factor, and all cross-loadings are set to zero. When this is not an accurate assumption and in fact the items load significantly onto multiple factors (whether due to substantive theory or to measurement issues), CFA models will demonstrate poor fit. Even more concerning is that when the congeneric model is misapplied, it results in inaccurate parameter estimates with inflated factor correlations. The inability of EFA to model method effects or other sources of error term covariance can also contribute to a misspecified model when evaluated with CFA (Asparouhov & Muthén, 2009; Marsh et al., 2009).

A new analytic technique was recently developed with the intention of combining the exploratory nature of EFA with the flexibility and advantages of CFA, providing a more streamlined assessment of the properties of a new measure. Exploratory structural equation modeling (ESEM) allows one to estimate all factor loadings freely, while also having the options of specifying error covariances, comparing multiple samples within the same model, and including a structural model with regression paths (for a mathematical account of ESEM, see Asparouhov

& Muthén, 2009). Thus ESEM more directly reveals cross-loadings and structural issues than do extensive post hoc and atheoretical adjustments in CFA guided by modification indices (i.e., indices showing paths that, if freed, would improve model fit). Mplus software (Muthén & Muthén, 1998–2012) currently includes syntax for conducting ESEM analyses.

One example of a commonly used measure that does not appear to fit the congeneric model is the NEO Five Factor Inventory (Costa & McCrae, 1992), a self-report measure that assesses the Big Five personality traits. Although the five-factor structure of this measure has been reported in many samples with EFA, it consistently shows poor fit when evaluated with CFA, likely because indicators of personality traits often have secondary loadings. However, when all factor loadings are estimated with ESEM and error covariances are allowed among similar items (i.e., items from the same "facet") within each factor, model fit has been very good in nonclinical and clinical samples (Marsh et al., 2010; Rosellini & Brown, 2011). Because ESEM was developed recently, it has not yet been used in published measure development studies, but the technique holds great promise for more efficiently and accurately modeling and refining the structure of new symptom or trait measures. In addition, CBT researchers should consider whether ESEM may be more appropriate than CFA/SEM for a given analysis, particularly when the structure of the measure is poorly understood or the structure is known to be complex (i.e., it does not conform to the congeneric model).

Two other techniques in the CFA family may be useful for examining certain complex measurement models. First, bifactor analysis is germane when items are hypothesized to load onto a general factor, as well as independent group factors. For example, an evaluation of the Inventory for Depression and Anxiety Symptoms indicated that all symptoms loaded on a general Distress factor, as well as specific symptom factors (e.g., generalized anxiety, appetite loss, irritability). In addition, symptoms differed as to how strongly they loaded on the general versus specific factors (Simms, Gros, & Watson, 2008). Second, Bayesian SEM (BSEM) is an alternative to traditional CFA that can also address many of the concerns discussed in reference to ESEM and is becoming more widespread among applied researchers. BSEM, which incorporates "priors" or likely parameter values based on previous data and/or theory, provides the option of allowing cross-loadings that approximate zero, rather than cross-loadings that are fixed strictly to zero. Such an approach is likely to be more realistic for many measures or constructs and is less prone to inflated factor correlations than traditional SEM. Furthermore, BSEM does not rely on large-sample theory and can model non-normal distributions flexibly. See Muthén and Asparouhov (2012) for a detailed description of BSEM and applied examples.

Assessment of Reliability and Information

Measure "reliability" is traditionally defined as the proportion of true score variance to total observed variance (i.e., true score variance plus error variance) in test scores (Lord & Novick, 1968). Thus reliability can be thought of as the ability of a scale to detect variance specific to the construct being measured. Cronbach's coefficient alpha is the standard index of reliability, where alpha is a function of the number of items in the scale and the average interitem correlation (Cronbach, 1951). However, it has been shown that alpha is inaccurate under at least two conditions. First, alpha underestimates reliability if tau equivalence does not hold; tau equivalence means that factor loadings on a given factor are the same across all items. In other words, every item on the scale must have the exact same relationship with the underlying construct—a condition that is not commonly met. Second, if a measure has correlated item error terms, alpha may either underestimate or overestimate reliability (Raykov, 2001a, 2001b, 2004).

To circumvent these problems, Raykov (2001a, 2004) put forth a formula that directly estimates scale reliability (i.e., proportion of true score variance) based on the CFA parameter estimates: reliability = squared sum of unstandardized factor loadings/(squared sum of unstandardized factor loadings + sum of unstandardized measurement error terms). This index may be calculated by hand from CFA parameters or by additional syntax programming in latent variable software programs such as Mplus and LISREL (in EQS, the scale reliability estimate can be generated by a single command option). Raykov (2004) compared this method of computing reliability with reliability as estimated by coefficient alpha for the Social Interaction Anxiety Scale in a large sample of psychiatric patients. In this case, coefficient alpha (.953) only slightly overestimated reliability relative to the formula above (.946), although Raykov noted that the difference would be larger for measures with larger error covariances among items. It is important to note that Raykov's method (like alpha) results in a point estimation of reliability that is sample-specific, rather than indicative of the true population value. However, it is possible to calculate the standard error for this estimate and construct confidence intervals around it, allowing for greater certainty regarding likely population values for reliability. This method has also been extended for more complex circumstances, such as binary outcomes, noncongeneric scales, and scales with a higher-order factor structure (see Brown, 2015).

IRT offers a different conception of reliability via the concept of "information," defined in this context as the inverse of the standard error of measurement. Unlike classically defined reliability, information for a given item or scale may vary among people, depending on their level of the latent construct being assessed (e.g., a scale may be less informative at low vs. high levels of depression). Thus information is a property not simply of the scale, but also of the value of the latent variable being assessed. In IRT information is additive, such that information for each item is summed to determine scale information. During the scale development process, one can then select items that maximize information for the values (or difficulty) of the latent trait of interest, or shorten the scale by omitting items that do not add substantial information (Thomas, 2011). IRT analyses have shown that many diagnostic or screening measures have information that peaks at high levels of severity (e.g., Cooke, Michie, Hart, & Hare, 1999). While this is beneficial if one is interested in a dichotomous cutoff (i.e., presence vs. absence of major depression), items that are informative at lower and moderate levels of severity also should be included for dimensional constructs such as cognitive vulnerabilities. For example, an IRT analysis of the Anxiety Sensitivity Index revealed that the measure is fairly informative across the full range of severity, with some items broadly contributing to information and others focused on the upper end of the underlying trait (Zvolensky, Strong, Bernstein, Vujanovic, & Marshall, 2009). Assessing measure reliability with these more nuanced methods in CFA or IRT during scale development would be likely to bolster both the efficiency and validity of new scales.

Multitrait–Multimethod Matrix with SEM

Campbell and Fiske (1959) first presented the "multitrait–multimethod matrix" as a means of evaluating convergent and discriminant validity for a measure; in other words, this approach assesses whether a particular measure is related to other measures and constructs as one would expect from theory and previous research. A multitrait–multimethod study includes the target measure, other measures of the target construct, and measures of distinct but related constructs (referred to here as different "traits"). Each trait is also measured with different methods (e.g., self-report, interview, other-report, neuroimaging, behavioral observation). A correlation matrix is then constructed among the different traits and methods, with particular interpretive focus on the heteromethod and monomethod blocks. Strong positive correlations along the validity diagonal (i.e., same trait, different method) are consistent with good convergent validity. Discriminant validity is supported when correlations for different constructs with different methods are weaker than the corresponding convergent correlations. Last, one can examine the influence of method effects by comparing the correlations of different traits with the same method versus different methods. This correlational approach to discriminant and convergent validity has several limitations, however. First, results may vary greatly, depending on the psychometric properties of the specific convergent and discriminant measures included. Second, the procedure is subjective, in that it is unclear how large the differences between correlations should be to support good convergent and discriminant validity.

Because CFA can directly model method effects, it can more cleanly separate and quantify method-driven variance in a way that facilitates interpretation of the multitrait–multimethod matrix. There are two ways to model method variance in CFA: "correlated methods" and "correlated uniqueness" (i.e., error terms) (Marsh & Grayson, 1995). For the correlated methods approach, there must be at least three traits and three methods, and each trait and method must have at least three indicators. In this model, each indicator loads on one trait factor and one method factor, without any other cross-loadings. In addition, correlations among trait factors and among method factors are freely estimated, but correlations between trait and method factors are fixed to zero. Indicator error terms cannot be correlated in this method. In contrast, the correlated uniqueness approach does not model method variance as latent variables, but rather by allowing correlations among error terms for indicators using the same method. For this model, at least two traits and three methods are necessary. One recent example using the correlated methods approach examined anxiety disorders in children (social phobia, generalized anxiety disorder, panic disorder, and separation anxiety disorder) assessed with three different methods (self-report, parent-report, and diagnostic interview), and found that the frequently observed disagreement among methods was not reflective of poor construct validity for the disorders (Langer, Wood, Bergman, & Piacentini, 2010).

When one is interpreting these multitrait–multimethod matrices in CFA, strong and significant factor loadings on the trait factors (which adjust for the effect of methods) provide evidence of convergent validity. Conversely, weak correlations among trait factors indicate good discriminant validity. The presence of method effects is indicated by strong and significant loadings on the method factor (correlated methods approach) or strong and significant correlations among error terms (correlated uniqueness approach) (Brown, 2015). In addition to examining convergent and discriminant validity with CFA, the models just described can be extended by embedding them in a larger structural model that includes outcome or external validators.

How does one decide whether to use the correlated methods or correlated uniqueness approach? Both have advantages and disadvantages. The correlated methods approach more directly models the ideas of Campbell and Fiske (1959) with separate trait and method factors, but the model is often underidentified and fails to converge (e.g., Kenny & Kashy, 1992; Marsh & Bailey, 1991). To resolve this identification problem, Eid and colleagues proposed a multitrait–multimethod model that is more likely to converge: the $M - 1$ model, which contains one less method factor than the number of methods in the study (see Eid, 2000, and Eid, Lischetzke, Nussbeck, & Trierweiler, 2003). Additional method effects beyond the method factors (such as reverse-keyed items) cannot be modeled with this approach. An example of this method as applied to clinical assessment is Kollman, Brown, and Barlow's (2009) examination of the construct validity of acceptance. They used multiple measures of acceptance and two related (but purportedly distinct) constructs: cognitive reappraisal and perceived emotional control. The results of the multitrait–multimethod CFA analyses suggested good convergent and discriminant validity for acceptance as a construct; however, acceptance demonstrated poor concurrent validity, in that it was unrelated to numerous psychological symptoms in this sample. In contrast to the $M - 1$ approach, the correlated uniqueness approach typically results in proper solutions, and one can model multiple sources of variance. However, interpretation may be less straightforward, as it is difficult to determine which method has the most method variance, and correlations cannot be specified among methods or between methods and traits.

Validation across Different Groups

One strength of CFA is the ability to directly compare parameters across two or more groups within a single model. Traditionally, measures are deemed to be valid across different populations when psychometric properties are strong in different types of samples (e.g., different genders, races, ages, clinical status); however, it is difficult to determine in this manner whether items have the same meaning across different samples. Multiple-groups CFA can flexibly test for differences across a variety of measurement and structural parameters. Invariance of measurement parameters (e.g., factor loadings and intercepts) can be directly tested in CFA, allowing one to determine whether the means, variance, and covariances are comparable across groups prior to interpreting any observed differences on structural parameters (Brown, 2015). Thus testing for differences among groups proceeds from the "bottom up" as described below.

First, a multiple-groups analysis is run to determine whether the groups have equal form (identical factor structure) by including both groups but allowing all parameters to vary across groups. Identical factor structure is supported if the model has a good fit to the data in all groups, and this model then serves as the baseline comparison model for more stringent comparisons of parameters across groups. Next, the equality of factor loadings is tested. This is especially important in measurement validation, as it determines whether the items have comparable relationships to the latent constructs across groups. To test this, a model that restricts the factor loadings for each indicator to be equal across groups is compared to the previous model of equal form. The models' chi-squared values are then compared; if the difference is significant, this indicates that constraining the factor loadings to be equal leads to a significant decrement in fit (see Brown, 2015, for more detail). In other words, a significant chi-squared difference test indicates that one or more of the factor loadings are not equal across groups and that the strength of the relationships between some of the indicators and the latent variables differs across groups, whereas a nonsignificant result is supportive of equal factor loadings. Similar model comparisons can be conducted to determine whether indicator intercepts are equal across groups; a noninvariant indicator intercept suggests that individuals in different groups at the same level of the latent trait have different predicted observed scores on that indicator. If invariance of latent form, factor loadings, and indicator intercepts is demonstrated, then one can conclude that the measure functions similarly across groups, such that a given observed score on the measure represents the same level of the construct in each group. It is important to note that full measurement invariance—meaning invariance of all factor loadings and all indicator intercepts—is not required for results to be interpretable and meaningful across groups. Rather, partial measurement invariance (i.e., when the majority of indicators on each factor are invariant) is sufficient to proceed with group comparisons (Brown, 2015).

There are several examples of measurement invariance evaluations in the CBT literature. For instance, South, Krueger, and Iacono (2009) evaluated whether the Dyadic Adjustment Scale, a commonly used measure of relationship satisfaction, is invariant across genders. They found evidence of partial measurement invariance, suggesting that differences between the scores of men and women on this measure are a function of true differences in relationship satisfaction, as opposed to measurement bias. Similarly, Gomez, Vance, and Gomez (2012) found that the Children's Depression Inventory (CDI) was fully invariant across children and adolescents with and without depressive disorders, even after they accounted for age, sex, and the presence or absence of anxiety disorders. Thus scores on the CDI may be interpreted uniformly regardless of a current depressive disorder.

In IRT, a related concept of "test bias" exists, in which bias is demonstrated when individuals from different groups but with the same standing on the latent variable have different probabilities of endorsing an item (similar to noninvariant indicator intercepts, as described previously). Such items display differential item functioning (DIF), and these analyses allow one to separate out whether observed differences are due to genuine differences in the latent variable versus test bias. In one recent DIF study, researchers found that differences on depression scores for boys and girls were attributable to true group differences rather than test bias (Carle, Millsap, & Cole, 2008). If some items are found to have DIF for a given group comparison, these items can be revised or removed from the measure to create a more generalizable scale that is valid for different populations.

Longitudinal Analyses: Trait–State–Occasion Model

Many questions of interest in CBT research involve a longitudinal design; for example, researchers may wish to track symptom change over the course of therapy or evaluate the temporal stability of trait-like vulnerability factors (e.g., anxiety sensitivity). In a seminal paper on this topic, Barnett and Gotlib (1988) reviewed the complexities of assessing how depression and related risk factors (e.g., negative cognitions, personality, social support, coping) are associated over time, given that such risk factors may vary in temporal stability and onset relative to depression (e.g., negative attributions may be antecedents, concomitants, or consequences of depression). Researchers have noted that nearly all psychological constructs contain two components: (1) stable "trait" variance that remains constant over time and (2) unstable "state" variance that changes on the basis of transient factors (e.g., current mood state, time of the day, true change processes) (e.g., Baltes, 1987). For example, an individual's scores on a Neuroticism scale may be divided into variance that is common across all assessment points and variance that is unique to each assessment point. Although most analytic techniques collapse these two sources of variance into a single estimate, it is best to use models that can statistically separate them (e.g., trait level of Neuroticism vs. changes in Neuroticism over time) if one source is particularly relevant to a research question.

Although several such models have been proposed in the past two decades (e.g., Kenny & Zautra, 1995; Steyer & Schmitt, 1994), David Cole and colleagues recently created an improved and elaborated model called the "trait–state–occasion" (TSO) model (Cole, Martin, & Steiger, 2005). The TSO model, formulated within the SEM framework, is built from two or more indicators of a construct that are each assessed at three or more time points. The latent variables formed from these indicators are referred to as "state" factors and represent the total observed variance for the construct as measured at a particular point in time. The variance for the state factors is then completely distributed into two sources: (1) a "trait" factor, on which all state factors load at unity and (2) "occasion" factors that are defined by each state factor (again, loading at unity). In this way, the trait factor represents the time-invariant, stable component shared across assessment points, whereas the occasion factors represent transient, time-variant components for each assessment not accounted for by the trait component. In addition, the occasion factors are autoregressive, with regression paths between subsequent time points (e.g., from Time 1 to Time 2) that model the stability of situational influences.

The TSO model can be used to examine consistency over time in latent variables, as well as to isolate particular components (i.e., time-variant or time-invariant) within a larger structural model with covariates and predictors. In one recent example, Prenoveau and colleagues (2011) evaluated the stability of depression, anxiety, and personality traits over the course of 3 years in an adolescent nonclinical sample, with the hypothesis that personality traits should be more stable than affective symptoms. Because the authors were interested in stability, they focused on the time-invariant portion of each construct in the TSO model, which provided a quantification and direct comparison of stabilities across constructs after sources of noise and change were removed. Prenoveau and colleagues found that anxiety symptoms and personality traits were very stable over 3 years (time-invariant component = 73–84% of the total variance), whereas depression symptoms were more episodic (time-invariant component = 46% of the total variance). We also describe a second study that used the TSO model (see "Application to Theoretical Issues in CBT: The Causal Status of Cognition").

Computer-Adaptive Testing

A final application of advanced measurement techniques to CBT assessment pertains to scale administration, rather than scale validation. Computer-adaptive testing (CAT) is an iterative technique derived from IRT analyses, in which an individual's answer to an item results in an initial estimation (calculated by a computer) of his or her standing on the latent trait. Using this estimation, the computer selects the next item to be maximally informative in more accurately determining the individual's level of the latent trait. In this way, the computer "zeroes in" on the true value of the latent trait, making adjustments based on each answer if necessary, in a minimal number of items (see Walter et al., 2007). Although CATs have primarily been created in ability and achievement tests, some CATs have also been designed for personality/psychopathology measures. For example, a CAT version of the Schedule for Nonadaptive and Adaptive Personality (Clark, 1993) was created that was more efficient than, and deemed preferable by participants to, the pencil-and-paper version (Simms & Clark, 2005). It is likely that CAT administrations of symptom measures will become more common in coming years, as the National Institute of Health is currently developing a large number of CATs for mental and physical health assessment for the Patient-Reported Outcomes Measurement Information System (Cella et al., 2010). A CAT administration of symptom questionnaires could greatly streamline clinical and research assessments in many contexts.

APPLICATION TO THEORETICAL ISSUES IN CBT: THE CAUSAL STATUS OF COGNITION

In addition to using advanced analytic techniques to enhance CBT measure development and assessment as described above, CBT researchers can also use these techniques to test certain hypotheses more powerfully and precisely. One perennial controversial issue in CBT research is the nature of the association between cognitions and affective symptoms. Many models of cognitive therapy posit that maladaptive schemas cause depressive or anxiety symptoms, and changing these schemas is therefore the target of cognitive therapy (see Garratt & Ingram, 2007, for a review of cognition in cognitive therapy for depression). If this assumption is accurate, then change in maladaptive schemas or cognitions should precede symptom reduction during cognitive therapy (or even during the natural course of recovery). Thus change in cognitions should mediate symptom change or treatment outcome. There is extensive support for the efficacy of CBT and for elements of the cognitive model (e.g., Garratt & Ingram, 2007), but less is understood regarding cognition as a real-time mechanism of symptom change. Furthermore, some dismantling studies have found that therapy for depression with only behavioral components performs as well as full CBT, suggesting at the least that an explicit focus on maladaptive thoughts is not necessary for symptom reduction (e.g., Jacobson et al., 1996). Next we describe two studies that used advanced measurement techniques in creative ways to assess whether change in cognitions leads to change in depression and anxiety symptoms.

LaGrange and Colleagues (2011)

LaGrange et al. (2011) focused on the temporal direction of prospective relations between maladaptive cognitions and depressive symptoms in a group of children ages 7–16, assessed annually over the course of 4 years.

They noted that previous longitudinal studies of the association between cognition and depression likely had limited power due to the low reliability of many cognition measures and to the relative short-term stability of depression, which results in a restriction of range. To address both concerns, the authors used the TSO model (Cole et al., 2005), a longitudinal autoregressive SEM model described in detail previously. LaGrange et al. created one TSO model for negative cognitions and one for depression symptoms, separating out the time-invariant and time-variant components of each. They then combined these two models into a parallel process model with cross-lagged paths between the time-variant (i.e., "occasion") components of each construct to evaluate temporal ordering of change. Thus the TSO model increased power to detect effects in two ways, as compared to previous studies: (1) by using latent variables that had less error variance, relative to single measures, and (2) by removing stable variance in each construct to focus analyses solely on the portion of the construct that changed over time (i.e., time-variant variance).

LaGrange et al. (2011) conducted multiple-groups analysis with the TSO model to examine prospective cognition–depression associations across three different age cohorts (second, fourth, and sixth graders). They first examined whether the time-variant component of depression was predicted by the time-variant component of maladaptive cognition at the preceding time point. They did not find support for a causal role of cognition, as only 3 of 28 paths from cognition to the subsequent assessment of depression were significant (and 2 of the associations were negative, counter to hypotheses). In contrast, 14 of the 28 paths from depression to the subsequent assessment of cognition were significant in the expected direction. Furthermore, multiple-groups analyses revealed that the prospective effect of depression on cognition was larger for later grade levels. Thus this study found that change in depressive symptoms leads to change in maladaptive cognitions, not vice versa as cognitive models would predict.

Woody, Whittal, and McLean (2011)

Woody and colleagues (2011) set out to test portions of a cognitive theory of obsessive–compulsive disorder (OCD), which hypothesizes that the meaning attributed to obsessive thoughts (e.g., that the thoughts are dangerous or must be controlled) is what leads to clinical distress (Salkovskis, 1985). They used both traditional mediation analysis and a type of latent difference scores (LDS) analysis (specifically, they used bivariate dual change scores or BDCS analysis), allowing for a comparison of results with the two analytic techniques. The traditional statistical approach to mediation has been outlined by Baron and Kenny (1986), in which mediation is supported if a series of regression analyses indicate that the association between the predictor and outcome is significantly reduced or eliminated after one has accounted for the mediator (along with an indirect effect that is significantly different from zero). In applied research, this approach is often implemented by using single indicators and with concurrent measurement of the mediator and outcome, precluding an evaluation of temporal precedence (i.e., the change in the mediator should precede change in the outcome) (Kraemer, Wilson, Fairburn, & Agras, 2002). In contrast, LDS analysis is a latent variable analysis derived from SEM that can easily account for temporal ordering. In the current study, LDS analysis was used to determine whether appraisals of obsessive thoughts are a precedent of subsequent change in obsessive symptoms, or vice versa. Each individual's latent trajectory (e.g., symptom change) has three components in this approach: the individual's rate of linear change; self-feedback coefficients (change in relation to a participant's previous latent score on the same variable; e.g., change in appraisals based on previous appraisals); and a coupling parameter (change in relation to a participant's previous latent score on the other variable; e.g., change in appraisals based on previous obsessive symptoms). For more detail regarding LDS and BDCS analyses, see McArdle (2009).

Woody et al.'s sample consisted of 73 individuals with OCD enrolled in a randomized controlled trial comparing CBT and stress management training. All participants had primary obsessions, with few or no compulsions. The severity of obsessive symptoms and OCD-related cognitions/appraisals was assessed prior to each of the 12 therapy sessions, as well as 6 and 12 months after completing treatment. Using traditional mediation analyses based on pre–post scores, the researchers found that, consistent with the cognitive model, OCD-related appraisals mediated reduction in obsessive thoughts following CBT. However, the LDS analyses, which used latent variables and took temporal precedence into account, found that a model with cognition preceding weekly changes in OCD symptoms was not consistent with the data (as indicated by fit indices). In contrast, a model in which prior OCD symptoms preceded change in cognitions was supported. Thus, although traditional mediation analyses supported OCD-related cognitions as a mediator of symptom change during treatment, this more sophisticated method found that the directionality of effects was reversed.

Although more research is needed to draw firm conclusions about the causal status of cognition in relation to symptom reduction (whether in therapy or during the natural course of the disorder), the LaGrange et al. (2011) and Woody et al. (2011) studies illustrate the value of longitudinal, latent variable analytic techniques and provide initial evidence that symptom change may affect subsequent cognitions, not vice versa.

APPLICATIONS AND FUTURE DIRECTIONS

Psychologists with different professional roles—whether practitioners, researchers, or educators—can all play an important part in enhancing measurement validation in CBT assessment and research. Educators and trainers can work to make these techniques accessible to general professional training and emphasize their relevance to practice in several ways. For example, methods classes that teach statistical analysis can regularly utilize applied examples that are of interest to students and allow students to complete practice assignments and papers with their own data when possible. In addition, for students who lack the time or interest to learn the mathematics behind latent variable modeling in detail, instructors can offer courses that are specifically designed to provide sufficient information to conduct these analyses, with a particular focus on learning to use the necessary statistical software. Last, nonstatistical graduate courses (e.g., clinical research methods, psychopathology) can strive to incorporate articles that utilize these advanced statistical approaches so that students have greater exposure to them in a variety of contexts. In particular, when students learn to conduct evaluations and therapy, trainers should initiate discussion of methodology and measures used to assess patient progress.

Practitioners frequently administer self-report or interview measures in the course of psychological evaluations and therapy. While it may not be feasible to research the psychometric properties and development of each measure, practitioners can try to select measures that were rigorously developed by consulting with researchers or referring to books for practitioners that compile data on measure properties (e.g., Antony, Orsillo, & Roemer, 2001). Utilizing CAT measures can also save administrative and scoring time for practitioners, perhaps facilitating greater use of empirical measures. In addition, practitioners should be mindful that they are truly interested in assessing underlying constructs, rather than a particular measure and its specific quirks; using multiple brief measures and different sources/methods when possible is much more likely to yield robust clinical data.

Researchers can focus on developing new measures and revising existing measures to maximize construct validity with advanced statistical methods. As reviewed in this chapter, CFA and IRT can be used to create measures with items and scales that are maximally informative, are reliable, are not biased across different demographic groups, and demonstrate strong convergent–discriminant validity (Brown, 2015; Thomas, 2011). These techniques can also be used to identify and eliminate method effects or other minor factors that are not substantively meaningful. In addition, issues of real-world feasibility should be considered in terms of the burden on the patients/participants and the clinician administering the measure; there should be a particular focus on keeping scales as short and understandable as possible without sacrificing information. Another important task for researchers is to clarify the associations among related constructs and measures by conducting more studies of construct validity with multitrait–multimethod matrices in SEM. For example, although there is much interest in constructs such as emotion regulation, distress tolerance, and mindfulness, it remains unclear exactly how they are related and to what extent there may be redundancies. In addition, because constructs are best assessed with multiple complementary methods in latent variable analyses, researchers should attempt to include not only different reporters (e.g., self, other, clinician) in their studies, but also neuroimaging and laboratory indices (e.g., skin conductance, event-related potentials) whenever possible.

In conclusion, advanced statistical methods such as CFA, SEM, and IRT have much to offer in improving measurement validation in CBT research, and can benefit psychologists in a variety of roles and settings. Such analytic methods provide greater flexibility and power to develop measures with strong properties and to test research hypotheses. As these techniques and statistical software are further developed, they are likely to become increasingly accessible and more frequently used, rather than appearing esoteric or intimidating. Ideally, this will result in a fuller understanding of the causal, maintaining, and effective therapeutic influences on psychopathology.

KEY POINTS

FOR PRACTITIONERS

- Consult with researchers or books on measurement of psychometric properties to select measures that were rigorously developed.
- Use multiple measures when possible in assessing patients.
- Utilize CAT measures when available to save time for both patients and clinicians.
- Keep in mind that *constructs* are of interest, not individual measures.

FOR RESEARCHERS

- Use advanced statistical techniques like SEM or IRT when creating new measures.
- Consider real-world feasibility, such as administration time and readability.
- Design studies to include multiple complementary methods (e.g., self-report, other-report, interview, neuroimaging, laboratory indices) for latent variable analyses.

- Use SEM to investigate the convergent–discriminant validity of related constructs to reduce redundancy among constructs and to clarify similarities and distinctions.

FOR STUDENTS AND EDUCATORS

- Read the results sections of articles carefully, and ask questions regarding unfamiliar terms and methods.
- Collaborate with more senior students with statistical expertise to learn new techniques.
- Seek out courses in advanced statistical analyses.
- For students who are less quantitatively oriented, provide advanced statistics courses that focus on applied examples, syntax and software, and opportunities to analyze students' own data.
- Nonstatistical courses should include articles with advanced statistical approaches to expose students to a range of analyses.
- When teaching clinical skills, include discussion of methodology and measures used to assess patient progress.

REFERENCES

Antony, M. M., Orsillo, S. M., & Roemer, L. (2001). *Practitioner's guide to empirically based measures of anxiety.* New York: Kluwer Academic/Plenum.

Asparouhov, T., & Muthén, B. (2009). Exploratory structural equation modeling. *Structural Equation Modeling, 16,* 397–438.

Baltes, P. B. (1987). Theoretical propositions of life-span developmental psychology: On the dynamics between growth and decline. *Developmental Psychology, 23,* 611–626.

Barnett, P. A., & Gotlib, I. H. (1988). Psychosocial functioning and depression: Distinguishing among antecedents, concomitants, and consequences. *Psychological Bulletin, 104,* 97–126.

Baron, R. M., & Kenny, D. A. (1986). The moderator–mediator variable distinction in social psychological research: Conceptual, strategic, and statistical considerations. *Journal of Personality and Social Psychology, 51,* 1173–1182.

Brown, T. A. (2003). Confirmatory factor analysis of the Penn State Worry Questionnaire: Multiple factors or method effects? *Behaviour Research and Therapy, 41,* 1411–1426.

Brown, T. A. (2015). *Confirmatory factor analysis for applied research* (2nd ed.). New York: Guilford Press.

Campbell, D. T., & Fiske, D. W. (1959). Convergent and discriminant validation by the multitrait–multimethod matrix. *Psychological Bulletin, 56,* 81–105.

Carle, A. C., Millsap, R. E., & Cole, D. A. (2008). Measurement bias across gender on the Children's Depression Inventory: Evidence for invariance from two latent variable models. *Educational and Psychological Measurement, 68,* 281–303.

Cella, D., Riley, W., Stone, A., Rothrock, N., Reeve, B., Yount, S., et al. (2010). Initial item banks and first wave testing of the Patient-Reported Outcomes Measurement Information System (PROMIS) network: 2005–2008. *Journal of Clinical Epidemiology, 63,* 1179–1194.

Clark, L. A. (1993). *The Schedule for Nonadaptive and Adaptive Personality (SNAP).* Minneapolis: University of Minnesota Press.

Cole, D. A., Martin, N. C., & Steiger, J. H. (2005). Empirical and conceptual problems with longitudinal trait–state models: Introducing a trait–state–occasion model. *Psychological Methods, 10,* 3–20.

Cooke, D. J., Michie, C., Hart, S. D., & Hare, R. D. (1999). Evaluating the screening version of the Hare Psychopathy Checklist—Revised (PCL:SV): An item response theory analysis. *Psychological Assessment, 11,* 3–13.

Costa, P. T., & McCrae, R. R. (1992). *NEO PI-R professional manual: Revised NEO Personality Inventory (NEO PI-R) and NEO Five-Factor Inventory (NEO-FFI).* Odessa, FL: Psychological Assessment Resources.

Cronbach, L. J. (1951). Coefficient alpha and the internal structure of a test. *Psychometrika, 16,* 297–334.

Cronbach, L. J., & Meehl, P. E. (1955). Construct validity in psychological tests. *Psychological Bulletin, 52,* 281–302.

de Ayala, R. J. (2009). *The theory and practice of item response theory.* New York: Guilford Press.

Eid, M. (2000). A multitrait–multimethod model with minimal assumptions. *Psychometrika, 65,* 241–261.

Eid, M., Lischetzke, T., Nussbeck, F. W., & Trierweiler, L. I. (2003). Separating trait effects from trait-specific method effects in multitrait–multimethod models: A multiple-indicator CT-C(M − 1) model. *Psychological Methods, 8,* 38–60.

Embretson, S. E., & Reise, S. P. (2000). *Item response theory for psychologists.* Mahwah, NJ: Erlbaum.

Fresco, D. M., Heimberg, R. G., Mennin, D. S., & Turk, C. L. (2002). Confirmatory factor analysis of the Penn State Worry Questionnaire. *Behaviour Research and Therapy, 40,* 313–323.

Garratt, G., & Ingram, R. E. (2007). Cognitive processes in cognitive therapy: Evaluation of the mechanisms of change in the treatment of depression. *Clinical Psychology: Science and Practice, 14,* 224–239.

Gomez, R., Vance, A., & Gomez, A. (2012). Children's Depression Inventory: Invariance across children and adolescents with and without depressive disorders. *Psychological Assessment, 24,* 1–10.

Grice, J. W. (2001). Computing and evaluating factor scores. *Psychological Methods, 6,* 430–450.

Jacobson, N. S., Dobson, K. S., Truax, P. A., Addis, M. E., Koerner, K., Gollan, J. K., et al. (1996). A component analysis of cognitive-behavioral treatment for depression. *Journal of Consulting and Clinical Psychology, 64,* 295–304.

Kenny, D. A., & Kashy, D. A. (1992). Analysis of the multitrait–multimethod matrix by confirmatory factor analysis. *Psychological Bulletin*, *112*, 165–172.

Kenny, D. A., & Zautra, A. (1995). The trait–state–error model for multiwave data. *Journal of Consulting and Clinical Psychology*, *63*, 52–59.

Kline, R. B. (2010). *Principles and practice of structural equation modeling* (3rd ed.). New York: Guilford Press.

Kollman, D. M., Brown, T. A., & Barlow, D. H. (2009). The construct validity of acceptance: A multitrait–multimethod investigation. *Behavior Therapy*, *40*, 205–218.

Kraemer, H. C., Wilson, T., Fairburn, C. G., & Agras, W. S. (2002). Mediators and moderators of treatment effects in randomized clinical trials. *Archives of General Psychiatry*, *59*, 877– 883.

LaGrange, B., Cole, D. A., Jacquez, F., Ciesla, J., Dallaire, D., Pineda, A., et al. (2011). Disentangling the prospective relations between maladaptive cognitions and depressive symptoms. *Journal of Abnormal Psychology*, *120*, 511–527.

Langer, D. A., Wood, J. J., Bergman, R. L., & Piacentini, J. C. (2010). A multitrait–multimethod analysis of the construct validity of child anxiety disorders in a clinical sample. *Child Psychiatry and Human Development*, *41*, 549–561.

Lord, F. M., & Novick, M. (1968). *Statistical theories of mental test scores*. Reading, MA: Addison-Wesley.

Marsh, H. W., & Bailey, M. (1991). Confirmatory factor analyses of multitrait–multimethod data: A comparison of alternative models. *Applied Psychological Measurement*, *15*, 47–70.

Marsh, H. W., & Grayson, D. (1995). Latent variable models of multitrait–multimethod data. In R. H. Hoyle (Ed.), *Structural equation modeling: Concepts, issues, and applications* (pp. 177–198). Thousand Oaks, CA: Sage.

Marsh, H. W., Lüdtke, O., Muthén, B., Asparouhov, T., Morin, A. J. S., Trautwein, U., et al. (2010). A new look at the Big Five factor structure through exploratory structural equation modeling. *Psychological Assessment*, *22*, 471–491.

Marsh, H. W., Muthén, B., Asparouhov, A., Lüdtke, O., Robitzsch, A., Morin, A. J. S., et al. (2009). Exploratory structural equation modeling, integrating CFA and EFA: Application to students' evaluations of university teaching. *Structural Equation Modeling*, *16*, 439–476.

McArdle, J. J. (2009). Latent variable modeling of differences and changes with longitudinal data. *Annual Review of Psychology*, *60*, 577–605.

Muthén, B., & Asparouhov, T. (2012). Bayesian SEM: A more flexible representation of substantive theory. *Psychological Methods*, *17*, 313–335.

Muthén, L. K., & Muthén, B. O. (1998–2012). *Mplus user's guide*. Los Angeles: Authors.

Prenoveau, J. M., Craske, M. G., Zinbarg, R. E., Mineka, S., Rose, R. D., & Griffith, J. W. (2011). Are anxiety and depression just as stable as personality during late adolescence?: Results from a three-year longitudinal latent variable study. *Journal of Abnormal Psychology*, *120*, 832–843.

Raykov, T. (2001a). Estimation of congeneric scale reliability using covariance structure analysis with nonlinear constraints. *British Journal of Mathematical and Statistical Psychology, 54,* 315–323.

Raykov, T. (2001b). Bias of Cronbach's alpha for fixed congeneric measures with correlated errors. *Applied Psychological Measurement, 25,* 69–76.

Raykov, T. (2004). Behavioral scale reliability and measurement invariance evaluation using latent variable modeling. *Behavior Therapy, 35,* 299–331.

Rosellini, A. J., & Brown, T. A. (2011). The NEO Five-Factor Inventory: Latent structure and relationships with dimensions of anxiety and depressive disorders in a large clinical sample. *Assessment, 18,* 27–38.

Salkovskis, P. M. (1985). Obsessional–compulsive problems: A cognitive-behavioral analysis. *Behaviour Research and Therapy, 23,* 571–583.

Simms, L. J., & Clark, L A. (2005). Validation of a computerized adaptive version of the Schedule for Nonadaptive and Adaptive Personality (SNAP). *Psychological Assessment, 17,* 28–43.

Simms, L. J., Gros, D. F., & Watson, D. (2008). Parsing the general and specific components of depression and anxiety with bifactor modeling. *Depression and Anxiety, 25,* E34–E46.

South, S. C., Krueger, R. F., & Iacono, W. G. (2009). Factorial invariance of the Dyadic Adjustment Scale across gender. *Psychological Assessment, 21,* 622–628.

Steyer, R., & Schmitt, T. (1994). The theory of confounding and its application in causal modeling with latent variables. In A. von Eye & C. C. Clogg (Eds.), *Latent variables analysis: Applications for developmental research* (pp. 36–67). Thousand Oaks, CA: Sage.

Strauss, M. E., & Smith, G. T. (2009). Construct validity: Advances in theory and methodology. *Annual Review of Clinical Psychology, 5,* 1–25.

Takane, Y., & de Leeuw, J. (1987). On the relationship between item response theory and factor analysis of discretized variables. *Psychometrika, 52,* 393–408.

Thomas, M. L. (2011). The value of item response theory in clinical assessment: A review. *Assessment, 18,* 291–307.

Walter, O. B., Becker, J., Bjorner, J. B., Fliege, H., Klapp, B. F., & Rose, M. (2007). Development and evaluation of a computer adaptive test for anxiety (Anxiety-CAT). *Quality of Life Research, 16,* 143–155.

Woody, S. R., Whittal, M. L., & McLean, P. D. (2011). Mechanisms of symptom reduction in treatment for obsessions. *Journal of Consulting and Clinical Psychology, 79,* 653–664.

Zvolensky, M. J., Strong, D., Bernstein, A., Vujanovic, A. A., & Marshall E. C. (2009). Evaluation of anxiety sensitivity among daily adult smokers using item response theory analysis. *Journal of Anxiety Disorders, 23,* 230–239.

13

Implicit Measures of Associations

A Case of Exaggerated Promises?

Anne Roefs, Jorg Huijding, Fren T. Y. Smulders,
Anita T. M. Jansen, and Colin M. MacLeod

Researchers in psychology have long sought ways to more fully understand human cognition and behavior that do not rely on self-report.
Investigators in the domain of psychopathology are no exception. Three
reasons are most often cited, harking back to the early critiques of introspection (see Boring, 1953): (1) Self-reports rely on introspection, yet we
know that people do not have introspective access to all of the mechanisms that underlie their behavior (Nisbett & Wilson, 1977); (2) self-
report measures are subject to socially desirable biases; and (3) people
may dismiss as irrelevant certain cognitions that actually are relevant
(Schwarz, 1999; Schwarz & Oyserman, 2001).

MacLeod (1993) even argued that accepting introspective self-
report measures as data would place psychopathology research "outside the boundaries of legitimate science" (p. 179). He convincingly
reasoned that the cognitive revolution in clinical psychology took quite
a different form than the cognitive revolution in experimental psychology did. In experimental psychology, cognition was allowed in the form
of hypothetical constructs in theories, but self-reported cognitions were
not accepted as data. The evaluation of theories relied only on directly
observable measures—that is, overt behaviors (e.g., response latencies).
In clinical psychology, cognitions were allowed in theory as well as
in data. So self-reports of cognition were accepted as data for testing

cognitive models of psychopathology. In a sense, this meant a return to the era before behaviorism. However, McNally (2001) has rightfully pointed out that it is neither possible nor right to dismiss introspection altogether, while also noting that introspection is not entirely absent in cognitive experimental psychology either, even when conducted in a neuroscience framework. Certain phenomena have no behavioral manifestation, are only accessible by introspection, and can only be reflected in verbal report (e.g., obsessions). He argues that researchers should be attentive to when introspection is useful and when it is not.

In psychopathology, research has focused for several decades on aspects of cognition such as biases in attention (e.g., Williams, Mathews, & MacLeod, 1996) and memory (e.g., Mitte, 2008), the goal being to better understand the dysfunctional cognitive architecture of patients. In the past couple of decades specifically, a different class of measurement procedures has gained popularity in psychopathology research. The most visible examples include the Implicit Association Test (IAT; Greenwald, McGhee, & Schwartz, 1998) and the affective priming paradigm (APP; Fazio, Sanbonmatsu, Powell, & Kardes, 1986). These measurement procedures have been designed to obtain implicit measures of psychological attributes (for a review, see Roefs et al., 2011). The goal has been to develop measures untainted by the flaws of introspection and self-report.

What makes a measure implicit? De Houwer, Teige-Mocigemba, Spruyt, and Moors (2009) have defined an "implicit" measure as "a measurement *outcome* that is causally produced by the to-be-measured attribute in the absence of certain goals, awareness, substantial cognitive resources, or substantial time" (p. 350; emphasis in original). It is, however, important to keep in mind that implicitness is not an all-or-none feature of a measure (Moors & De Houwer, 2006). For example, a measure can be labeled as implicit in the sense that people are unaware of the existence of their association, or of its origin, or cannot control the process that leads to the measurement outcome. It is likely that not all implicit measures possess the same features of implicitness, and the degree to which a measure is implicit is to a large extent an empirical question. De Houwer and colleagues (De Houwer, 2006, 2009; De Houwer et al., 2009) provide extensive reviews of the degree to which various implicit measures meet the criteria for implicitness.

MEASUREMENT PROCEDURES

Quite a variety of measurement procedures have been used in the realm of psychopathology to obtain implicit measures of associations, with the

IAT (including variants on this procedure; Greenwald et al., 1998) and to a lesser extent the APP (Fazio et al., 1986) being the main ones (see Roefs et al., 2011). These paradigms are considered *indirect* measurement procedures. That is, participants are not asked to report directly on their thoughts or attitudes; instead, these are inferred from a pattern of response latencies. The *measurement outcomes* of these paradigms are considered *implicit measures* of associations. It is informative to try one of these procedures: IATs for a large number of topics can be found online (*https://implicit.harvard.edu/implicit*). Having taken the time to perform an IAT, it is then reasonable to consider these questions: (1) "Were you aware of what was being assessed?", (2) "Were you aware that you held the associations that the test identified?", and (3) "Do you agree that these associations reflect your attitude?" After taking a test once and reviewing your results, it would also be informative to try to "fake" the results by trying to appear different on the task the second time than you did the first time.

In this type of paradigm, participants are usually presented with single stimuli representing disorder-relevant targets (e.g., "spider") and attributes (e.g., "afraid"), and are instructed to respond as quickly as possible to these stimuli. As is common in cognitive measures, response latency and accuracy are the main dependent variables. The general idea behind these paradigms is that a certain pattern of response latencies and error percentages can serve as an index of the strength of target–attribute associations. Because they are the two most frequently used paradigms, the APP and the IAT are now explained in some detail.

In the APP (Fazio et al., 1986), two stimuli are presented in quick succession: a "prime" followed by a "target" (a stimulus onset asynchrony of 150 ms is typical). Prime stimuli represent the concepts of interest (e.g., spiders vs. butterflies), and target stimuli represent the attributes (e.g., positive vs. negative). A participant can ignore the prime, but must respond to the target as quickly as possible either by evaluating it as positive or negative or by naming it. The purpose of this paradigm is to assess the extent to which the prime presentation influences the response to the target. The critical idea is that affectively congruent prime–target pairs (e.g., "spider–awful") should lead to shorter response latencies than should affectively incongruent prime–target pairs (e.g., "spider–happy"). Mismatches should slow down responses. To the degree that such a pattern of response latencies is observed, it is taken to reflect the person's evaluation of the prime (e.g., spiders).

In the IAT (Greenwald et al., 1998), the participant is instructed to categorize each presented stimulus as quickly and as accurately as possible according to a target dimension (e.g., high-fat vs. low-fat foods) or an attribute dimension (e.g., positive vs. negative). In the two critical combination phases of the IAT, the participant performs a double-categorization task; that is, he or she is instructed to make a binary decision for stimuli from two dimensions, with the dimension that is to be used to categorize the stimulus alternating on each trial. The two combination phases differ in the types of attribute and target stimuli that are mapped onto one response. So, for example, in a first combination phase, the participant presses the left button for high-fat foods and positive words, and the right button for low-fat foods and negative words. In a second combination phase, the response assignment for the target dimension is reversed (e.g., press the left button for low-fat foods and positive words; press the right button for high-fat foods and negative words). The IAT effect is typically computed as the difference in average response latency (and/or percentage of errors) between these two combination phases (see Greenwald, Nosek, & Banaji, 2003, for an alternative scoring algorithm, the D-measure). The logic behind the IAT is that people perform better when two associated targets/attributes share a response key than when two unassociated targets/attributes share a response key. So, in the current example, if participants are better at responding with the combination "high-fat and positive" versus "low-fat and negative" than when the combination is reversed, the conclusion will be that participants have a more positive association with high-fat foods than with low-fat foods.

COGNITIVE THEORY

In psychopathology research, an implicit measure is often assumed to reflect the strength of association between a disorder-relevant target (e.g., the self in depression) and an attribute (e.g., negative). Thus, for example, when depressed an individual would see him- or herself in a more negative light. These targets and attributes are usually derived from the proposed dysfunctional beliefs held by those with the disorder. These dysfunctional beliefs are, on the one hand, often apparent from the characterization of the disorder as specified in the fifth edition of the *Diagnostic and Statistical Manual of Mental Disorders* (DSM-5; American Psychiatric Association, 2013); on the other hand, they are specified in the principal cognitive theories, often based on Beck's cognitive approach to psychopathology (e.g., Beck & D. A. Clark, 1997; Beck, Freeman, & Davis, 2004; Beck, Rush, Shaw, & Emery, 1979).

For some disorders, not surprisingly, multiple competing cognitive models exist, and these are often more specific than Beck's schema model. Examples include D. M. Clark and Wells's (1995) model of social phobia; the impaired-cognitive-control account of depression (Joormann, Yoon,

& Zetsche, 2007); Ingram's (1984) information-processing analysis of depression; and the framework of Williams, Watts, MacLeod, and Matthews (1997) for depression. Similarly, Segal (1988) argues that for proving the existence and crucial role of negative self-schemas in depression, it is important to move beyond a heuristic use of the term "schemas" and a reliance of self-reports to test them. The conceptualization and testing of schemas should fit with current theorizing and methodologies of cognitive science.

In fact, however, much of the cognitive psychological research into the bases of psychopathology does not test more specific models and is (implicitly) based on Beck's schema model, which does not really address issues relating to the exact structure and function of schemas (Segal, 1988). In essence, the schema model proposes that a patient has a dysfunctional schema—that is, a cognitive assembly of associated knowledge that guides information processing in both automatic and controlled ways (see, e.g., Bartlett, 1932; Rumelhart, 1980). Therefore, information processing is thought to be biased, as reflected in measurable attention, memory, and interpretation biases in patient populations that differ from those of the general population. Implicit measures of associations were designed—and are believed—to have the capacity to reveal aspects of these dysfunctional schemas that explicit measures cannot reveal.

IMPLICIT MEASURES OF ASSOCIATION IN PSYCHOPATHOLOGY RESEARCH

We recently reviewed studies that obtained implicit measures of associations in various forms of psychopathology (Roefs et al., 2011). In the following paragraphs, then, rather than repeat this extensive summary, we limit ourselves to the general conclusions and most striking results from this review. The first thing to realize is that a large number of studies using implicit measures have provided evidence converging with that obtained with explicit measures. That is, in this set of studies, both types of measures have pointed in the same direction. For example, in patients suffering from spider phobia, implicit measures have generally indicated negative associations with spiders (e.g., Huijding & de Jong, 2007). In another set of studies, quite consistent evidence has been marshaled for implicit measures' going in the opposite direction of explicit measures. For example, in people suffering from depressive disorder, implicit measures quite consistently have reflected positive associations with the self (e.g., De Raedt, Schacht, Franck, & De Houwer, 2006); this is not consistent with the clinical picture and cognitive theory (e.g., D. A. Clark,

Beck, & Alford, 1999), where negative self-esteem is typically postulated. In a third set, implicit measures of associations with craved substances (food, alcohol, nicotine, and drugs) have reflected both the positive (e.g., "High-fat foods taste good") and the negative (e.g., "Alcohol can give you a hangover") aspects of these substances (e.g., Houben & Wiers, 2006; Roefs & Jansen, 2002). The picture is a complex one.

Consider the case of alcohol. Although both positive and negative associations with alcohol have been observed, multiple-regression analyses showed that only the positive associations proved to be predictive of drinking behavior (e.g., Houben & Wiers, 2008). In other disorders, implicit measures have shown incremental predictive validity, explaining a range of behavioral measures beyond those explained by explicit measures. This was the case, for example, with performance on a spider behavioral avoidance test (e.g., Teachman & Woody, 2003), panic symptoms (e.g., Teachman, Smith-Janik, & Saporito, 2007), mirror avoidance (Clerkin & Teachman, 2009), and food choice (e.g., Perugini, 2005). Thus, to take one example in a little more detail, an IAT measure of spider associations predicted variance of performance on a spider behavioral avoidance test, beyond what was explained by self-reported spider fear (e.g., Teachman & Woody, 2003).

In addition, in keeping with dual-process models of information processing (e.g., Fazio & Towles-Schwen, 1999), which typically posit two types of cognitive processes (automatic vs. controlled), some evidence has been found for the idea that implicit measures are specifically predictive of *spontaneous* types of behavior. The argument is that when more elaborative processing is possible, then behavior will be more in line with explicit measures. People then have the possibility to consciously consider both their cognitions and their behavior. Examples include the startle response in the context of specific phobia (Huijding & de Jong, 2006) and immediate affective reactions in the context of depression (Haeffel et al., 2007). Also in keeping with dual-process models are the findings that implicit measures have been shown to be predictive of behavior only when cognitive resources were limited either by an experimental manipulation (such as a depletion manipulation; e.g., Hofmann, Rauch, & Gawronski, 2007) or by an individual differences factor (e.g., Hofmann, Friese, & Roefs, 2009). This evidence for incremental predictive power demonstrates the added value that implicit measures can provide.

Though the experimental approach—that is, *manipulating* the theorized determinants of implicit measures—may be especially revealing, relatively few studies have taken this approach. Those that have done so generally have found the expected effect of the manipulation on the implicit measure(s). For example, a negative mood induction led to reduced self–positive associations in formerly depressed participants (e.g., Gemar, Segal, Sagrati, & Kennedy, 2001), and inductions of craving and hunger positively affected associations with food in both healthy and eating-disordered participants (e.g., Seibt, Häfner, & Deutsch, 2007). On the one hand, this is evidence for the construct validity of the implicit measure; on the other hand, it is potentially problematic for the assessment of presumably stable dysfunctional schemas that these measures are so readily influenced by "acute" experimental manipulations.

Finally, a few studies have addressed the effect of treatment on disorder-relevant implicit measures, an area that surely warrants more attention. For specific phobia, social phobia, pain disorder, and panic disorder, successful exposure therapy or cognitive-behavioral therapy (CBT) was associated with significant improvements on implicit measures of disorder-relevant associations (e.g., Grumm, Erbe, von Collani, & Nestler, 2008; Teachman & Woody, 2003). For obesity and alcohol dependence, no or very small effects of treatment on implicit measures were observed (Craeynest, Crombez, Deforche, Tanghe, & De Bourdeaudhuij, 2008; Thush et al., 2009; Wiers, van de Luitgaarden, van den Wildenberg, & Smulders, 2005). Interestingly, for panic disorder, cognitive changes preceded symptom reduction (Teachman, Marker, & Smith-Janik, 2008)—suggesting, but not proving with certainty, that the cognitive changes may actually be the cause of the clinical improvement. The results of this latter study notwithstanding, an important question that remains for further research is whether observed changes in implicit measures after treatment are causally related to genuine symptom improvement or merely constitute an epiphenomenon, in that implicit measures may just fluctuate along with the experienced clinical symptoms. Another important question is whether certain implicit measures can predict symptom onset.

INFERENTIAL CONFUSION: THE DUBIOUS CONSTRUCT VALIDITY OF IMPLICIT MEASURES

The popularity of paradigms to obtain implicit measures, and in particular of the IAT, no doubt derives in large part from the discipline-wide usage of cognitive science methods and focus on indirect measurement procedures for cognition, as in the domains of implicit learning (see Stadler & Frensch, 1998) and implicit memory (see Roediger & Geraci, 2005). But it also rests in part on the promises that are made about what these paradigms can reveal. For example, the website of Project Implicit (*http://projectimplicit.net/index.html*) states that "Project Implicit investigates thoughts and feelings outside of conscious awareness and control," and the website of Project Implicit Mental Health (*https:// implicit.harvard.edu/implicit/user/pimh/background.html*) states that "implicit measures assess implicit attitudes, identities and beliefs that people are either unwilling or unable to report." These claims go beyond the definition provided by De Houwer et al. (2009), who have reserved and defined the term "implicit" for the measurement outcome, not for a mental construct (e.g., attitude or belief), and who state that "the implicitness of a measure says little about how the underlying attribute is represented. For instance, it is difficult to determine whether different attributes underlie implicit and explicit measures or whether both measures reflect the same attributes under different conditions" (p. 351). This more narrow definition by De Houwer and colleagues is much more warranted, given the current state of empirical evidence

These statements that appear on the websites about implicit measures are also reflected in research applying the IAT. For example, Asendorpf, Banse, and Mücke (2002, p. 392) concluded, "Just as free associations in psychoanalytic settings provide a window to the unconscious, implicit association tests provide another, probably more reliable window." Often the measurement outcome of an IAT or APP has been equated with a mental construct, such as an implicit attitude or belief. Examples include "implicit attractiveness beliefs" (e.g., Buhlmann, Teachman, & Kathmann, 2011) and "implicit self-esteem" (e.g., Franck, De Raedt, Dereu, & Van den Abbeele, 2007). Even our own early work made references to attitudes—that is, "implicit attitudes towards high-fat foods" (Roefs & Jansen, 2002). When the measurement outcome of a certain paradigm is equated with a mental construct, every time evidence is obtained with a certain paradigm (e.g., an IAT effect), this is interpreted as evidence for the existence of the mental construct (e.g., an implicit attitude) (De Houwer, 2011). Although such claims are provocative, they are not backed by empirical evidence regarding the implicitness of these measures, let alone regarding the existence of a separate implicit construct (e.g., an "implicit attitude"). Despite implicit measures' not presupposing introspection, this does not imply that the constructs reflected by implicit measures are indeed unconscious/unavailable for introspection. In other words, though the participant is not asked to engage in introspection when performing an IAT-like measure, this does not mean that the construct the IAT measurement outcome is taken to reflect is not *available* for introspection (Gawronski, LeBel, & Peters, 2007).

VALIDITY ISSUES

The IAT and APP derived initial validity from studies showing that these paradigms can reflect affective associations with stimuli that most people normatively evaluate negatively or positively (e.g., Fazio, 2001; Greenwald et al., 1998). Also, providing stronger support for their validity, both the APP and IAT reflected associations that were newly created in a classical conditioning procedure while participants showed no contingency awareness (Olson & Fazio, 2001, 2002). However, there are also validity problems with these measures. In the worst case, three "interpretation leaps" are made: (1) that measurement outcomes reflect associations; (2) that associations reflect mental constructs such as attitudes, stereotypes, or beliefs; and (3) that these mental constructs are implicit/unconscious. Doubts surround each of these assumptions.

Measurement Outcomes Reflect Associations

Although there is certainly evidence that the IAT and APP can reflect associations, no measure is process-pure (see the arguments of Jacoby, 1991). In the case of the IAT, other sources of effects have been identified (Fiedler, Messner, & Bluemke, 2006), such as salience asymmetries in the target and attribute dimensions (Rothermund & Wentura, 2004), extrapersonal knowledge (Olson & Fazio, 2004), and cognitive abilities (McFarland & Crouch, 2002; Mierke & Klauer, 2003). We briefly consider each of these.

Salience asymmetries arise because unfamiliar and negative information is typically more salient than is familiar and positive information (see Rothermund & Wentura, 2004, for a review of the evidence). In a series of experiments, Rothermund and Wentura (2004) found that participants were faster to respond when the two salient (e.g., old–nonword) and the two nonsalient (e.g., young–word) categories shared a response key than when the salient and nonsalient categories were mixed. Moreover, valence-free variants of the IAT—that is, IAT variants with attribute categories that have no valence (e.g., word–nonword)—correlated with explicit measures of attitudes. This was of course not an expected result, considering that valence-free IAT variants are not informative regarding attitudes at all. Considering that valence associations and salience asymmetries are typically confounded in applications of the IAT, caution is needed in interpreting these results.

Olson and Fazio (2004) proposed another source of IAT effects: "extrapersonal associations." These are associations that are available in memory but are not relevant to someone's personal evaluation of a certain attitude object. For example, a person who is allergic to chocolate may know that people generally are very fond of chocolate. This knowledge may affect the person's performance on an IAT assessing associations with chocolate. Relevant to this point is the surprising finding that African American participants do not show an in-group bias on the IAT (Nosek, Banaji, & Greenwald, 2002), which may be best explained by their knowledge of the often negative portrayal of African Americans in the mass media. Although Olson and Fazio (2004) agree that an individual necessarily is part of a culture, and that it is difficult to see how an individual would not be influenced by society (see Banaji, 2001), their main argument is that one's personal attitude can deviate from the cultural norm or the attitude of other people. Knowledge about the cultural norm and other people's attitudes can influence IAT performance. Note, however, that Nosek and Hansen (2008) have argued against culture as a contaminating influence on the IAT, and consider the attempt to separate cultural from personal influences on the IAT to be futile (for an elaborate discussion of this issue, see Olson, Fazio, & Han, 2009).

A third identified source of IAT effects is cognitive skill. Supporting the influence of cognitive skill on the IAT effect, one study found that IATs aimed at assessing prejudice and self-esteem correlated with control IATs with nonsocial and irrelevant dimensions (McFarland & Crouch, 2002). Moreover, an IAT that relied on similarities in the superficial stimulus characteristics of stimulus size and color correlated not only with a second administration of this IAT, but also with an IAT assessing flower–insect preferences (Mierke & Klauer, 2003)—a conceptual dimension. This is suggestive of an underlying cognitive skill. In later research, it appeared that the influence of the cognitive skill confound almost disappeared when the alternative scoring algorithm (D-measure) proposed by Greenwald and colleagues (2003) was used (Cai, Siriam, Greenwald, & McFarland, 2004). However, most recent evidence suggests that the D-measure does not protect completely against the cognitive skill confound, as cognitive control still correlated with IAT performance (Klauer, Schmitz, Teige-Mocigemba, & Voss, 2010), even when the role of attitude was factored out (Siegel, Dougherty, & Huber, 2012). In addition, by experimentally manipulating cognitive control (e.g., by manipulating awareness of the IAT's goal), it was shown that cognitive control is not merely a correlate of IAT effects, but plays a causal role in it (Siegel et al., 2012). This remaining effect of cognitive skill on the IAT effect may be due to qualitative differences among participants in the type of strategy that is employed to "solve" the sorting task, which cannot be corrected for by a scoring algorithm (Fiedler et al., 2006).

One way to explain most of the alternative sources of IAT effects discussed in the preceding paragraphs is to use the similarity account (De Houwer, Geldof, & De Bruycker, 2005). The central idea of this account is that IAT effects are not restricted to reflect associations in semantic memory (as the IAT was devised to test), but that participants can take advantage of any type of similarity in the stimulus dimensions to perform the task as quickly as possible, including similarities in salience and perceptual characteristics. If associations are broadly defined (see Greenwald, Nosek, Banaji, & Klauer, 2005)—that is, not restricted to associations in a *semantic* network—then the similarity account is not incompatible with the idea that the IAT measures associations. This broadening does, however, quite radically change the conceptualization of the IAT.

Importantly, as Rothermund and Wentura (2004) pointed out, as soon as participants develop a conscious strategy regarding how best to perform the IAT (i.e., how to take advantage of the observed similarity of presented stimuli), the IAT measurement outcome cannot be considered implicit (see also Fiedler et al., 2006). So if participants can easily recode the task by using only one dimension (e.g., pleasant vs. unpleasant) instead of two (e.g., pleasant vs. unpleasant, peaceful vs. violent) to categorize the stimuli in the compatible phase, and can then apply this strategy consciously, it is certainly reasonable to question whether the measurement outcome is implicit in the sense of reflecting spontaneous associations. It is worth noting in this regard that Greenwald et al. (2005) do not take a position regarding the involvement of controlled processes in the strategy use of participants in a typical IAT. Interesting in this respect is the finding in one study that APP effects relied on so-called "embodied" processes (i.e., activation of the corrugator and zygomatic facial muscles; Foroni & Semin, 2012), whereas IAT effects did not. To the extent that the activation of these facial muscles can be interpreted as automatic affective responses, this pattern is also suggestive of more strategic involvement in the IAT.

Associations Reflect Mental Constructs Such as Attitudes and Beliefs

It is often assumed that implicit measures can be considered the implicit equivalents of explicit dysfunctional beliefs (comparable to attitudes in social psychology); for example, implicit measures of "spider–negative" associations presumably reflect spider-related dysfunctional beliefs (e.g., Huijding & de Jong, 2005). However, can dysfunctional beliefs really be reduced to these simpler associations captured by implicit measures? It may turn out that certain constructs, such as self-esteem, cannot be reduced to simple associations with the self (Buhrmester, Blanton, & Swann, 2011). An illustration would be implicit measures of self-esteem, which are often obtained in research on depressive disorders on the assumption that they reflect dysfunctional depressive beliefs (e.g., De Raedt et al., 2006; Gemar et al., 2001). The assessment of simpler associations is of course not necessarily problematic or of less relevance, but considering them to be the implicit equivalent of explicit dysfunctional beliefs is likely to be problematic.

Another issue concerns the stability of the dysfunctional schemas on the one hand and the stability of the implicit measures on the other hand. Cognitive models in psychopathology typically assume that dysfunctional schemas are deep-rooted and relatively stable (e.g., Beck & D. A. Clark, 1997; Beck et al., 1979, 2004). Valid measures of these schemas should therefore possess a fair amount of stability over time and situations. However, there is a wealth of evidence indicating the opposite—that implicit measures are highly malleable by the momentary context and short-term manipulations (e.g., Karpinski & Hilton, 2001; Roefs et al., 2006; for reviews, see Blair, 2002; Gawronski et al., 2007). For example, an APP measure of valence associations with food was more sensitive to a short-term manipulation emphasizing health versus taste than to weight status (obese vs. healthy weight) of the participants (Roefs et al., 2006). Often self-report measures prove to be less influenced by these experimental manipulations than implicit measures are (for a review, see Gawronski et al., 2007).

The fact that implicit measures are highly specific—that is, very much influenced by short-term circumstances—may partly account for another frequently mentioned problem, their frequent low test–retest reliability (e.g., Fazio & Olson, 2003; LeBel & Paunonen, 2011), posing problems for their validity and replicability. Test–retest reliability for the IAT is moderately good (median r = .56; De Houwer et al., 2009; Nosek, Greenwald, & Banaji, 2007), but the APP findings are less consistent. Some studies on the APP have reported low test–retest reliability (.08–.28; Bosson, Swann, & Pennebaker, 2000), whereas another study, which corrected for measurement error, showed substantially higher test–retest reliability (stability estimate = .68; Cunningham, Preacher, & Banaji, 2001).

Similar problems have been reported regarding internal consistency, which is moderately good for the IAT (r/alpha = .7–.9), but low for the APP (e.g., Bosson et al., 2000: alpha =–.16–.49; Olson & Fazio, 2003: r = .04), except when a correction for measurement error is included (alpha = .64; Cunningham et al., 2001). The lower-than-ideal reliability estimates also contribute to the problem of low convergent validity over implicit measures (e.g., Bosson et al., 2000; Cunningham et al., 2001), which is notably improved when a latent variable approach is used (Cunningham et al., 2001).

The reliability of implicit measures has been the subject of concern in other research domains (e.g., memory) as well. Indeed, Buchner and Wippich (2000) suggest that the frequently reported dissociation of implicit and explicit memory tests, wherein an effect evident on an explicit test is not seen on an implicit test, is very often due to the unreliability of the implicit test. This unreliability concern leads to the recommendation that because individual response latencies fluctuate over trials (due, for example, to fatigue, practice, and sequence effects), researchers should strive to include as many trials per condition as feasible for response latency measures. In fact, the improved reliability of the IAT over the APP may be caused by strategic influences on the IAT, as well as associations with categories of stimuli instead of with individual stimuli (Olson & Fazio, 2003). Both of these influences would likely lead to less variability over trials. Naturally, the same reasoning could be applied to self-report instruments, where higher reliability may be inflated because participants often have a tendency to be consistent.

Mental Constructs Are Implicit

As discussed previously, De Houwer et al. (2009) restrict the definition of "implicit" to the measurement outcomes and do not extend it to the mental constructs that are supposedly reflected by these outcomes. In general, it appears doubtful whether implicit measures reflect representations to which participants do not have introspective access (Gawronski et al., 2007). Indeed, even when one limits the discussion to the implicitness of the measurement outcomes, there remains much room for discussion. De Houwer and colleagues (De Houwer, 2006, 2009; De Houwer et al., 2009) provide extensive reviews of the degree to which various implicit measures meet the criteria for implicitness, to which the interested reader is referred. It is important to keep in mind is that participants are not necessarily unaware of what is being assessed (e.g., Monteith, Voils, & Ashburn-Nardo, 2001) and are not necessarily unable to control responses (Gawronski et al., 2007), especially when they have experience with, for example, the IAT (e.g., Fiedler & Bluemke, 2005). This effect of IAT experience on controllability poses obvious problems for designs with repeated testing, especially when combined with the observation that the IAT effect generally decreases with repeated administration (e.g., Huijding & de Jong, 2007; Robusto, Cristante, & Vianello, 2008).

PROS AND CONS OF A PARADIGM APPROACH TO RESEARCH

In a paradigm approach, much research is focused on the specifics of a certain paradigm. Currently we seem to have the situation that a behavioral effect (i.e., a difference in response latencies) obtained with a certain indirect measurement procedure (e.g., the IAT or APP) is equated with a mental process or construct (e.g., an unconscious attitude or dysfunctional belief). Although IAT and APP effects are often interpreted as reflecting attitudes to which participants lack introspective access, the empirical evidence reviewed thus far raises doubts about this assertion. The obvious risk, then, is that, in attempting to validate theoretical models by findings from a specific paradigm, a researcher may not have the right experimental proxy for the mental construct of interest. Put another way, other mental processes/constructs may well also be able to account for the obtained effects (De Houwer, 2011). Yet it is true that this paradigm-oriented research approach dominates most of experimental psychology (Meiser, 2011). Although Meiser admits that it is a typical characteristic of "normal science," he points to the danger of limiting research to the specific features of a certain paradigm without sufficient attention to converging evidence from other paradigms or unifying models that integrate findings from different paradigms.

On the positive side, experimental paradigms have the important function of broadening the range of phenomena that can be measured, and consequently can and do lead to new theories (Greenwald, 2012; Meiser, 2011). A highly illustrative example, provided by Meiser, concerns the four-card Wason selection task (Wason, 1966). Although the Wason task was originally designed to study deductive reasoning, it became evident that the task actually does not assess deductive reasoning. Nevertheless, research with the task continued and inspired new theoretical and empirical approaches. Just one example concerns the effects of content on human reasoning (Cheng & Holyoak, 1985). Individuals use pragmatic reasoning schemas to solve the card selection task. That is, people can solve the task better when it relates to rules in realistic situations with which they have experience.

When we apply this realization to the topic of this chapter, we conclude that although implicit measures may not reflect dysfunctional beliefs or attitudes to which people lack introspective access, this does not mean that research with the IAT and APP is meaningless. As became evident from the review of findings in the field of psychopathology research (see also Roefs et al., 2011), implicit measures have shown incremental predictive validity, and outcomes with these paradigms have sometimes yielded findings that were the opposite of those obtained with explicit measures (e.g., self-esteem questionnaires vs. implicit measures of associations with the self). So these paradigms reflect something potentially interesting and worthy of further study. Put simply, such dissociations are provocative and lead us to new interpretations and to new research approaches.

WHERE TO NEXT?

To avoid the problems created by treating implicit measures as the implicit equivalents of explicit attitudes and beliefs, researchers should in their interpretation of results remain true to what has actually been assessed by the experimental task. In a sense, it is quite surprising that researchers did not initially do that, considering that they have done so more often in research that adapted paradigms from cognitive psychology directed at other cognitive processes and constructs, such as attention (e.g., Field, Munafo, & Franken, 2006) and memory (e.g., Mitte, 2008). In research on attention bias, for instance, effects in paradigms such as the dot-probe task (e.g., Bradley, Mogg, & Lee, 1997) have been interpreted in terms of attention processes, and not directly extended to attitudes or beliefs. Thus the interpretation is closer to the phenomena that are assessed by the paradigm, involving less inference to mental constructs.

Rather than making leaps from measurement outcomes, via associations, to implicit dysfunctional beliefs or attitudes, it would seem better to restrict interpretations of APP and IAT results to a tendency to associate certain concepts more strongly than others, which might be termed "association bias." It remains for further research to ascertain which paradigm is best suited to capturing such an association bias. It may be that the APP comes closer to assessing spontaneous associations than the IAT, as the IAT is an inherently more complex task that elicits strategy use in at least some participants. So, from a cognitive perspective, on the one hand researchers should focus on the paradigm that is best capable of assessing the theoretical construct of interest, and on the other hand they should strive for convergence of results across various paradigms. It should be noted that convergence may be expected only when paradigms are structurally similar, not just similar in the goal of obtaining implicit measures. When we consider De Houwer's (2003) structural analysis of the APP and the IAT (among other paradigms), it is no longer surprising that the results obtained in these paradigms do not necessarily correlate highly.

To be able to design the best paradigm to study dysfunctions in cognitions, cognitive models should be formulated in specific terms. As we have noted at the outset, much of the research with implicit measures has relied on Beck's schema model (e.g., Beck & D. A. Clark, 1997; Beck et al., 1979, 2004). As Van den Hout (1999) has argued, the heuristic value of the belief concept is undeniable, and it is undoubtedly true that dysfunctional beliefs play an important role in psychopathology. Manipulations of these beliefs lead to changes in psychopathology. To gain a more profound understanding of specific cognitive dysfunctions in psychopathology, though, it certainly will be beneficial to specify cognitive models of psychopathology in greater detail, beyond just proposing a dysfunctional schema. As Segal (1988) has argued, it will be important to learn from theoretical progress regarding knowledge representations in cognitive science, and to incorporate this learning in the conceptualization of dysfunctional schemas. While it is true that such models do already exist for certain disorders, as noted earlier in this chapter, they have not formed the basis for research with implicit measures. When an explanation is more specific about the precise mental process that is disturbed, more focused paradigms can be developed that also permit more effective use of converging measures. Although this issue is certainly not unique to the domain of psychopathology, it is also certainly very relevant in this domain. Good paradigms tend to develop, and to produce reliable data, when they are based on well-specified theories (Strauss & Smith, 2009).

One way to design more specific theoretical models is to combine the cognitive approach with a functional approach, as recently argued by De Houwer (2011):

> A functional approach to psychology is the practice of defining behavioral effects exclusively in terms of elements in the environment [p. 204]. . . . The functional approach is concerned mainly with the question of when certain elements in the environment influence behavior. The cognitive approach addresses the question of how those elements in the environment influence behavior. It does so by describing the mental processes/representations that are assumed to mediate the effect of the environment on behavior [p. 205]. . . . The more we know about when a behavioral effect occurs, the more precise we can be about the mental constructs that mediate this effect [p. 205]. . . . Vice versa, mental explanations can generate new hypotheses about the conditions under which behavioral effects occur [pp. 205–206].

For example, if it is consistently found (in different paradigms) that participants with depressive disorder when required to give a speeded response, respond faster when the concepts of "me" and "failure" are paired than when the concepts of "me" and "success" are paired (functional description), this may provide boundary conditions for the structure of the mental representation of this knowledge (cognitive description).

As has become evident in the part of this chapter on validity issues, it seems safe to conclude that personal attitudes or beliefs can be a source of IAT and APP effects. In contrast, the reverse inference is considerably more problematic: IAT and APP effects cannot with certainty be interpreted as evidence for the mental constructs of (unconscious) attitudes or beliefs, or for the existence of latent schemas. Yet it is certainly the case that evidence obtained with these paradigms has been interpreted as evidence for theories postulating unconscious attitudes, which is of course problematic if effects obtained with these paradigms do not prove to be valid mental proxies. We believe that future research would benefit from a combined functional and cognitive approach. This approach would start by describing and studying IAT and APP effects in functional terms, which could then lead to a more specific description of the mental constructs—the cognitive processes—potentially responsible for these effects.

Table 13.1 (inspired by De Houwer's [2011] Table 1) makes it clear that the cognitive and functional approaches yield quite different descriptions. The same approach could be taken for other experimental tasks that are often used to test cognitive models of psychopathology, probing functions like attention and memory. When this approach is taken, diverging results from different paradigms—constituting a lack of convergent validity in a cognitive approach—are not problematic, and are even to be expected, given that tasks are never process-pure. What results is a more detailed and complete *functional picture* of a disorder. Convergence can then be striven for at this functional level. This functional perspective can then be used to form the basis of a well-informed specific cognitive model for different forms of psychopathology.

TABLE 13.1. Cognitive versus Functional Approaches to IAT and APP

Element	Cognitive approach	IAT functional approach	APP functional approach
Definition	Differential response speed due to associations in memory/ unconscious attitudes or dysfunctional beliefs	Slower response speed when less similar categories are combined under one response button	Slower response speed with less similar prime–target combinations
Explanandum[a]	IAT and APP effect	Differential response speed in the two combined phases	Differential response speed with different types of prime–target combinations
Explanans[b]	Unconscious attitudes and dysfunctional beliefs	Combinations of categories	Prime–target combinations

[a]Explanandum, what needs to be explained.

[b]Explanans, that which is used to explain.

CONCLUSION

In this chapter, we have proposed that researchers should refrain from straying too far from the phenomena when making interpretations of what is actually measured in the experimental task. Researchers using paradigms like the IAT and the APP tend to go from measurement outcome via association to implicit attitude or dysfunctional belief, assuming that this is a shorter inferential route than is actually the case. It is important to note that this has not been the case so much with paradigms capturing other constructs that are deemed of relevance in cognitive theories of psychopathology, such as attention and memory biases. Restricting the interpretation of IAT and APP results to an *association bias* is probably more justified. Taking this to the next level is the functional approach (De Houwer, 2011), thereby preventing problems inherent with a cognitive approach that uses behavioral proxies for mental constructs. The cognitive approach clearly will benefit from the detailed specific results from the functional approach, and the functional approach will be inspired by cognitive theories.

KEY POINTS

FOR PRACTITIONERS

- Implicit measures are useful as a research tool for theory development, but are not ready for individual diagnosis or clinical practice, due to incomplete knowledge regarding their validity and reliability and to their frequent low reliability.
- However, implicit measures may *eventually* provide useful insights into clinical disorders that may call for changes in therapy.

FOR RESEARCHERS

- Researchers should in their interpretation of results remain true to what has actually been assessed by the experimental task. Therefore, the interpretation of implicit measures should be restricted to *association bias*, instead of extending it to implicit attitudes or beliefs.
- There is insufficient empirical evidence regarding the existence of a separate implicit construct (e.g., an "implicit attitude"), nor is there enough evidence regarding the implicitness of these measures.
- A behavioral effect (e.g., an IAT effect) should not be equated with a mental process or construct (e.g., an unconscious attitude or dysfunctional belief).
- Psychopathology research that departs from a cognitive perspective is

likely to benefit from keeping an eye on the state-of-the-art theorizing and methodologies from cognitive science.

FOR STUDENTS AND EDUCATORS

- Avoid gaining/teaching an oversimplified view of implicit measures, but instead include discussion on the validity of implicit measures.
- Think carefully, or have students think carefully, about what implicit measures really reflect. Do not simply accept the interpretations that are provided in research articles.

REFERENCES

American Psychiatric Association. (2013). *Diagnostic and statistical manual of mental disorders* (5th ed.). Arlington, VA: Author.

Asendorpf, J. B., Banse, R., & Mücke, D. (2002). Double dissociation between implicit and explicit personality self-concept: The case of shy behavior. *Journal of Personality and Social Psychology, 83*, 380–393.

Banaji, M. R. (2001). Implicit attitudes can be measured. In H. L. Roediger & J. S. Nairne (Eds.), *The nature of remembering: Essays in honor of Robert G. Crowder* (pp. 117–150). Washington, DC: American Psychological Association.

Bartlett, F. C. (1932). *Remembering: A study in experimental and social psychology.* Cambridge, UK: Cambridge University Press.

Beck, A. T., & Clark, D. A. (1997). An information processing model of anxiety: Automatic and strategic processes. *Behaviour Research and Therapy, 35*, 49–58.

Beck, A. T., Freeman, A., & Davis, D. D. (Eds.). (2004). *Cognitive therapy of personality disorders* (2nd ed.). New York: Guilford Press.

Beck, A. T., Rush, A. J., Shaw, B. F., & Emery, G. (1979). *Cognitive therapy of depression.* New York: Guilford Press.

Blair, I. V. (2002). The malleability of automatic stereotypes and prejudice. *Personality and Social Psychology Review, 6*, 242–261.

Boring, E. G. (1953). A history of introspection. *Psychological Bulletin, 50*, 169–189.

Bosson, J. K., Swann, W. B., & Pennebaker, J. W. (2000). Stalking the perfect measure of implicit self-esteem: The blind men and the elephant revisited? *Journal of Personality and Social Psychology, 79*, 631–643.

Bradley, B. P., Mogg, K., & Lee, S. C. (1997). Attentional biases for negative information in induced and naturally occurring dysphoria. *Behaviour Research and Therapy, 35*, 911–927.

Buchner, A., & Wippich, W. (2000). On the reliability of implicit and explicit memory measures. *Cognitive Psychology, 40*, 227–259.

Buhlmann, U., Teachman, B. A., & Kathmann, N. (2011). Evaluating implicit attractiveness beliefs in body dysmorphic disorder using the go/no-go association task. *Journal of Behavior Therapy and Experimental Psychiatry, 42*, 192–197.

Buhrmester, M. D., Blanton, H., & Swann, W. B. (2011). Implicit self-esteem: Nature, measurement, and a new way forward. *Journal of Personality and Social Psychology, 100*(2), 365–385.

Cai, H., Siriam, N., Greenwald, A. G., & McFarland, S. G. (2004). The Implicit Association Test's D measure can minimize a cognitive skill confound: Comment on McFarland and Crouch (2002). *Social Cognition, 22*, 673–684.

Cheng, P. W., & Holyoak, K. J. (1985). Pragmatic reasoning schemas. *Cognitive Psychology, 17*, 391–416.

Clark, D. A., Beck, A. T., & Alford, B. A. (1999). *Scientific foundations of cognitive theory and therapy of depression.* New York: Wiley.

Clark, D. M., & Wells, A. (1995). A cognitive model of social phobia. In R. G. Heimberg, M. R. Liebowitz, D. A. Hope, & F. R. Schneier (Eds.), *Social phobia: Diagnosis, assessment, and treatment* (pp. 69–93). New York: Guilford Press.

Clerkin, E. M., & Teachman, B. A. (2009). Automatic and strategic measures as predictors of mirror gazing among individuals with body dysmorphic disorder symptoms. *Journal of Nervous and Mental Disease, 197*, 589–598.

Craeynest, M., Crombez, G., Deforche, B., Tanghe, A., & De Bourdeaudhuij, I. (2008). The role of implicit attitudes towards food and physical activity in the treatment of youth obesity. *Eating Behaviors, 9*, 41–51.

Cunningham, W. A., Preacher, K. J., & Banaji, M. R. (2001). Implicit attitude measurement: Consistency, stability, and convergent validity. *Psychological Science, 12*, 163–170.

De Houwer, J. (2003). A structural analysis of indirect measures of attitudes. In J. Musch & K. C. Klauer (Eds.), *The psychology of evaluation: Affective processes in cognition and emotion* (pp. 219–244). Mahwah, NJ: Erlbaum.

De Houwer, J. (2006). What are implicit measures and why are we using them? In R. W. Wiers & A. W. Stacy (Eds.), *The handbook of implicit cognition and addiction* (pp. 11–28). Thousand Oaks, CA: Sage.

De Houwer, J. (2009). Comparing measures of attitudes at the functional and procedural level: Analysis and implications. In R. E. Petty, R. H. Fazio, & P. Brinol (Eds.), *Attitudes: Insights from the new implicit measures* (pp. 361–390). New York: Erlbaum.

De Houwer, J. (2011). Why the cognitive approach in psychology would profit from a functional approach and vice versa. *Perspectives on Psychological Science, 6*, 202–209.

De Houwer, J., Geldof, T., & De Bruycker, E. (2005). The Implicit Association Test as a general measure of similarity. *Canadian Journal of Experimental Psychology, 59*, 228–239.

De Houwer, J., Teige-Mocigemba, S., Spruyt, A., & Moors, A. (2009). Implicit measures: A normative analysis and review. *Psychological Bulletin, 135*, 347–368.

De Raedt, R., Schacht, R., Franck, E., & De Houwer, J. (2006). Self-esteem and depression revisited: Implicit positive self-esteem in depressed patients? *Behaviour Research and Therapy, 44*, 1017–1028.

Fazio, R. H. (2001). On the automatic evaluation of associated evaluations: An overview. *Cognition and Emotion, 15*, 115–141.

Fazio, R. H., & Olson, M. A. (2003). Implicit measures in social cognition research: Their meaning and use. *Annual Review of Psychology, 54*, 297–327.

Fazio, R. H., Sanbonmatsu, D. M., Powell, M. C., & Kardes, F. R. (1986). On the automatic activation of attitudes. *Journal of Personality and Social Psychology, 50*, 229–238.

Fazio, R. H., & Towles-Schwen, T. (1999). The MODE model of attitude–behavior processes. In S. Chaiken & Y. Trope (Eds.), *Dual-process theories in social psychology* (pp. 97–116). New York: Guilford Press.

Fiedler, K., & Bluemke, M. (2005). Faking the IAT: Aided and unaided response control on the Implicit Association Test. *Basic and Applied Social Psychology, 27*, 307–316.

Fiedler, K., Messner, C., & Bluemke, M. (2006). Unresolved problems with the "I," the "A," and the "T": A logical and psychometric critique of the Implicit Association Test (IAT). *European Review of Social Psychology, 17*, 74–147.

Field, M., Munafo, M. R., & Franken, I. H. (2009). A meta-analytic investigation of the relationship between attentional bias and subjective craving in substance abuse. *Psychological Bulletin, 135*, 589–607.

Foroni, F., & Semin, G. R. (2012). Not all implicit measures of attitudes are created equal: Evidence from an embodiment perspective. *Journal of Experimental Social Psychology, 48*, 424–427.

Franck, E., De Raedt, R., Dereu, M., & Van den Abbeele, D. (2007). Implicit and explicit self-esteem in currently depressed individuals with and without suicidal ideation. *Journal of Behavior Therapy and Experimental Psychiatry, 38*, 75–85.

Gawronski, B., LeBel, E. P., & Peters, K. R. (2007). What do implicit measures tell us?: Scrutinizing the validity of three common assumptions. *Perspectives on Psychological Science, 2*, 181–193.

Gemar, M. C., Segal, Z. V., Sagrati, S., & Kennedy, S. J. (2001). Mood-induced changes on the Implicit Association Test in recovered depressed patients. *Journal of Abnormal Psychology, 110*, 282–289.

Greenwald, A. G. (2012). There is nothing so theoretical as a good method. *Perspectives on Psychological Science, 7*, 99–108.

Greenwald, A. G., McGhee, D. E., & Schwartz, J. L. K. (1998). Measuring individual differences in implicit cognition: The Implicit Association Test. *Journal of Personality and Social Psychology, 74*, 1464–1480.

Greenwald, A. G., Nosek, B. A., & Banaji, M. R. (2003). Understanding and using the Implicit Association Test: I. An improved scoring algorithm. *Journal of Personality and Social Psychology, 85*, 197–216.

Greenwald, A. G., Nosek, B. A., Banaji, M. R., & Klauer, K. C. (2005). Validity of the salience asymmetry interpretation of the Implicit Association Test:

Comment on Rothermund and Wentura (2004). *Journal of Experimental Psychology: General, 134,* 420–425.

Grumm, M., Erbe, K., von Collani, G., & Nestler, S. (2008). Automatic processing of pain: The change of implicit pain associations after psychotherapy. *Behaviour Research and Therapy, 46,* 701–714.

Haeffel, G. J., Abramson, L. Y., Brazy, P. C., Shah, J. Y., Teachman, B. A., & Nosek, B. A. (2007). Explicit and implicit cognition: A preliminary test of a dual-process theory of cognitive vulnerability to depression. *Behaviour Research and Therapy, 45,* 1155–1167.

Hofmann, W., Friese, M., & Roefs, A. (2009). Three ways to resist temptation: The independent contributions of executive attention, inhibitory control, and affect regulation to the impulse control of eating behavior. *Journal of Experimental Social Psychology, 45,* 431–435.

Hofmann, W., Rauch, W., & Gawronski, B. (2007). And deplete us not into temptation: Automatic attitudes, dietary restraint, and self-regulatory resources as determinants of eating behavior. *Journal of Experimental Social Psychology, 43,* 497–504.

Houben, K., & Wiers, R. W. (2006). Assessing implicit alcohol associations with the Implicit Association Test: Fact or artifact? *Addictive Behaviors, 31,* 1346–1362.

Houben, K., & Wiers, R. W. (2008). Implicitly positive about alcohol?: Implicit positive associations predict drinking behavior. *Addictive Behaviors, 33,* 979–986.

Huijding, J., & de Jong, P. J. (2005). A pictorial version of the extrinsic affective Simon task: Sensitivity to generally affective and phobia-relevant stimuli in high and low spider fearful individuals. *Experimental Psychology, 52,* 289–295.

Huijding, J., & de Jong, P. J. (2006). Specific predictive power of automatic spider-related affective associations for controllable and uncontrollable fear responses toward spiders. *Behaviour Research and Therapy, 44,* 161–176.

Huijding, J., & de Jong, P. J. (2007). Beyond fear and disgust: The role of (automatic) contamination-related associations in spider phobia. *Journal of Behaviour Therapy and Experimental Psychiatry, 38,* 200–211.

Ingram, R. E. (1984). Toward an information-processing analysis of depression. *Cognitive Therapy and Research, 8,* 443–477.

Jacoby, L. L. (1991). A process dissociation framework: Separating automatic from intentional uses of memory. *Journal of Memory and Language, 30,* 513–541.

Joormann, J., Yoon, K. L., & Zetsche, U. (2007). Cognitive inhibition in depression. *Applied and Preventive Psychology, 12,* 128–139.

Karpinski, A., & Hilton, J. L. (2001). Attitudes and the Implicit Association Test. *Journal of Personality and Social Psychology, 81,* 774–788.

Klauer, K. C., Schmitz, F., Teige-Mocigemba, S., & Voss, A. (2010). Understanding the role of executive control in the Implicit Association Test: Why flexible people have small IAT effects. *Quarterly Journal of Experimental Psychology, 63,* 595–619.

LeBel, E. P., & Paunonen, S. V. (2011). Sexy but often unreliable: The impact of unreliability on the replicability of experimental findings with implicit measures. *Personality and Social Psychology Bulletin, 37*, 570–583.

MacLeod, C. (1993). Cognition in clinical psychology: Measures, methods or models? *Behaviour Change, 10*, 169–195.

McFarland, S. G., & Crouch, Z. (2002). A cognitive skill confound on the Implicit Association Test. *Social Cognition, 20*, 483–510.

McNally, R. J. (2001). On the scientific status of cognitive appraisal models of anxiety disorder. *Behaviour Research and Therapy, 39*, 513–521.

Meiser, T. (2011). Much pain, little gain?: Paradigm-specific models and methods in experimental psychology. *Perspectives on Psychological Science, 6*, 183–191.

Mierke, J., & Klauer, K. C. (2003). Method-specific variance in the Implicit Association Test. *Journal of Personality and Social Psychology, 85*, 1180–1192.

Mitte, K. (2008). Memory bias for threatening information in anxiety and anxiety disorders: A meta-analytic review. *Psychological Bulletin, 134*, 886–911.

Monteith, M. J., Voils, C. I., & Ashburn-Nardo, L. (2001). Taking a look underground: Detecting interpreting, and reacting to implicit racial bias. *Social Cognition, 19*, 395–417.

Moors, A., & De Houwer, J. (2006). Automaticity: A theoretical and conceptual analysis. *Psychological Bulletin, 132*, 297–326.

Nisbett, R. E., & Wilson, T. D. (1977). Telling more than we can know: Verbal reports on mental processes. *Psychological Review, 84*, 231–259.

Nosek, B. A., Banaji, M. R., & Greenwald, A. G. (2002). Harvesting implicit group attitudes and beliefs from a demonstration website. *Group Dynamics, 6*, 101–115.

Nosek, B. A., Greenwald, A. G., & Banaji, M. R. (2007). The Implicit Association Test at age 7: A methodological and conceptual review. In J. A. Bargh (Ed.), *Automatic processes in social thinking and behaviour* (pp. 265–292). New York: Psychology Press.

Nosek, B. A., & Hansen, J. J. (2008). The associations in our heads belong to us: Searching for attitudes and knowledge in implicit evaluation. *Cognition and Emotion, 22*, 553–594.

Olson, M. A., & Fazio, R. H. (2001). Implicit attitude formation through classical conditioning. *Psychological Science, 12*, 413–417.

Olson, M. A., & Fazio, R. H. (2002). Implicit acquisition and manifestation of classically conditioned attitudes. *Social Cognition, 20*, 89–104.

Olson, M. A., & Fazio, R. H. (2003). Relations between implicit measures of prejudice: What are we measuring? *Psychological Science, 14*, 636–639.

Olson, M. A., & Fazio, R. H. (2004). Reducing the influence of extrapersonal associations on the Implicit Association Test: Personalizing the IAT. *Journal of Personality and Social Psychology, 86*, 653–667.

Olson, M. A., Fazio, R. H., & Han, H. A. (2009). Conceptualizing personal and extrapersonal associations. *Social and Personality Psychology Compass, 3*, 152–170.

Perugini, M. (2005). Predictive models of implicit and explicit attitudes. *British Journal of Social Psychology, 44*, 29–45.

Robusto, E., Cristante, F., & Vianello, M. (2008). Assessing the impact of replication on Implicit Association Test effect by means of the extended logistic model for the assessment of change. *Behavior Research Methods, 40,* 954–960.

Roediger, H. L., III, & Geraci, L. (2005). Implicit memory tasks in cognitive research. In A. Wenzel & D. Rubin (Eds.), *Cognitive methods and their application to clinical research* (pp. 129–151). Washington, DC: American Psychological Association.

Roefs, A., Huijding, J., Smulders, F. T. Y., MacLeod, C. M., de Jong, P. J., Wiers, R. W., et al. (2011). Implicit measures of association in psychopathology research. *Psychological Bulletin, 137,* 149–193.

Roefs, A., & Jansen, A. (2002). Implicit and explicit attitudes toward high-fat foods in obesity. *Journal of Abnormal Psychology, 111,* 517–521.

Roefs, A., Quaedackers, L., Werrij, M. Q., Wolters, G., Havermans, R., Nederkoorn, C., et al. (2006). The environment influences whether high-fat foods are associated with palatable or with unhealthy. *Behaviour Research and Therapy, 44,* 715–736.

Rothermund, K., & Wentura, D. (2004). Underlying processes in the Implicit Association Test: Dissociating salience from associations. *Journal of Experimental Psychology: General, 133,* 139–165.

Rumelhart, D. E. (1980). Schemata: The building blocks of cognition. In R. J. Spiro, B. C. Bruce, & W. F. Brewer (Eds.), *Theoretical issues in reading comprehension* (pp. 33–58). Hillsdale, NJ: Erlbaum.

Schwarz, N. (1999). Self-reports: How the questions shape the answers. *American Psychologist, 54,* 93–105.

Schwarz, N., & Oyserman, D. (2001). Asking questions about behavior: Cognition, communication, and questionnaire construction. *American Journal of Evaluation, 22,* 127–160.

Segal, Z. V. (1988). Appraisal of the self-schema construct in cognitive models of depression. *Psychological Bulletin, 103,* 147–162.

Seibt, B., Häfner, M., & Deutsch, R. (2007). Prepared to eat: How immediate affective and motivational responses to food cues are influenced by food deprivation. *European Journal of Social Psychology, 37,* 359–379.

Siegel, E. F., Dougherty, M. R., & Huber, D. E. (2012). Manipulating the role of cognitive control while taking the Implicit Association Test. *Journal of Experimental Social Psychology, 48,* 1057–1068.

Stadler, M. A., & Frensch, P. A. (Eds.). (1998). *Handbook of implicit learning.* Thousand Oaks, CA: Sage.

Strauss, M. E., & Smith, G. T. (2009). Construct validity: Advances in theory and methodology. *Annual Review of Clinical Psychology, 5,* 1–25.

Teachman, B. A., Marker, C. D., & Smith-Janik, S. B. (2008). Automatic associations and panic disorder: Trajectories of change over the course of treatment. *Journal of Consulting and Clinical Psychology, 76,* 988–1002.

Teachman, B. A., Smith-Janik, S. B., & Saporito, J. (2007). Information processing biases and panic disorder: Relationships among cognitive and symptom measures. *Behaviour Research and Therapy, 45,* 1791–1811.

Teachman, B. A., & Woody, S. R. (2003). Automatic processing in spider phobia: Implicit fear associations over the course of treatment. *Journal of Abnormal Psychology, 112*, 100–109.

Thush, C., Wiers, R. W., Ames, S. L., Grenard, J. L., Sussman, S., & Stacy, A. W. (2007). Apples and oranges?: Comparing indirect measures of alcohol-related cognition predicting alcohol use in at-risk adolescents. *Psychology of Addictive Behaviors, 21*, 587–591.

Van den Hout, M. (1999). Armies of idiots and idiosyncrasies: On reductions in experimental psychopathology. *Behaviour Research and Therapy, 37*, S135–S145.

Wason, P. C. (1966). Reasoning. In B. M. Foss (Ed.), *New horizons in psychology* (pp. 135–151). Harmonsworth, UK: Penguin Books.

Wiers, R. W., van de Luitgaarden, J., van den Wildenberg, E., & Smulders, F. T. (2005). Challenging implicit and explicit alcohol-related cognitions in young heavy drinkers. *Addiction, 100*, 806–819.

Williams, J. M. G., Mathews, A., & MacLeod, C. (1996). The emotional Stroop task and psychopathology. *Psychological Bulletin, 120*, 3–24.

Williams, J. M. G., Watts, F. N., MacLeod, C., & Mathews, A. (1997). *Cognitive psychology and emotional disorders*. Chichester, UK: Wiley.

14

Advances in Construct Validity Theory

Implications for Cognitive-Behavioral Therapy Assessment

Leila Guller and Gregory T. Smith

The intent of this chapter is to review recent advances in construct validity theory that are likely to be relevant to assessment in cognitive-behavioral therapy (CBT), and to relate those advances to current challenges in the CBT field. In important ways, the validity of CBT-related assessment has progressed in ways highly consistent with advances in construct validity theory. Also, as is true in any field, there are cautionary tales of the problems resulting from insufficiently rigorous application of validation principles to measure development. We begin with a brief review of the history of construct validity theory and recent advances in this field. In this overview, we highlight four issues: (1) the ongoing, iterative nature of theory development and construct validation; (2) the challenge of developing informative programs of validation research; (3) the challenge of construct representation in measures; and (4) the importance of assessing homogeneous constructs. We then discuss these issues as relevant to assessment tools commonly used in CBT. We conclude by applying our discussion to the provision of general guidelines for measure development, as well as for the evaluation of measures by practitioners.

A BRIEF HISTORY OF VALIDATION
EFFORTS IN CLINICAL PSYCHOLOGY

Early Measure Development and Validity

A milestone in the history of both validity theory and psychopathology research was the development of the Woodworth Personal Data Sheet (WPDS) in 1919—and, in particular, the general lack of success of the measure. The WPDS was developed in World War I as a tool to screen out recruits who might be more susceptible than others to "shell shock" or "war neurosis," as it was intended to measure emotional stability (Garrett & Schneck, 1928). Woodworth constructed the test by creating 116 dichotomous items on rational grounds (drawing content from case histories of patients identified as "neurotic") as well as empirical grounds (deleting items that were endorsed by 50% or more of a "normal" test group) (Garrett & Schneck, 1928).

Despite these scientifically appropriate efforts, the WPDS was far from successful. Total WPDS score did not differentiate dysfunctional from functional individuals, as evidenced by its inability to discriminate between college freshmen (an elite group in the early 1900s) and "avowed psychoneurotics" (Garrett & Schneck, 1928), as well as its lack of correlation with teacher ratings of students' emotional stability (Flemming & Flemming, 1929). In an attempt to explain its failure, researchers considered the multifaceted nature of the item content on the WPDS (Garrett & Schneck, 1928; Laird, 1925) and indeed found a diverse range of items. Sample items included "Have you ever lost your memory for a time?", "Can you sit still without fidgeting?", "Does it make you uneasy to have to cross a wide street or an open square?", and "Does some particular useless thought keep coming into your mind to bother you?" Regarding the diversity of mental complaints that went into the computation of an overall score, Garrett and Schneck (1928) concluded: "It is this fact, among others, which is causing the present-day trend away from the concept of mental disease as an entity. Instead of saying that a patient has this or that disease, the modern psychiatrist prefers to say that the patient exhibits such and such symptoms" (p. 465).

This thinking led the researchers to investigate the predictive success of individual items, rather than of the test as a whole; furthermore, they sought to identify covariation between individual item responses and specific diagnoses, rather than membership in a global "mentally ill" category. In this early study, Garrett and Schneck recognized the need to avoid combining items of different content. Their approach thus anticipated two important advances. First, their use of an empirical item–person classification produced very different results from prior rational classifications (Laird, 1925), thus indicating the importance of empirical validation and anticipating criterion-keying methods of test construction.

Second, they anticipated the more recent appreciation for construct homogeneity, with its emphasis on unidimensional traits and unidimensional symptoms as the proper objects of theoretical study and measure validation (Edwards, 2001; McGrath, 2005; Smith, McCarthy, & Zapolski, 2009; Strauss & Smith, 2009). From the standpoint of today's more sophisticated understanding of psychopathology, the WPDS items combined several different forms of dysfunction into a single measure that produced a single score. As we discuss further, this approach undermines efforts to validate measures and test theory.

Criterion-Related Validity and the Rise of Construct Validity Theory

Following the WPDS, much of the remainder of the first half of the 20th century was characterized by using purely criterion-keying approaches in the validation of psychological measures. In this method, any item distinguishing between a clinical group and a comparison group is included in a measure, regardless of the item's content. Thus, in a sense, the validity of a measure is built in by the method of item selection. From this perspective, a test is valid only to the extent that it can predict a given criterion, or, as Anastasi (1950) wrote, "It is only as a measure of a specifically defined criterion that a test can be objectively validated at all. . . . To claim that a test measures anything over and above its criterion is pure speculation" (p. 67).

This approach did indeed yield two of the most widely used measures in psychological testing: the Minnesota Multiphasic Personality Inventory–2 (MMPI-2; Butcher, 1990) and the California Psychological Inventory (CPI; Gough, 1968; Megargee, 2008). The MMPI-2 has provided valid distinctions among psychiatric inpatients and outpatients, and has been useful when employed in treatment planning (Butcher, 1990; Greene, 2006). It has also proved useful in work with nondisabled populations (Butcher, 2002), head-injured populations (Gass, 2002), and individuals in correctional facilities (Megargee, 2006). The CPI has also validly predicted a wide range of criteria (Gough & Bradley, 1996). The success of criterion-keyed tests made it possible to make important predictions that affected people's lives with improved validity.

Despite these important successes, there are two limitations in focusing solely on criterion-related validity, or the ability of a test to predict a circumscribed criterion. First, the method requires the assumption that the criterion measure is itself valid (Bechtoldt, 1951). To return to the WPDS, it now seems clear that an enormous limitation to validating the measure was the relative absence of sound criteria, given the absence of a sound, well-validated model of psychopathology. At the time, many important distinctions among different forms of psychological distress were not yet recognized. The criterion of being "neurotic" seems, by today's standards, poorly defined and inadequately measured (Strauss & Smith, 2009).

The second problem is that when tests are developed for the specific intent of predicting a circumscribed criterion, and when they are only validated with respect to that predictive task, the process adds little to basic theory. In the absence of developing theory, the clinician lacks a foundation for proposing new possible relationships among variables. Criterion-validated tests are not well suited for use in testing theories describing relationships among psychological processes, such as among risk factors, precipitating events, and dysfunction.

In reaction to these limitations, Meehl and Challman, working as part of the American Psychological Association Committee on Psychological Tests, introduced the concept of construct validity in the 1954 Technical Recommendations (American Psychological Association, 1954). However, the concept of construct validity truly gained recognition as a result of Cronbach and Meehl's (1955) classic paper and was further developed by researchers similarly looking to build theory about unobservable entities (Campbell & Fiske, 1959; Loevinger, 1957). A core idea of construct validity is that one can develop a measure so that variation in scores on the measure represent individual differences in an underlying, unobserved, inferred construct.

The idea of construct validity changed the way researchers approached psychological functioning, in that it allowed for the study of unobservable attributes that are inferred to be real entities. Theories about constructs are tested by developing measures of these inferred entities and testing whether these measures relate to measures of other inferred entities. As described by Smith (2005), if we develop a measure of hypothetical construct A, we can only validate our measure if we have some theoretical argument that, for instance, A relates positively to B, but is unrelated to C. If we have such a theory, and if we have measures of constructs B and C, we can test whether our measure of A performs as predicted by our theory. Thus the construct validation process requires the prior development of theories. More than that, the process simultaneously involves testing the validity of a measure and the validity of the theory of which the measured construct is a part. Construct validation is also theory validation.

ADVANCES IN CONSTRUCT VALIDITY

The Iterative Nature of Construct Validation

It follows that the construct validation process is indeterminate. If our measure of A performs as expected, then we are likely to have increased confidence in both our theory and our measure of A. However, we cannot be certain both that our theory is correct and that our measure is accurate. Suppose, instead, our new measure of A inadvertently overlaps with B (which is known not to correlate with C), and our supportive results are really due to the fact that the measures of A and B partly reflect the same construct. Thus positive results increase our confidence in our measure and in our theory, but they do not constitute either proof of a theory or full validation of a measure.

Similarly, if our measure of A does not perform as expected by theory, we must consider whether the measure, the theory, both, or neither, lack validity. Suppose A relates to both B and C. We have no certain basis for determining whether (1) our theory was accurate but our measure of A was inadequate; (2) our theory was incorrect and our measure of A was adequate; or (3) our theory was correct, and our measure of A was adequate, but our measure of C was inadequate. There are, of course, other possibilities as well, which include issues of research design as well as measurement.

Clinical psychologists often measure inferred constructs, and the validity of any measure is inextricably related to the validity of the theory that led to the measure. One of the realities of this process is that it does not yield definitive, final results. This reality does not reflect a relative weakness in psychological science as compared to other scientific disciplines; on the contrary, the ongoing process of improving theory and hence revisitation of construct validity issues is a typical part of the scientific process across disciplines.

Application to CBT-Related Assessment

One way in which our understanding of the construct validity of measures tends continually to change is that researchers can identify multiple dimensions in what had previously been thought to be unidimensional constructs. When that occurs, there is a whole new set of construct validity challenges. The recent history of the measurement of anxiety sensitivity provides a good example of construct validity issues as they change in response to scientific advances (see Olatunji & Wolitzky-Taylor, 2009). The Anxiety Sensitivity Index (ASI; Reiss, Peterson, Gursky, & McNally, 1986) was initially developed under the assumption that anxiety sensitivity, as a construct, was unidimensional. Specifically, anxiety sensitivity was conceptualized as a broad vulnerability to misin-terpreting bodily sensations as danger cues, thus leading to heightened levels of anxiety (Reiss, 1991; Reiss & McNally, 1985). Development of the ASI (Reiss et al., 1986) reflected the belief that anxiety sensi-tivity was a unitary construct. However, as reviewed by Olatunji and Wolitzky-Taylor (2009), understanding of the construct of anxiety sen-sitivity changed over time, requiring changes in the assessment tools used to measure it. Specifically, factor analyses of the original ASI sug-gested that there appear to be several factors within anxiety sensitivity: (1) physical symptoms, (2) public observable anxiety symptoms, and (3) cognitive dyscontrol. These findings led to the development of the ASI—Revised (Taylor & Cox, 1998b). However, content issues in the ASI-R led Taylor and Cox (1998a) to develop the Anxiety Sensitivity Profile (ASP), which aimed to capture a six-factor solution to measure anxiety sensitivity. Yet the ASP was not without its shortcomings, and its use has been limited (Olatunji & Wolitzky-Taylor, 2009). Ultimately, the ASI-3 (Taylor et al., 2007), which was designed to measure physical, cognitive, and social concerns, was developed in response to various difficulties with ASI-R and the ASP; to date, it has appeared to be more valid than previous versions of anxiety sensitivity measures.

This process highlights important psychometric developments that often take place in response to demands guided by validity theory. There is reason to anticipate that this process will be ongoing, as advances in theoretical and psychometric knowledge lead to a new and differ-ent understanding of the nature and dimensions of anxiety sensitivity. For example, Osman et al. (2010) argue for the presence of both a gen-eral anxiety sensitivity factor and the three specific factors, and their analysis raises the issue of whether the general factor is the most useful. Researchers will weigh their findings against other findings reflecting discriminant validity among the subscales, and over time, theory and measurement will continue to improve. Change of this kind reflects the ongoing process of improving theory and improving measurement of theoretical constructs.

Strong, Weak, and Informative Programs of Construct Validation Research

A second advance addresses Cronbach and Meehl's (1955) classic idea of the "nomological network," or set of lawful relations among entities. One difficulty with this concept is that the idea that one can define constructs by their place in a lawful network of relationships assumes a theoretical precision that is generally not present in the social sciences. Typically, psychopathology researchers are faced with the task of validating their measures and theories, despite the absence of a set of precisely definable, expected lawful relations among constructs and the measures that represent them. Cronbach (1988) attempted to address this issue by contrasting strong and weak programs of construct validity. Strong programs, which were advocated by Cronbach, fit with the nomological network ideal of lawful relationships. Alternately, weak programs stem from less fully articulated theories and construct definitions. In the absence of carefully articulated theory, virtually any correlation between a target measure and another measure, of any magnitude, can be described as validation evidence (Cronbach, 1988). In the absence of a commitment to precise construct definitions and specific theories, validation research can have an ad hoc, opportunistic quality (Kane, 2001), in which sets of correlations with readily available measures are cobbled together as evidence of construct validity.

As argued by Smith (2005) and Strauss and Smith (2009), researchers are not stuck between the unattainable ideal of strong validation programs and inadequate, weak validation programs. It is perhaps more accurate to understand the validation process as a developmental enterprise. There is an iterative process in which tests of partially developed theories provide information that leads to theory refinement and elaboration, which in turn provide a sounder basis for subsequent validation research and more precise construct and theory validation tests. Cronbach and Meehl (1955) referred to this "bootstrapping" process and to the inductive quality of construct definition and theory articulation. Thus, as Smith (2005) has suggested, the standard for evaluating validation research should not be described in terms of "strong" versus "weak" testing, but instead should focus on how *informative* validation tests are. The informative nature of these tests depends on their satisfactory answers to the following questions. To what degree does a hypothesis involve direct criticism of a theory, or direct comparison between two alternative theoretical explanations? To what degree does a hypothesis involve a direct response to a criticism of a theory? To what degree does a hypothesis involve a claim that, if supported, would undermine criticism of one's theory? To what degree does a hypothesis involve a claim that, if not supported, would cast real doubt on one's theory? Given the state of development of any one theory, tests of this kind may or may not constitute strong programs of construct validation, but they do not represent weak validation programs. They address questions that will clarify the validity of theories and the measures used to test them. Because of the iterative nature of theory and measure development and validation, theoretical tests of this kind are likely to provide useful information.

A second difficulty with the nomological network concept is that it is perhaps too closely related to a philosophy of science described by Bartley (1962) and others as "justificationist": Theories can either be fully justified or fully disproved on the basis of observation or empirical evidence. The classic idea of a critical experiment, the results of which could demonstrate that a theory is false, is an example of justificationism (Duhem, 1914/1991; Lakatos, 1968). Logical positivism (Blumberg & Feigl, 1931), with its belief that theories are straightforward derivations from observed facts, is one example of justificationist philosophy of science. Under justificationism, one could imagine the validity of a theory and its accompanying measures being fully and unequivocally established as a result of a series of critical experiments.

In recent decades, historians of science and philosophers of science have moved away from justificationism, endorsing instead what is referred to as "nonjustificationism" (Bartley, 1987; Feyerabend, 1970; Kuhn, 1970; Lakatos, 1968; Rorer & Widiger, 1983; Weimer, 1979). Nonjustificationism refers to the concept that scientific theories are neither fully justified nor definitively disproven by individual, empirical studies. It is based on the following considerations. The test of any theory presupposes the validity of several other theories (often referred to as "auxiliary theories"), including theories of measurement, that also influence the empirical test (Lakatos, 1999; Meehl, 1978, 1990). Consider the brief example we have presented above, in which we refer to measures of constructs A, B, and C. To test our theory of A, we must rely on the validity of the theory of how construct B operates; the validity of the measure of construct B; the validity of the theory of how construct C operates; the validity of the measure of construct C; and the validity of the theory that B is unrelated to C. Empirical results that are negative for A may reflect the failure of any number of theories other than the validity of our measure of construct A: It could be due to problems with our measure of A, but it may also be due to problems with our theories of either B or C, or both; with our measure of B; with our measure of C; with both measures; and/or with our theory that B and C are unrelated. In short, there are many possible explanations for the findings of any study. In part for this reason, no theory is ever fully proved or disproved; hence the term "nonjustificationism."

Because science appears to operate in this way (Weimer, 1979)— and because this process is inevitably developmental in nature, such that each new study provides information concerning the validity of existing theories and measures—Smith (2005) has argued against the use of static concepts such as strong and weak construct validity tests. Instead, it is more useful to consider how informative any study is with respect to the validity of relevant theories and the measures used to test them.

Application to CBT-Related Assessment

Segal's (1988) appraisal of the self-schema construct in cognitive models of depression raises issues that tie into the concepts of strong, weak, and informative programs of construct validation. Segal discusses difficulties with the construct of negative self-schemas believed to be part of depression by reviewing methodological and theoretical short-comings of the construct. According to the theory underlying a nega-tive self-schema, depression is explained in terms of "differences in the interconnectedness of personal constructs between depressed and non-depressed people," with episodes of depression characterized by "acti-vation of a self-structure that is negative in content," and episodes of remission characterized by a remittance in the dominance of the negative self-structure (Segal, 1988, p. 151). However, there are important meth-odological challenges associated with validating this argument. Specifi-cally, Segal (1988) argues that depressed versus nondepressed episodes are characterized by fluctuations in negative verbalizations, therefore making paper-and-pencil measurement of this construct more a reflec-tion of such fluctuations than of the schema itself (Coyne & Gotlib, 1986). Segal (1988, p. 147) argues that "the strategy of relying on nega-tive self-reports to validate a construct whose operation is intended to explain these self-reports becomes increasingly circular unless additional external referents can be provided to demonstrate schematic processing" (Segal & Shaw, 1986). Indeed, the absence of external referents to the schematic processing could be understood to reflect a weakness in this program of construct validation.

There are other difficulties as well. Segal (1988) discusses the Dys-functional Attitude Scale (DAS; Weissman, 1979), which was designed to assess negative schemas typical in depression, and posits two rela-tionships that should be present, given Beck's (1967) cognitive model of depression. First, schemas measured by the DAS should correlate with other measures of cognitive distortions. This requirement, as dis-cussed by Segal, has been supported by various studies of the correlation between the DAS and other measures of cognitive distortions, including the Cognitive Style Test (Blackburn, Jones, & Lewin, 1987), the Cogni-tive Response Test (Giles & Rush, 1983), and the Automatic Thoughts Questionnaire (Hollon, Kendall, & Lumry, 1986). Second, elevated scores on the DAS found during a depressed episode should continue to be elevated during remission, which would offer support for the ongo-ing influence of depressogenic schemas. However, Segal notes several studies that seem to counter this argument: Scores on the DAS often return to the mean range after depressed episodes remit, or do not show elevations during the depressed episode in the first place (Blackburn et al., 1987; Dobson & Shaw, 1986; Eaves & Rush, 1984; Giles & Rush, 1983). One implication of this combination of findings is that the DAS may measure negative verbalizations rather than underlying negative self-schemas. Segal (1988) concludes his evaluation of the DAS construct by stating that "paper-and-pencil inventories of schematic processes are not capable of providing the type of evidence necessary for demonstrating cognitive structure" (p. 152).

One might argue that the attempt to measure negative self-schemas through self-reports understood to vary as a function of depressive symptom level does not offer a sound enough basis for evaluating the validity of the construct of negative self-schemas. As a result, validation tests using this method may not prove as informative as is desirable. One cannot be sure that correlations between paper-and-pencil measures of negative self-schemas and other constructs reflect the operation of the inferred schemas or instead reflect transient mood states. An absence of expected correlations may be a function of problems with the measurement approach rather than with the validity of the intended construct.

Just as there are problematic construct validation programs of inquiry, there are also clearly informative programs of construct validation operating in CBT-related assessment. As discussed earlier, when conceptualization of the construct of anxiety sensitivity changed over time, so did the measures used to assess it. Specifically, what started as the ASI (Reiss et al., 1986) eventually evolved into the ASI-3 (Taylor et al., 2007) through a process of theory informing measurement, construct validation procedures in turn informing theory, and so on. Informative programs of construct validation research will thus tend to have an iterative quality, as theory and measurement inform each other and improve over time.

Of course, informative construct validity research has important implications for the clinical utility of measures as well. The ASI-3 can inform what specific types of anxiety sensitivity concerns need to be addressed in therapy. For example, an individual who presents with elevated physical concerns, but average cognitive and social concerns, may benefit from exposure-type therapy. However, someone with primarily cognitive concerns may benefit more from completing thought records and challenging cognitive distortions.

Construct Representation

Strauss and Smith (2009) have discussed a growing emphasis among construct validity researchers on what is known as "construct representation." This concept was first used in cognitive psychology to refer to a theory concerning response processes that result in a score (such as accuracy or reaction time) in the performance of cognitive tasks (Embretson, 1998; Whitely, 1983). In other words, construct representation reflects the psychological processes that determine responses in an experiment. The reason for the emphasis on this concept is that many investigators develop "home-grown" measures that are thought to reflect a given cognitive process, but do not provide systematic empirical evidence that a given measure actually reflects the target process. More precisely, there has historically been little research designed to address the question of how much variance in responses to a measure reflects variance in the target construct.

Application to CBT-Related Assessment

To extend this concept more broadly to clinically relevant assessment tools, the question that arises is: To what degree do items in an assessment tool accurately represent the intended target construct? This concern is not oriented toward face validity or even content validity, but rather toward systematic analyses to determine what percentage of variance in participant responses reflects variation in the target construct. Consider, for example, the constructs of anxiety and anxiety sensitivity. When a new construct, anxiety sensitivity, is introduced, it is important to specify how it is different from related constructs, such as anxiety. One can test directly how much variance in anxiety sensitivity measures is reliable but independent of variance in anxiety. For example, Kemper, Lutz, Bähr, Rüddel, and Hock (2012) found that global anxiety sensitivity (on the ASI-3) had good internal consistency (alpha = .92) and correlated with the State–Trait Anxiety Inventory (r = .61). Because 92% of the variance in the global score is reliable and 36% of its variance is shared with a measure of general anxiety, it follows that 92 – 36 = 56% of the variance in global anxiety sensitivity does not overlap with general anxiety. This analysis does not necessarily indicate that 56% of the variance in the global score reflects anxiety sensitivity; rather, it indicates that up to 56% of the variance reflects that construct. It is necessary to study the associations among scores on the ASI-3 and scores reflecting different types of clinical symptoms to determine the construct validity of the ASI-3. To that end, the replicated finding that different subscales of anxiety sensitivity play different roles in relation to different types of anxiety syndromes speaks to the validity of the construct measure. For example, the physical concerns subscale of the ASI-3 relates uniquely to panic symptoms; the Cognitive Concerns subscale relates uniquely to depressive symptoms; and both Social Concerns and Cognitive Concerns relate to fear and avoidance symptoms (Olthuis, Watt, & Stewart, 2014).

Construct Homogeneity

The process of construct validation requires rigorous definitions of target constructs and a clear statement of anticipated relationships among constructs. One important implication of this reality is this: scales that produce single scores representing multiple dimensions on a construct may obscure relationships among the underlying constructs, and thus may compromise the construct validation process (Edwards, 2001; Hough & Schneider, 1996; McGrath, 2005; Paunonen, 1998; Paunonen & Ashton, 2001; Schneider, Hough, & Dunnette, 1996; Smith et al., 2009; Strauss & Smith, 2009). This negative effect can occur for two related reasons. First, with a single score that reflects multiple dimensions, one cannot be certain how each dimension contributes to that score. For example, one dimension may be highly correlated with the criterion, and another dimension not correlated at all—but, taken together, these two dimensions may correlate moderately with a criterion. The second source of uncertainty lies in the fact that different combinations of elevations on different dimensions can yield the same overall score. To give a simplified example, if a person scores a 10 on dimension A, and a 2 on dimension B, and the overall score is represented by $A + B$, this person will get a score of 12 on that measure. However, a person with completely flipped scores—that is, 2 on dimension A and 10 on dimension B—will also receive a score of 12. These two people are very different on these two dimensions and could well be experiencing different psychopathological processes, but their final scores are identical. If a single score is used, they are not differentiated. It follows that correlations of such a single score with measures of other constructs have unclear meaning. Fortunately, this problem is easily avoided by using subscale scores rather than total scores.

Application to CBT-Related Assessment

Construct homogeneity, of course, plays an important role in the measurement of constructs relevant to CBT. As reviewed by Berle and Starcevic (2005), "thought–action fusion" (TAF) can be broken up into two related but distinct constructs: (1) "TAF morality," or the belief that unacceptable thoughts are equally immoral as overt unacceptable action, and (2) "TAF likelihood," or the belief that certain thoughts can increase the likelihood of particular events. Measurement of TAF has relied almost exclusively on the TAF Scale (Shafran, Thordarson, & Rachman, 1996), a self-report measure consisting of 12 TAF morality and 7 TAF likelihood items. Psychometric properties of these two scales offer good evidence for their reliability and validity, thus supporting the presence of two separate, homogeneous constructs. The two scales have demonstrated alphas above .80, and they correlate modestly ($r = .44$) with each other (Shafran et al., 1996; Rassin, Merkelbach, Muris, & Schmidt, 2001); the two are thus estimated to share 19.4% of their variance.

The two scales have different and complex relationships with measures of specific aspects of obsessive–compulsive disorder (OCD). For example, Rassin et al. (2001) found that the TAF likelihood scale was significantly correlated with cleaning behaviors, as measured by the Maudsley Obsessional–Compulsive Inventory (Hodgson & Rachman, 1977), and fantasy proneness, as measured by the Creative Experiences Questionnaire (Merckelbach, Muris, Schmidt, Rassin, & Horselenberg, 1998), while the TAF morality scale was not; interestingly, the TAF morality scale did not demonstrate any unique correlations with OCD-related measures. More recently, Siev, Chambless, and Huppert (2010) published findings that may clarify the role of TAF morality in relation to OCD. They found that (1) Christians endorsed higher levels of TAF morality than did Jews, independently of OCD symptoms; (2) religiosity was correlated with TAF morality for Christians but not for Jews (Christian religious adherence is related to beliefs about the moral import of thoughts); and (3) TAF morality was related to OCD symptoms only in Jews. Thus for Christians, TAF morality was related to religiosity but not OCD symptoms, whereas for Jews, the reverse was true. The authors concluded that TAF morality may only be a marker of pathology when such beliefs are not culturally normative (Siev et al., 2010).

This finding suggests that the use of a total TAF score in populations characterized by a Christian rather than Jewish heritage may involve averaging the effects of one predictive construct (TAF likelihood) with one nonpredictive construct (TAF morality). Indeed, in a Netherlands sample (the population of the Netherlands is 0.18% Jewish and over 50% Christian), Muris, Meesters, Rassin, Merckelbach, and Campbell (2001) found that for each of 10 anxiety and depression syndromes (e.g., OCD, generalized anxiety, panic), the correlation between the total score and the criterion was intermediate between the higher correlation for TAF likelihood and the lower correlation for TAF morality. For this sample, use of the total score would underestimate the predictive importance of TAF likelihood and overestimate the predictive importance of TAF morality.

The focus on construct homogeneity is likely to be particularly important for practitioners, who have the task of assessing specific problem areas to be addressed in treatment. Indeed, CBT approaches and the assessment procedures used to guide them clearly focus on specific, homogeneous domains of functioning. For example, a commonly used

CBT manual, *Mind over Mood* (Greenberger & Padesky, 1995), contains several handouts that encourage the client to target specific areas of dysfunction. One finds chapters titled "Alternative or Balanced Thinking" (often used to reduce negative affect) and "Experiments and Action Plans" (often used to increase positive affect) listed in the table of contents. Although diagnostic systems such as the *Diagnostic and Statistical Manual of Mental Disorders*, fifth edition (DSM-5) and many researchers often focus on assessing broad, multidimensional constructs such as depression, treatment-oriented professionals need instead to assess and treat specific problems, such as high negative affect or low positive affect (both of which contribute to the broad construct of depression). In the long run, perhaps research diagnosticians can learn a great deal from the unidimensional assessment focus that is often characteristic of CBT. In the short run, it is of course true that CBT practitioners must work within the DSM-5 framework. In the relative absence of evidence for the construct validity of many diagnoses (Smith et al., 2009), we encourage practitioners to focus attention on the valid assessment of homogeneous constructs within broader DSM-5 diagnoses. Valid assessment of homogeneous constructs can facilitate accurate treatment planning and also contribute to DSM-5 diagnosis.

MEASURE DEVELOPMENT AND EVALUATION

There are a number of resources for effective measure development that include very specific recommendations on how to proceed (e.g., Clark & Watson, 1995; Smith, Fischer, & Fister, 2003). We would like to add to this literature by emphasizing the centrality of the four issues we have addressed in this chapter. First, it is important to keep in mind that the development of measures is an ongoing process. In a real sense, one never fully completes the development and validation of a measure. It is better to view measure development and validation as a developmental process by which each new study provides further information about the validity of a theory and the measure used to represent it, such that both theoretical and psychometric revisions are expected parts of an ongoing advance in scientific and clinical understanding. Revisions are to be embraced, not resisted. Second, it is important to document carefully that there is reliable variance in a new measure that is independent of variance in other, related measures. A rigorous focus on incremental validity, followed by convergent and discriminant validity, is necessary to achieve this aim. It is never appropriate to assume that a measure reflects the construct by which it is named; instead, one must demonstrate empirically how much of the variance in the construct measure is unique, and then demonstrate that the unique variance relates to other construct measures as predicted by theory. Third, support for construct homogeneity must be emphasized. We recommend including only items that are judged, through systematic content validation analysis (Haynes, Richards, & Kubany, 1995), to be prototypic of a target construct. Inclusion of items that, although they correlate with the target construct, are not prototypic of the construct and instead reflect a different construct is to invite unwanted heterogeneity and scientific uncertainty. Content validity analysis, as well as exploratory and confirmatory factor analysis, are useful tools in this regard. We believe that to the degree that researchers maintain these three areas of focus, their efforts to validate their measures will be informative. Last, although discussion of this issue is beyond our scope, it is important to validate a measure on samples that fairly represent the clinical populations with whom the measure will be used.

The previous discussion highlights the potentially daunting task practitioners must face when considering use of new measures in clinical settings. We therefore suggest that they pose the following questions to themselves when evaluating the validity of new assessment tools:

1. Is the definition of the construct clear to you, and does it relate to a recognizable clinical phenomenon?
2. Does the validity evidence indicate that the new measure provides information that is not yet readily accessible?
3. How strong is the validity evidence? Are the effects of sufficient magnitude to differentiate among clinical phenomena? Would use of the measure increase your confidence in the conclusions you draw clinically?
4. Are the clients with whom you would use the measure similar to the individuals on whom the measure was validated on cultural and demographic variables, such as sex, culture, race, age, education level, and nature of psychopathology? If not, there is the caution that the measure is not fully validated for use with a particular clientele.

SUMMARY

We have provided a brief historical overview of validation efforts in psychology, in the hope that appreciation of this history can be of benefit to researchers attempting to sharpen construct validity procedures within CBT-related assessment. We have also discussed recent advances in construct validity theory, and we have highlighted four issues of particular relevance to CBT-related assessment: (1) the ongoing, iterative nature of theory development and construct validation; (2) the challenge of developing informative programs of validation research; (3) construct representation in measures; and (4) the importance of assessing homogeneous constructs. We have then provided examples from the CBT literature to illustrate both challenges and successes in the CBT field and general guidelines for measure development and for the evaluation of measures by practitioners. In our view, CBT-related assessment is continually evolving, as is characteristic of active, productive programs of theory and construct validation research. The practical focus in this field on the assessment of specific dimensions of functioning, rather than aggregate concepts, serves CBT well and sets something of an example for the field of clinical psychology.

KEY POINTS

FOR PRACTITIONERS

- When using measures in clinical assessment, practitioners should seek measures that were developed in accordance with the major principles of construct validation. That is, measure development should (1) be iterative, in that measures change as the field advances; (2) include tests of validity that are informative about their clinical use; and (3) focus on assessment of single or homogeneous constructs.
- Practitioners can ask themselves several questions to ascertain the validity of a new assessment tool under consideration for use in clinical practice: (1) Is the construct clearly defined and recognizable?, (2) Does the new measure provide information that is not yet readily accessible?, (3) Is it supported by relevant empirical validity evidence?, (4) Has it been validated in a population with characteristics similar to those of clients with whom the measure will be used?
- Practitioners should continue to focus on unidimensional constructs in clinical practice, rather than aim to assess specific DSM-5 diagnoses.

FOR RESEARCHERS

- Researchers working on the development of new measures assessing psychopathology should adhere to the major principles of construct validity. That is, constructs should be developed in an iterative, informative, representative, and homogeneous manner.
- Rather than focus on strong versus weak construct validity tests, researchers should focus on how informative studies are with respect to the validity of relevant theories and the measures used to test them.
- Research diagnosticians should consider the needs of treatment-oriented

professionals: Instead of targeting broad, multidimensional diagnoses, researchers should target specific, unidimensional forms of dysfunction, as this may have greater utility in clinical practice.

FOR STUDENTS AND EDUCATORS

- It is important in both research and clinical practice to use measures with good evidence for construct validity.
- Evidence for construct validity is acquired when a measure is developed through an iterative, informative process and captures constructs that are both representative and homogeneous in nature.
- It is particularly important to consider construct validity of tools used in CBT assessment, given that these measures have real-life implications for treatment of individuals who are experiencing distress. Use of measures with weak validity evidence can lead to the implementation of ineffective or even harmful intervention strategies in clinical practice.

REFERENCES

American Psychological Association. (1954). Technical recommendations for psychological tests and diagnostic techniques. *Psychological Bulletin, 51,* 201–238.

Anastasi, A. (1950). The concept of validity in the interpretation of test scores. *Educational and Psychological Measurement, 10,* 67–78.

Bartley, W. W., III. (1962). *The retreat to commitment.* New York: Knopf.

Bartley, W. W., III. (1987). Philosophy of biology versus philosophy of physics. In G. Radnitzky & W. W. Bartley III (Eds.), *Evolutionary epistemology, rationality, and the sociology of knowledge* (pp. 7–46). La Salle, IL: Open Court.

Bechtoldt, H. P. (1951). Selection. In S. S. Stevens (Ed.), *Handbook of experimental psychology* (pp. 1237–1266). New York: Wiley.

Beck, A. T. (1967). *Depression: Clinical, experimental and theoretical aspects.* New York: Harper & Row.

Berle, D., & Starcevic, V. (2005). Thought–action fusion: Review of the literature and future directions. *Clinical Psychology Review, 25,* 263–284.

Blackburn, I. M., Jones, S., & Lewin, R. J. P. (1987). Cognitive style in depression. *British Journal of Clinical Psychology, 25,* 241–251.

Blumberg, A. E., & Feigl, H. (1931). Logical positivism. *Journal of Philosophy, 28,* 281–296.

Butcher, J. N. (1990). *Use of the MMPI-2 in treatment planning.* New York: Oxford University Press.

Butcher, J. N. (2002). *Clinical personality assessment: Practical approaches* (2nd ed.). New York: Oxford University Press.

Campbell, D. T., & Fiske, D. W. (1959). Convergent and discriminant validation by the multitrait–multimethod matrix. *Psychological Bulletin, 56,* 81–105.

Clark, L. A., & Watson, D. (1995). Constructing validity: Basic issues in objective scale development. *Psychological Assessment*, 7, 309–319.

Coyne, J. C., & Gotlib, I. H. (1986). Studying the role of cognition in depression: Well trodden paths and cul-de-sacs. *Cognitive Therapy and Research*, 10, 794–812.

Cronbach, L. J. (1988). Five perspectives on validation argument. In H. Wainer & H. Braun (Eds.), *Test validity* (pp. 3–17). Hillsdale, NJ: Erlbaum.

Cronbach, L. J., & Meehl, P. E. (1955). Construct validity in psychological tests. *Psychological Bulletin*, 52, 281–302.

Dobson, K. S., & Shaw, B. F. (1986). Cognitive assessment with major depressive disorders. *Cognitive Therapy and Research*, 10, 13–29.

Duhem, P. (1991). *The aim and structure of physical theory* (P. Weiner, Trans.). Princeton, NJ: Princeton University Press. (Original work published 1914)

Eaves, G., & Rush, A. J. (1984). Cognitive patterns in symptomatic and remitted unipolar major depression. *Journal of Abnormal Psychology*, 93, 31–40.

Edwards, J. R. (2001). Multidimensional constructs in organizational behavior research: An integrative analytical framework. *Organizational Research Methods*, 4, 144–192.

Embretson, S. E. (1998). A cognitive design system approach for generating valid tests: Approaches to abstract reasoning. *Psychological Methods*, 3, 300–396.

Feyerabend, P. (1970). Against method. In M. Radner & S. Winokur (Eds.), *Minnesota studies in the philosophy of science: Vol. 4. Analyses of theories and methods of physics and psychology* (pp. 17–130). Minneapolis: University of Minnesota Press.

Flemming, E. G., & Flemming, C. W. (1929). The validity of the Mathews' revision of the Woodworth Personal Data Questionnaire. *Journal of Abnormal and Social Psychology*, 23, 500–506.

Garrett, H. E., & Schneck, M. R. (1928). A study of the discriminate value of the Woodworth Personal Data Sheet. *Journal of General Psychology*, 1, 459–471.

Gass, C. (2002). Personality assessment of neurologically impaired patients. In J. N. Butcher (Ed.), *Clinical personality assessment: Practical approaches* (2nd ed., pp. 208–224). New York: Oxford University Press.

Giles, D. E., & Rush, A. (1983). Cognitions, schemas, and depressive symptomatology. In M. Rosenbaum, C. M. Franks, & Y. Jaffe (Eds.), *Perspectives on behavior therapy in the eighties* (pp. 184–199). New York: Springer.

Gough, H. G. (1968). An interpreter's syllabus for the California Psychological Inventory. In P. McReynolds (Ed.), *Advances in psychological assessment* (Vol. 1, pp. 55–79). Palo Alto, CA: Science and Behavior Books.

Gough, H. G., & Bradley, P. (1996). *Manual for the California Psychological Inventory* (3rd ed.). Palo Alto, CA: Consulting Psychologists Press.

Greenberger, D., & Padesky, C. A. (1995). *Mind over mood: A cognitive therapy treatment manual for clients*. New York: Guilford Press.

Greene, R. L. (2006). Use of the MMPI-2 in outpatient mental health settings. In J. N. Butcher (Ed.), *MMPI-2: A practitioner's guide* (pp. 253–272). Washington, DC: American Psychological Association.

Haynes, S. N., Richards, D. C. S., & Kubany, E. S. (1995). Content validity in psychological assessment: A functional approach to concepts and methods. *Psychological Assessment, 7*, 238–247.

Hodgson, R. J., & Rachman, S. S. (1977). Obsessional–compulsive complaints. *Behaviour Research and Therapy, 15*, 389–395.

Hollon, S. D., Kendall, P. C., & Lumry, A. (1986). Specificity of depressotypic cognitions in clinical depression. *Journal of Abnormal Psychology, 95*, 52–59.

Hough, L. M., & Schneider, R. J. (1996). Personality traits, taxonomies, and applications in organizations. In K. R. Murphy (Ed.), *Individuals and behavior in organizations* (pp. 31–88). San Francisco: Jossey-Bass.

Kane, M. T. (2001). Current concerns in validity theory. *Journal of Educational Measurement, 38*, 319–342.

Kemper, C. J., Lutz, J., Bähr, T., Rüddel, H., & Hock, M. (2012). Construct validity of the Anxiety Sensitivity Index–3 in clinical samples. *Assessment, 19*, 89–100.

Kuhn, T. S. (1970). *The structure of scientific revolutions* (2nd ed.). Chicago: University of Chicago Press.

Laird, D. A. (1925). A mental hygiene and vocational test. *Journal of Educational Psychology, 16*, 419–422.

Lakatos, I. (1968). Criticism and the methodology of scientific research programs. *Proceedings of the Aristotelian Society, 69*, 149–186.

Lakatos, I. (1999). Lectures on scientific method. In I. Lakatos & P. Feyerabend (Eds.), *For and against method* (pp. 19–112). Chicago: University of Chicago Press.

Loevinger, J. (1957). Objective tests as instruments of psychological theory. *Psychological Reports, 3*(Monograph Suppl.), 635–694.

McGrath, R. E. (2005). Conceptual complexity and construct validity. *Journal of Personality Assessment, 85*, 112–124.

Meehl, P. E. (1978). Theoretical risks and tabular asterisks: Karl, Ronald, and slow progress of soft psychology. *Journal of Consulting and Clinical Psychology, 46*, 806–834.

Meehl, P. E. (1990). Appraising and amending theories: The strategy of Lakatosian defense and two principles that warrant it. *Psychological Inquiry, 1*, 108–141.

Megargee, E. (2006). Use of the MMPI-2 in correctional settings. In J. N. Butcher (Ed.), *MMPI-2: A practitioner's guide* (pp. 327–360). Washington, DC: American Psychological Association.

Megargee, E. (2008). The California Psychological Inventory. In J. N. Butcher (Ed.), *Oxford handbook of personality assessment* (pp. 323–335). New York: Oxford University Press.

Merckelbach, H., Muris, P., Schmidt, H., Rassin, E., & Horselenberg, R. (1998). De Creatieve Ervaringen Vragenlijst als maat voor "fantasy proneness" [The Creative Experiences Questionnaire (CEQ) as a measure of fantasy proneness]. *De Psycholoog, 33*, 204–208.

Muris, P., Meesters, C., Rassin, E., Merkelbach, H., & Campbell, J. (2001).

Thought–action fusion and anxiety disorders symptoms in normal adolescents. *Behaviour Research and Therapy, 39,* 843–852.

Olatunji, B. O., & Wolitzky-Taylor, K. B. (2009). Anxiety sensitivity and the anxiety disorders: A meta-analytic review and synthesis. *Psychological Bulletin, 135,* 974–999.

Olthuis, J. V., Watt, M. C., & Stewart, S. H (2014). Anxiety Sensitivity Index (ASI-3) subscales predict unique variance in anxiety and depressive symptoms. *Journal of Anxiety Disorders, 28*(2), 115–124.

Osman, A., Gutierrez, P. M., Smith, K., Fang, Q., Lozano, G., & Devine, A. (2010). The Anxiety Sensitivity Index–3: Analyses of dimensions, reliability estimates, and correlates in nonclinical samples. *Journal of Personality Assessment, 92,* 45–52.

Paunonen, S. V. (1998). Hierarchical organization of personality and prediction of behavior. *Journal of Personality and Social Psychology, 74,* 538–556.

Paunonen, S. V., & Ashton, M. C. (2001). Big Five factors and facets and the prediction of behavior. *Journal of Personality and Social Psychology, 81,* 524–539.

Rassin, E., Merkelbach, H., Muris, P., & Schmidt, H. (2001). The Thought–Action Fusion Scale: Further evidence for its reliability and validity. *Behaviour Research and Therapy, 39,* 537–544.

Reiss, S. (1991). Expectancy model of fear, anxiety, and panic. *Clinical Psychology Review, 11,* 141–153.

Reiss, S., & McNally, R. J. (1985). The expectancy model of fear. In S. Reiss & R. R. Bootzin (Eds.), *Theoretical issues in behavior therapy* (pp. 107–121). Orlando, FL: Academic Press.

Reiss, S., Peterson, R. A., Gursky, D. M., & McNally, R. J. (1986). Anxiety sensitivity, anxiety frequency and the predictions of fearfulness. *Behaviour Research and Therapy, 24,* 1–8.

Rorer, L. G., & Widiger, T. A. (1983). Personality structure and assessment. *Annual Review of Psychology, 34,* 431–463.

Schneider, R. J., Hough, L. M., & Dunnette, M. D. (1996). Broadsided by broad traits: How to sink science in five dimensions or less. *Journal of Organizational Behavior, 17,* 639–655.

Segal, Z. V. (1988). Appraisal of the self-schema construct in cognitive models of depression. *Psychological Bulletin, 103,* 147–162.

Segal, Z. V., & Shaw, B. F. (1986). When cul-de-sacs are more mentality than reality: A rejoinder to Coyne and Gotlib. *Cognitive Therapy and Research, 10,* 813–826.

Shafran, R., Thordarson, D. S., & Rachman, S. (1996). Thought–action fusion in obsessive–compulsive disorder. *Journal of Anxiety Disorders, 10,* 379–391.

Siev, J., Chambless, D. L., & Huppert, J. D. (2010). Moral thought–action fusion and OCD symptoms: The moderating role of religious affiliation. *Journal of Anxiety Disorders, 24,* 309–312.

Smith, G. T. (2005). On construct validity: Issues of method and measurement. *Psychological Assessment, 17,* 396–408.

Smith, G. T., Fischer, S., & Fister, S. M. (2003). Incremental validity principles in test construction. *Psychological Assessment, 15*(4), 467–477.

Smith, G. T., McCarthy, D., & Zapolski, T. (2009). On the value of homogeneous constructs for construct validation, theory testing, and the description of psychopathology. *Psychological Assessment, 21,* 272–284.

Strauss, M., & Smith, G. (2009). Construct validity: Advances in theory and methodology. *Annual Review of Clinical Psychology, 5,* 25–51.

Taylor, S., & Cox, B. J. (1998a). Anxiety sensitivity: Multiple dimensions and hierarchic structure. *Behaviour Research and Therapy, 36,* 37–51.

Taylor, S., & Cox, B. J. (1998b). An expanded Anxiety Sensitivity Index: Evidence for a hierarchic structure in a clinical sample. *Journal of Anxiety Disorders, 12,* 463–483.

Taylor, S., Zvolensky, M. J., Cox, B. J., Deacon, B., Heimberg, R. G., Ledley, D. R., et al. (2007). Robust dimensions of anxiety sensitivity: Development and initial validation of the Anxiety Sensitivity Index–3. *Psychological Assessment, 19,* 176–188.

Weimer, W. B. (1979). *Notes on the methodology of scientific research.* Hillsdale, NJ: Erlbaum.

Weissman, A. N. (1979). The Dysfunctional Attitude Scale: A validation study (Doctoral dissertation, University of Pennsylvania, 1978). *Dissertation Abstracts International, 40,* 1389B–1390B.

Whitely, S. E. (1983). Construct validity: Construct representation versus nomothetic span. *Psychological Bulletin, 93,* 179–197.

CONCLUSION

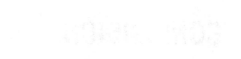

15

Fresh Pools or Stagnant Streams?

Current Status of
Cognitive Clinical Assessment

Gary P. Brown and David A. Clark

It has been said many times that cognitive-behavioral therapy (CBT) and the theory underlying it have come of age. An original impetus for CBT assessment was to establish cognition as a key target of clinical efforts that needed to be measured validly. That battle has long since been decided; as early as 1986, Ingram and Kendall felt able to declare, "The cognitive revolution is over" (Ingram & Kendall, 1986). Cognitive constructs are part of the fabric of mainstream thinking across mental health. There is little dispute that cognitive phenomenology is a part of the general clinical picture, and cognitive variables are integral to many official diagnoses. CBT has established itself as an empirically supported therapy for a variety of disorders; it is now considered a critical component of training programs in clinical psychology, psychiatry, and even family practice; and the general public in most developed countries is not only aware of its efficacy, but requesting access to services. However, there are still many critical issues to be resolved in CBT, particularly concerning improved access to treatment, therapist training and competence, and the critical elements of the therapy responsible for its effectiveness.

Among the many questions that clamor for our attention, it is surprising that the issue of assessment is so easily drowned out by other research agendas and clinical interests. In fact, research on cognitive assessment has been given faint lip service in the past 20 years, despite considerable focus on this topic during the early years of the "cognitive revolution." Within the clinical literature, considerable attention has been given to case formulation, but even here relatively little is said about the assessment of thoughts and beliefs. Moreover, the emerging trends noted in the foregoing chapters (e.g., transdiagnostic approaches, imagery work) and others that are equally promising but not focused upon here (e.g., so-called "third way" therapies) all presuppose underlying mechanisms that need to be measurable in order to be studied and confirmed as functionally related to worsening or improvement in clinical status; without relevant measurement, we can only suppose but not demonstrate. And so it is not surprising that with regard to measurement and assessment, there is an often unspoken sense of dissatisfaction. Previous reviews (e.g., Clark, 1997) reflected the hope, if not confidence, that higher standards of measurement would be met. In light of the essential stasis of the field since the last major set of reviews, it is difficult to be as sanguine today.

The objective of this book has been to address the "assessment gap" in CBT research and clinical literature. The preceding 14 chapters have delved into specific issues in cognitive clinical assessment, with particular focus on what has been learned and what remains to be determined about these issues. In this concluding chapter, we offer a critical overview of the current status of cognitive clinical assessment as delineated in the previous chapters. We first focus on theoretical or research issues, in which we identify a series of themes that recur across the chapters. This is followed by an examination of clinical considerations. We conclude the chapter by suggesting a way forward that could once again bring assessment back into the CBT spotlight.

RESEARCH IN COGNITIVE CLINICAL ASSESSMENT

Reliance on Inference

One of the most obvious problems that continue to stymie advances in cognitive clinical assessment is the overreliance on retrospective self-report questionnaires to measure thought and belief content. This is noted in Chapter 1 of this volume (Clark & Brown), and Chapter 2 (Brown & Clark) reports that the vast majority of studies still adopt a monomethod approach to assessment. Admittedly, cognitive clinical researchers have increased their use of experimental information-processing paradigms to tap into cognitive structure and process, but retrospective self-report measures still predominate. This is not to say that such measures have no place in the armamentarium of cognitive assessment, but there is a need to redress the imbalance. More research is needed that takes a multimethod approach to cognitive assessment, in which endorsement, production, and experimental methods are compared in the same research study.

At the same time, as discussed in several chapters (Brown & Clark, Chapter 2; Haaga & Solomon, Chapter 3; Hawkes & Brown, Chapter 11), cognitive self-report's tendency to involve inference is the main source of doubts about its validity. In Chapter 2, we discuss the limits of retrospective self-report measures with particular attention to veridicality—that is, whether item endorsement on a questionnaire reflects the actual thought content experienced by the respondent. We also argue that not all variables measured by self-report are equally susceptible to inference-based responding. Where respondents are asked to report on enduring beliefs that are presumed to be held continuously, rather than trying to remember actual occurrences of thought content, they do not need to rely as much on inference to introspect and report on their degree of agreement. So the Dysfunctional Attitude Scale (DAS) may be a better indicator of actual negative belief, whereas the Automatic Thoughts Questionnaire (ATQ) may not indicate negative cognitions with the same degree of accuracy. This conclusion rests on the assumption that respondents endorse questionnaire items on the basis of what they assume they think or believe. Hawkes and Brown take up this theme further in Chapter 11, noting that the item wording of many cognitive questionnaires is infused with symptom or affect terms that further threaten their validity. At the very least, we can say that "one size does not fit all." Thus the dramatic shift toward greater emphasis on information processing to investigate more complex constructs such as cognitive vulnerability (see Evraire, Dozois, & Hayden, Chapter 5) or schematic organization is a tacit recognition of this problem of veridicality (MacLeod, 1993).

Against the background of the shortcomings of endorsement methods, Haaga and Solomon (Chapter 3) provide a detailed discussion of the pros and cons of production methods of assessment. These methods elicit responses to stimuli with only a few seconds at most between actual thought occurrence and self-report of the thought, thus relying less on recall and inference than endorsement methods do. By virtue of this advantage, there are likely to be many situations in which production methods of cognitive assessment will be superior to endorsement methodology, at least as far as veridicality is concerned. Think-aloud, thought-sampling, and thought simulation methods, such as the articulated thoughts in simulated situations (ATSS) paradigm (Davison, Navarre, & Vogel, 1995), may provide a more valid and precise representation of individuals' moment-by-moment thought content, but these methods suffer from questions of reliability and low convergence with other methods of cognitive assessment. This weakness is the price that is paid for the flexibility in response format that confers their advantages over endorsement methods, which rely on fixed item content and response formats. However, the fixed format of endorsement items, for all its limitations, affords a clearer basis for comparing responses between respondents than is true of production methods. Haaga and Solomon offer an interesting rapprochement between production and endorsement, in which production methods are used in the preliminary stages of scale development, enhancing the content validity of the resulting endorsement measures with content originating in respondents' reports of their actual thoughts. Hawkes and Brown discuss just such an approach entailing the use of techniques such as cognitive interviewing, which elicit verbal protocols of response processing similar to those provided by production methods, as a means for bridging the apparent dichotomy between methods that rely on post hoc judgments and those that more directly tap into online processing. Haaga and Solomon also note that the development of automated coding methodology might encourage the uptake of production methods in cognitive research.

As problematic as self-report methods may be, the assumption that salvation is to be found in experimental methods also needs to be tempered. As Roefs and colleagues (Chapter 13) argue, less direct and implicit means of operationalizing strength of beliefs are plagued by their own shortcomings. The validity of these approaches is based at least in part on limiting the possibility of inference by the respondent. However, experimental paradigms have their own inference issues, except that here it is the researcher who is susceptible. As Roefs and colleagues point out with regard to the Implicit Association Test (IAT), there has been a tendency to equate the measurement outcome with a mental construct, such as an implicit attitude or belief—a conclusion not supported by the evidence. They cast doubt on the possibility that constructs such as dysfunctional beliefs and self-esteem can be reduced to the simpler associations captured by implicit measures, and they urge researchers to limit their inferences to what is actually observed in experimental tasks. For example, tasks involving a shift in attentional resources should be inferred as relating to attention rather than schematic processing. To the extent that no convincing alternative exists to self-report for variables that are only available to introspection, then self-report, with all its limitations, may need to suffice.

Categories and Dimensions

Uliaszek, Alden, and Zinbarg (Chapter 7) discuss the complementary advantages and disadvantages of diagnostic and dimensional approaches to assessment, noting that diagnosis provides a concise summary that aids communication and clarifies treatment decisions, that it can increase reliability relative to the dimensional approach, and that it is particularly suited to addressing specific issues, such as etiological questions. However, categorical distinctions can be arbitrary and, with regard to research, can decrease statistical power and preclude the use of many useful analytic methods. Dimensional assessment provides a less concise basis for communication, but it is more flexible and suitable to a broader range of research approaches. There appears to be a convergence forming around a dual-track approach to the question of diagnosis within the mental health field, according to which categorical diagnoses and dimensional assessment are conducted jointly, either in sequence or in parallel. This has been the practice within CBT since its inception, and it typically entails the administration of diagnosis-specific measures of automatic thoughts and enduring beliefs to supplement assigning a diagnosis. The *Diagnostic and Statistical Manual of Mental Disorders*, fifth edition (DSM-5; American Psychiatric Association, 2013) advocates a hybrid categorical–dimensional framework that is a subject for further research and will potentially spur a more sophisticated understanding of how these diagnoses and dimensional assessments complement each other in research and in practice. Although DSM-5 was supposed to move psychiatric nosology closer to a dimensional nomenclature, the DSM-5 Task Force has indicated that a hybrid dimensional–categorical nomenclature is definitely the future of psychiatric diagnosis. So the emphasis on dimensionality in cognitive assessment is well placed to make a significant and noteworthy contribution to the future direction of psychiatric diagnosis.

Assessment within CBT practice is guided by the cognitive content-specificity hypothesis (CCSH). The CCSH, which is discussed in comprehensive detail by Baranoff and Oei (Chapter 8), centers on the claim that disorders can be characterized and distinguished from each other on the basis of their characteristic cognitive content. Baranoff and Oei usefully distinguish between a "sensitivity" aspect (i.e., the extent to which cognition is a meaningful marker of a particular affective state) and a "specificity" aspect (relating to the question of whether particular cognitive content is distinct to a particular order and not found in other disorders). They find more empirical support for the cognitive content hypothesis than for content specificity. That is, thoughts of loss/failure and threat/danger appear to characterize depressive and anxious states, respectively, but support for the more stringent hypothesis of a specific and unique cognitive profile for each disorder is less conclusive. Moreover, specificity may be stronger for loss/failure than for threat/danger, although the authors warn that this could be due to the insensitivity of the measures themselves. A related line of research follows from a growing body of evidence that our current approaches to cognitive assessment may be much better suited for assessing the common than the specific features of psychopathology. Smith, Ratcliff, and Norton's conclusion in Chapter 9 on transdiagnostic CBT that existing cognition measures could be used in transdiagnostic research and treatment implies that current cognition measures are tapping into the common processes underlying psychopathological states more than they are assessing the unique and specific features of disorders. In this connection, Harvey, Watkins, Mansell, and Shafran (2004, p. 271) suggest three possible bases according to which diagnoses differ from each other despite sharing underlying common transdiagnostic processes: The disorders differ in their characteristic concerns; the disorders differ in their balance of common processes; and processes that are distinct to a disorder (i.e., nontrasndiagnostic processes) may account for the difference between disorders. Continued efforts to work out the implications of the complex relationships among dimensional constructs and the complex system of diagnostic categorization is clearly warranted and has important implications for assessment and research.

Blending Nomothetic and Idiographic Approaches

The nomothetic and idiographic approaches to assessment can be usefully thought of as lying along a continuum. As discussed in Chapter 2 (Brown & Clark), construction of instruments such as the ATQ, geared to the nomothetic aim of characterizing the ongoing thought processes of depressed individuals as a group, flowed naturally from the idiographic clinical technique of eliciting and recording thoughts with the Daily Record of Dysfunctional Thoughts (DRDT; see also Haaga & Solomon, Chapter 3, for a discussion of DRDTs as production-based assessments). The central challenge of assessment is how to make use of group-wise nomothetic knowledge in regard to a given individual. As Bieling and Key (Chapter 10) note, the area of cognitive case formulation has largely developed as a guide to how to proceed when seeking to translate nomothetic cognitive theory and research into idiographic treatment. Scores on assessment instruments, formal diagnoses, and manualized treatment guidelines provide a starting reference for the clinician delivering psychotherapy to specific individuals. To take one typical example, if a particular psychotherapy client has been diagnosed with obsessive–compulsive disorder (OCD), he or she might be asked to complete a measure of enduring beliefs, such as the Obsessive Beliefs Questionnaire (OBQ), which produces a set of subscale scores. As Uliaszek et al. (Chapter 7) discuss, taxometric methods could be used to determine if it is justified to use cutoff points on the OBQ subscales to define belief-based subgroups of OCD, for which different treatment approaches might be structured. In the absence of such evidence, an idiographic approach in which sets of scores are considered separately for each individual is appropriate (although because the OBQ subscales do not represent distinct constructs or dimensions [Woods, Tolin, & Abramowitz, 2004], it may be that only use of a total score is supported). In a similar vein, Chapter 2 (Brown & Clark) describes a common practice within CBT of identifying salient items from a scale (e.g., those with relative elevations) to focus upon in further clinical investigation. In addition, several chapters mention a complementary trend for new methods appearing that pursue idiographic aims through using formal measurement approaches and, in certain instances, experimental techniques tailored to the individual (e.g., Bornstein, 2011; Cervone, 2004; Mumma, 2011).

Convergence across Methods

A central consideration in assessment research is the degree of convergence across assessment modes and experimental methods. Further research that sheds light on reasons for the low convergence between different methods of cognitive assessment is needed. Although we have known for years that different assessment methods show low convergence, we have made little progress in determining the parameters that affect level of convergence. There is typically an even greater lack of consistency between self-report and experimental paradigms. As Roefs et al. (Chapter 13) note, although findings with implicit measures often converge with those of explicit measures, other findings go in the opposite direction, and findings in still other areas are mixed. Haaga and Solomon (Chapter 3) argue that low convergent validity provides an opportunity for exploring the conditions under which one method may be more valid than another. Another possible avenue of research would be to determine the conditions that might influence convergence. For example, would measures of cognition show higher convergence during periods of heightened negative emotion or when underlying maladaptive schemas have been primed? Might convergence be higher in clinical samples experiencing an acute state of a disorder? Could there be individual differences in convergence—with, for example, individuals with higher self-consciousness or introspective ability showing greater convergence than individuals low in these personality characteristics? Clearly, it is time to move on from simply documenting poor convergent validity to more informative research that seeks to illuminate the low convergent validity of cognitive assessment methods.

For a generation, the multitrait–multimethod matrix (MTMM;

Campbell & Fiske, 1959) has been at the heart of validation research into the degree of convergence between methods, and newer analytic methods continue to provide means for fully exploiting the approach. Naragon-Gainey and T. A. Brown (Chapter 12) provide a useful summary of the rationale for the approach and note that structural equation models improve upon the traditional correlational approach, in particular through directly modeling shared variance among multiple measures by using latent variables (i.e., factors). This can serve as a corrective where measures in a particular domain are overreliant on a particular methodology. High loadings on the trait factors indicate convergence of evidence from different methods and measures. Conversely, MTMM matrices can help clarify whether putatively different but similar constructs such as emotion regulation, distress tolerance, and mindfulness are empirically distinct or whether they substantially overlap. When there is lack of consistency of evidence across methods, it is possible that either one of the contributory methods is flawed, or it could be the case that there are third-variable moderators or mediators that need to be taken into account. As Guller and Smith (Chapter 14) discuss, "strong theory"-based validation (Cronbach, 1988) is usually an unrealistic standard with regard to the type of latent constructs that are the targets of psychological measurement. However, the level of knowledge of basic cognitive processes involved in producing responses to assessment and experimental procedures (attention, memory, etc.) is sufficiently developed to allow for considerable progress to be made in understanding what underlies the convergent and divergent results with different methods.

Enduringness and Etiology

A central challenge in making progress on etiological questions has been to develop valid measures, whether self-report or based on experimental paradigms, that are capable of indexing ongoing and enduring risk factors for developing emotional difficulties outside of symptomatic periods. In this respect, assessment may be a much more dynamic process than the founders of CBT initially assumed it to be. That is, the context or conditions in which assessment takes place may greatly influence the accuracy of the assessment. This theme is taken up by Evraire and colleagues (Chapter 5) in their discussion of cognitive vulnerability. Early research on cognitive vulnerability was not particularly supportive of the CBT model, since scores on measures such as the DAS appeared to covary with symptom level. As Evraire et al. note, "The finding that cognitive vulnerability waxes and wanes along with symptom fluctuations calls into question whether such markers are best conceptualized as trait-like vulnerabilities or simply epiphenomena of disorder" (p. 96). This led some prominent researchers to conclude that negative cognitions and beliefs are consequences rather than causes of disturbed emotions (e.g., Coyne & Gotlib, 1983). Later research, however, has found that priming may be critical in cognitive vulnerability assessment. Priming methods have provided more consistent support for cognitive vulnerability, especially when vulnerability is assessed by endorsement measures (i.e., the DAS) or information-processing tasks like the dot-probe or emotional Stroop color-naming tasks. However, what are missing from the cognitive priming research are (1) application to production methods of assessment and (2) a better understanding of the parameters under which priming is or is not necessary for detecting cognitive vulnerability. In addition, we point out (Brown & Clark, Chapter 2) that the results of priming studies do not eliminate the plentiful counterevidence that appears consistent with the idea that the constructs measured by such scales as the DAS are consequences or epiphenomena of the emotional difficulties they are meant to predict. Naragon-Gainey and T. A. Brown (Chapter 12) discuss the studies recently appearing that have employed the latest structural equation modeling techniques specifically suited for temporal relationships between cognition and symptoms, and these all support the cognitions-as-consequences account. Finally, as Roefs and colleagues (Chapter 13) point out with regard to implicit measures, the susceptibility of variables to momentary experimental manipulation is at odds with the idea of a stable underlying vulnerability. It could be similarly argued that priming manipulations reflect a level of reactivity at odds with the argument that they are revealing underlying enduring vulnerabilities.

Functional Outcomes and Intervening Mechanisms

Critics of self-report within CBT (e.g., MacLeod, 1993) were proponents of addressing intervening mechanisms experimentally while preserving the methodological strictness of traditional behaviorism. The chapters of the present volume also touch upon a diverse set of reasons suggesting that self-report should also not be regarded as presumptively invalid. Among these are, first, as discussed extensively in Chapter 2 (Brown & Clark), systems have been developed (e.g., Ericsson & Simon's [1980] framework) for distinguishing valid and invalid verbal reports. Second, certain phenomena of interest either are only ascertainable through introspection, or, in the case of beliefs, are isomorphic with (i.e., correspond to) the phenomenon of interest. As discussed by Roefs and colleagues (Chapter 13), whereas certain experimental paradigms might identify constructs that moderate and mediate beliefs, they cannot fully replace self-report. Moreover, with regard to phenomena such as images, as discussed by Hales and colleagues (Chapter 4), verbal report can only be adjunctive. It is difficult to envisage a paradigm that would provide an alternate route to imagery that procedures like the IAT provide for verbal phenomena. Third, emerging concepts of validity place central emphasis on documenting the intervening mechanisms that give rise to an eventual response to a test item. In this regard, it is plausible that these emerging validity theories will benefit CBT research and assessment. The prevailing construct validity paradigm (Cronbach & Meehl, 1955), while not behaviorist in essence, was developed in an environment in which behaviorism dominated and so, unsurprisingly, was constructed in a way that obviated the necessity of accounting for intervening mechanisms. Broadening the concept of validity so that it emphasizes intervening mechanisms may give rise to additional techniques for gathering evidence for the operation of intervening mechanisms; this can only benefit areas such as CBT research and assessment, which are premised on the operation of such mechanisms. Finally, as Roefs et al. note in Chapter 13, when an explanation is more specific about the precise mental process that is disturbed, more focused experimental paradigms can be developed that also permit more effective use of converging measures.

CLINICAL CONSIDERATIONS

Never before have CBT practitioners had at their disposal such a wide array of measures to assess specific cognitive content, structures, and processes known to be integral in the etiology, persistence, and treatment of psychological disorders. It would be hard to find a DSM-5 disorder for which there are no measures of relevant thought content. And yet at the same time, clinical utilization of and training in formal cognitive assessment are at an all-time low. We have noted (Clark & Brown, Chapter 1) several surveys that indicate a decline in the proportion of time clinicians spend in diagnosis/assessment activities, as well as a corresponding decline in assessment competence as training programs reduce their assessment courses. There is no reason to believe that CBT practitioners are more versed in clinical assessment than clinicians of other theoretical persuasions. Many of the reasons for a neglect of cognitive assessment in CBT practice have been addressed in this book.

First, it is likely that many CBT clinicians take a rather naïve approach to cognitive assessment. We rely almost exclusively on clinical interview data and assume that a client's retrospective report of cognitions in past distressing situations is valid. At most, we might assign a thought record and encourage clients to record their cognitions at the time of occurrence, but we have no way of determining its veridicality. Aside from interview and thought records, most CBT clinicians rarely employ other cognitive assessment measures, even more standardized cognition questionnaires. This overreliance on a single method (i.e., the interview) will lead to incomplete information and biased clinical decision making (Meyer et al., 2001). There are several approaches that could be taken to rectify this situation. We need practice-based research that measures the negative effects of monomethod cognitive assessment in clinical practice. This could be followed by studies that delineate the optimal mix of cognitive assessment approaches that would significantly improve clinical decision making. Another approach would be actually training clinicians on how to get the most from a thought record. As Haaga and Solomon comment (Chapter 3), thought records are a form of production methodology—but when was the last time any of us saw formal training on "how to use a thought record"? We suspect that most clinicians are not getting the most clinical utility from their thought records because they have never been trained in their interpretation. The challenge to develop an evidence-based practice must include a more systematic, empirically driven approach to cognitive assessment as well (see Hunsley & Elliott, Chapter 6).

Second, many clinicians may see a diminishing return on treatment utility with increased emphasis on cognitive assessment. Today there is tremendous emphasis placed on efficiency, with the average treatment duration involving fewer and fewer contact hours. CBT is now delivered with significant effect online, through apps, and in various low-intensity face-to-face treatment formats (e.g., Richards & Borglin, 2011; Williams & Andrews, 2013). The emergence of these quick, minimal-contact interventions not only raises questions about whether there is a role for assessment, but casts doubt more generally on the treatment utility of a more protracted approach to cognitive assessment. At this point, the treatment utility and incremental validity of cognitive assessment within clinical practice has not been demonstrated. But it is worth raising the question whether the effectiveness of our interventions might be diminished by our relative neglect of cognitive assessment.

Third, although there has been much emphasis on case formulation in CBT training, Bieling and Key note that the empirical evidence for case formulation is found wanting. So is this heavy emphasis on case formulation justified? If so, why have advocates for cognitive case formulation shown such disregard for cognitive assessment? Surely the proverbial phrase "A chain is only as strong as its weakest link" applies to the link between cognitive assessment and case formulation. Cognitive assessment is the "feeder" for case formulation. If validity and veridicality are threatened by our approach to cognitive assessment, how can a valid and clinically useful case formulation flow from a faulty assessment? When discussing cognitive case formulation, clinical researchers and trainers need to focus much more intently on the assessment–formulation relationship.

And finally, treatment evaluation has always been an important element of CBT, and in the current environment of health care cost containment, the ability to demonstrate clinically significant outcomes is paramount. Cognitive assessment plays a central role in laying the foundation for treatment evaluation. It is not enough for CBT practitioners to document symptom reduction or improved quality of life with intervention. In addition, practitioners need to show that changes in specific cognitive content, structures, and processes have occurred because of treatment. Training in treatment evaluation is critical, as is the use of highly reliable and valid measures of cognition. In this era of the "dodo bird effect," it is incumbent on CBT practitioners to demonstrate cognitive mediation—that is, to show that their cognitive interventions lead to changes in cognition, which in turn mediate symptom reduction. The ability to detect cognitive mediation requires highly sensitive and specific measures of cognition that are applied in a skilled and contextualized fashion. In the final analysis, advances in CBT treatment, dissemination, and improved access depend in part on a renewed emphasis on the importance of cognitive assessment.

CHARTING A NEW COURSE

The chapters in the current book provide an overview of the state of CBT assessment that can be a starting point for considering what future directions research and practice in CBT assessment might take. There are obvious concerns, but also reasons to be hopeful. A clear initial priority is for assessment once again to be a central focus; that it has not been for the last 20 or so years has clearly been detrimental. To date, even the most established cognitive assessment measures fail to meet the highest validation standards—and, as we note (Clark & Brown, Chapter 1), incremental validity has rarely been addressed in cognition measures. We further contend (Brown & Clark, Chapter 2) that questions of content validity are prominent, since most cognition measures are contaminated with irrelevant items that increase error variance. Hunsley and Elliott (Chapter 6) point out that no clinical cognition measures are available with established norms and cutoff values, so their contribution to evidence-based practice is limited. More generally, Guller and Smith's (Chapter 14) characterization of the low standard of what is acceptable in research in the field has a ring of truth: "In the absence of carefully articulated theory, virtually any correlation between a target measure and another measure, of any magnitude, can be described as validation evidence . . . [and] sets of correlations with readily available measures are cobbled together as evidence of construct validity" (p. 322).

At the same time, it is important to recognize that many of the challenges facing CBT assessment and research are endemic in the field at large. Among the most prominent of these are the problems of measuring phenomena only available to introspection and reconciling the nomothetic–idiographic, categorical–dimensional, and cognitive–functional dichotomies. A particular strength of CBT research has been the tradition of promptly capitalizing on and applying advances in associated areas, and so CBT is in a position to benefit from the notable progress that has been made on all of these perennial issues and can also contribute to further progress. Traditionally, CBT research has naturally looked to experimental cognitive and behavioral research; however, given the widespread use of self-report scales, staying abreast of and assimilating developments in psychometrics and validity theory, survey research, and personality science would be likely to benefit and enrich the field.

Nearly 20 years ago, Clark (1997) concluded a review by stating, "The future of cognitive assessment very much depends on whether cognitive–clinical researchers pick up the 'gauntlet of assessment' and begin to directly address many of the methodological and conceptual issues raised" (p. 999). The inescapable conclusion from the present volume is that the challenge has not been met, and unless a conscious effort is undertaken, it is entirely possible that another 20 years will pass without a more rapid pace of progress. How can we know if the trend is beginning to shift? It is entirely likely that future changes will not be possible to anticipate, but based on perception of the field as it exists today, we propose the following indicative set of progress benchmarks for the next decade.

- Progress will have been made in systematically incorporating assessment information into case formulations and, through this, into treatment delivery.
- More cognitive assessment instruments will have formally published norms.
- Research will increasingly combine the aims of traditional construct validation in the Cronbach and Meehl tradition with those of construct representation and delineating intervening mechanisms.

- The standard approach to scale development will increasingly give appropriate emphasis to evidence based on content, process, and structure, as well as relationships among constructs.
- New instruments will be developed to convincingly operationalize constructs from imagery work, transdiagnostic assessment, and various "third way" approaches that do not recapitulate the shortcomings of the last generation of assessment instruments.
- Means for measuring etiological factors will be appropriately stable and nonreactive and will otherwise demonstrate that they are antecedents rather than concomitants or consequences of emotional problems.

CBT has been an incomparable success across the field of mental health and in virtually all areas of the world. That it has attained its current standing while neglecting the seemingly central issues covered in the current volume suggests that it has only begun to exploit its potential. If even modest progress is made on a portion of the issues identified in the current volume, CBT will move closer to fully realizing the promise of the revolution in psychotherapy that it began a generation ago.

REFERENCES

American Psychiatric Association. (2013). *Diagnostic and statistical manual of mental disorders* (5th ed.). Arlington, VA: Author.

Bornstein, R. F. (2011). Toward a process-focused model of test score validity: Improving psychological assessment in science and practice. *Psychological Assessment, 23*(2), 532–544.

Campbell, D. T., & Fiske, D. W. (1959). Convergent and discriminat validation by the multitrait–multimethod matrix. *Psychological Bulletin, 56*, 81–105.

Cervone, D. (2004). Personality assessment: Tapping the social-cognitive architecture of personality. *Behavior Therapy, 35*(1), 113–129.

Clark, D. A. (1997). Twenty years of cognitive assessment: Current status and future directions. *Journal of Consulting and Clinical Psychology, 65*(6), 996–1000.

Coyne, J. C., & Gotlib, I. H. (1983). The role of cognition in depression: A critical appraisal. *Psychological Bulletin, 94*, 474–505.

Cronbach, L. J. (1988). Five perspectives on validation argument. In H. Wainer & H. Braun (Eds.), *Test validity* (pp. 3–17). Hillsdale, NJ: Erlbaum.

Cronbach, L. J., & Meehl, P. E. (1955). Construct validity in psychological tests. *Psychological Bulletin, 52*, 281–302.

Davison, G. C., Navarre, S. G., & Vogel, R. S. (1995). The articulated thoughts in simulated situations paradigm: A think-aloud approach to cognitive assessment. *Current Directions in Psychological Science, 4*(1), 29–33.

Ericsson, K. A., & Simon, H. A. (1980). Verbal reports as data. *Psychological Review, 87*(3), 215–251.

Harvey, A., Watkins, E., Mansell, W., & Shafran, R. (2004). *Cognitive behavioural processes across psychological disorders: A transdiagnostic approach to research and treatment.* Oxford, UK: Oxford University Press.

Ingram, R. E., & Kendall, P. C. (1986). Cognitive clinical psychology: Implications of an information processing perspective. In R. E. Ingram (Ed.), *Information processing approaches to clinical psychology* (pp. 3–21). Orlando, FL: Academic Press.

MacLeod, C. (1993). Cognition in clinical psychology: Measures, methods or models? *Behaviour Change, 10,* 169–195.

Meyer, G. J., Finn, S. E., Eyde, L. D., Kay, G. G., Moreland, K. L., Dies, R. R., et al. (2001). Psychological testing and psychological assessment: A review of evidence and issues. *American Psychologist, 56,* 128–165.

Mumma, G. H. (2011). Validity issues in cognitive-behavioral case formulation. *European Journal of Psychological Assessment, 27*(1), 29–49.

Richards, D. A., & Borglin, G. (2011). Implementation of psychological therapies for anxiety and depression in routine practice: Two year prospective cohort study. *Journal of Affective Disorders, 133,* 51–60.

Williams, A. D., & Andrews, G. (2013). The effectiveness of internet cognitive behavioural therapy (iCBT) for depression in primary care: A quality assurance study. *PLoS One, 8,* e57447, 1–6.

Woods, C. M., Tolin, D. F., & Abramowitz, J. S. (2004). Dimensionality of the Obsessive Beliefs Questionnaire (OBQ). *Journal of Psychopathology and Behavioral Assessment, 26,* 113–125.

Index